Neurology
of the
Visual System

Seventh Printing

Neurology

of the

Visual System

By

DAVID G. COGAN, M.D.

Henry Willard Williams
Professor of Ophthalmology
Harvard Medical School
Chief of Ophthalmology
Massachusetts Eye and Ear Infirmary
Boston, Massachusetts

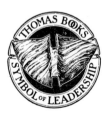

CHARLES C THOMAS • PUBLISHER
Springfield • Illinois • U.S.A.

Published and Distributed Throughout the World by
CHARLES C THOMAS • PUBLISHER
BANNERSTONE HOUSE
301-327 East Lawrence Avenue, Springfield, Illinois, U.S.A.

© 1966, by CHARLES C THOMAS • PUBLISHER
ISBN O-398-00322-X
Library of Congress Catalog Card Number: 64-8131

First Printing, 1966
Second Printing, 1967
Third Printing, 1968
Fourth Printing, 1970
Fifth Printing, 1972
Sixth Printing, 1974
Seventh Printing, 1976

With THOMAS BOOKS careful attention is given to all details of
manufacturing and design. It is the Publisher's desire to present books
that are satisfactory as to their physical qualities and artistic possibilities
and appropriate for their particular use. THOMAS BOOKS will be true
to those laws of quality that assure a good name and good will.

Printed in the United States of America
H-2

PREFACE

THIS VOLUME, intended to be companion to *Neurology of the Ocular Muscles* presents, it is hoped, the salient clinical aspects of the ocular sensory system as briefly as is consistent with a reasonably comprehensive coverage of the subject. The problem has been what to exclude rather than what to include. So vast is the field and so rich in speculation that it does not make for easy assimilation. While the book heavily represents the author's point of view—and he must take responsibility for the sins of omission and misguided emphases—it contains references of supportive and contradictory nature to which the reader must turn for more detailed information and discussion. Hopefully, judicious sampling with particular reference to recent articles may compensate for whatever violence has been done by incomplete coverage of the literature.

The subject matter is divided into retina, optic nerve, chiasm, optic tracts, lateral geniculate body, geniculostriate radiations, and cortical visual centers. It is neither ophthalmology nor neurology but that overlapping field of specialization which attempts to incorporate the language and experience of both. While mention is made of basic investigations, the prime orientation has been toward clinical applicability. Extensive experimental investigations are omitted unless they have obvious bearing on the living functions of man.

As was the case with the previous volume, I have incurred great debts in the writing of this. I owe much to those students, colleagues and members of my family who have patiently listened to my expostulations on the subject and criticized the text. I have also specific indebtedness to those who have participated intimately in the labors of its editing, typing, reference checking, and proof reading. I should most particularly like to thank Mrs. B. L. Young for her indefatigable editorial assistance, Mr. Jerome Glickman and Mr. John Jope for their help in illustrations, Dr. David D. Donaldson and Miss Inez M. Berry and the departments of Neuropathology and Radiology at the Massachusetts General Hospital (Dr. Paul New) for source material, Dr. Toichiro Kuwabara for preparation of histologic material, several persons (Drs. James Mount, Jack Goldstein, John Andrews, and Arthur Asbury) who read and criticized a penultimate version of the text and Miss Elisabeth Lavoie for typing and retyping. These have been pleasant companions in the venture of book-writing. Finally, I want to acknowledge the patient understanding and technical assistance of the publisher, Payne Thomas, who encouraged but never pushed me and always stood ready to give valuable guidance from a publisher's point of view.

DAVID G. COGAN, M.D.

CONTENTS

Neurology
of the
Visual System

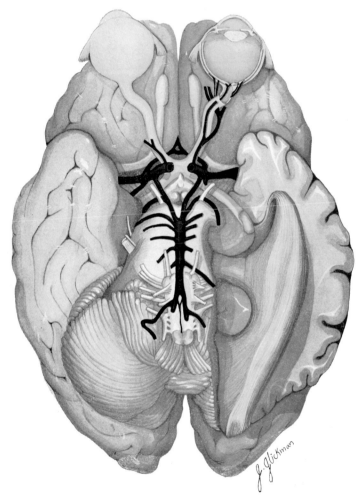

Frontispiece. Drawing of inferior surface of brain illustrating visual pathways from the eye to the occiput.

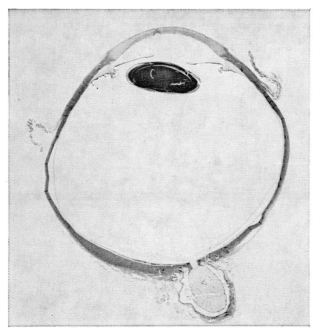

Routine cross section of eye, stained by Masson's trichrome method. Enlarged
3 times.

CHAPTER I

RETINA: Anatomy, Physiology, and Developmental Abnormalities

A. ANATOMY AND PHYSIOLOGY

THE RETINA, which comprises the seeing portion of the eye, is that innermost membrane about which all other ocular structures are functionally subordinate (Figure 1). The vitreous bounds it anteriorly and the pigment epithelium posteriorly. Although processes of the pigment epithelium interdigitate intimately with the rods and cones, the retina is firmly secured to the eye only at the nerve head (posteriorly) and at the ora serrata (anteriorly). It is a wonder that the retina does not regularly separate from the outer layers of the

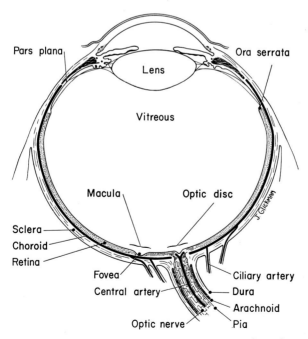

FIGURE 1. Diagram representing the horizontal section of an eye.

[5]

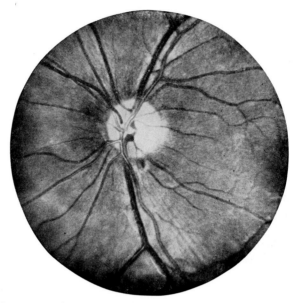

FIGURE 2. Ophthalmoscopic appearance of a normal fundus, magnified 10 x from actual size. The optic disc is actually about 1½ mm in diameter. The central retinal artery has a lumen 50-100 micra and is, therefore, in the arteriolar range. The retinal vein is at least one half wider than the artery and the contained blood is darker. The retina itself is normally invisible to the ophthalmoscope because of its transparency. The macular area represented at the extreme right of the photograph is about 3 mm in diameter and can be distinguished by the darker shade of the underlying pigment layer.

Although widely variable, highlights from the surface of the retina are commonly present and are illustrated in the present case along the major retinal vessels and the proximal nerve fibers.

eye. That it does not is attributable largely to the vitreous gel holding it in place from within.

(a) *Analogy with nervous system.* Embryologically the retina is an ectopic portion of the primitive forebrain and never does lose its similarity to the central nervous system. Thus, the inner layers of the retina show throughout life a lamination comparable to that of gray matter in the cortex, while the optic nerves show the same compartmentalization by pia and absence of sheaths of Schwann as characterize white matter in the brain.

The rods and cones are the photosensitive end organs. They are situated, paradoxically, in the outermost portion of the retina and face outward (Figure 5). These rods and cones, together with their cell bodies, constitute what is called the neuroectodermal layer of the retina analogous to sensory receptors in skin. Their nuclei form the outer nuclear layer consisting of cone nuclei adjacent to the external limiting membrane and rod nuclei deeper in the retina.

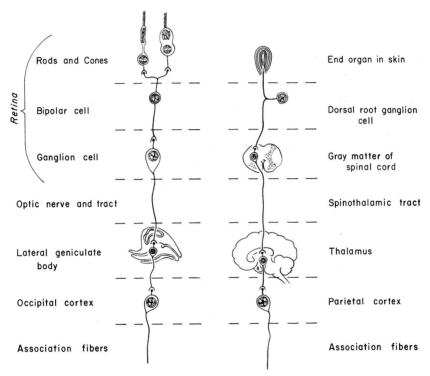

FIGURE 3. Analogy of the visual neuronal hierarchy with that of the general sensory system.

The bipolar cell layer forms the middle cellular lamina in the retina and serves chiefly to relay neural impulses from the neuroectodermal layer to the innermost neurones of the retina. The bipolar cells are thus the counterpart of the dorsal-root ganglia cells in the rest of the sensory nervous system. The bipolar cell layer also contains glial cell bodies which will be described subsequently.

The innermost cell lamina contains the retinal ganglion cells which correspond to neurones having cell bodies in the gray matter of the spinal cord and the primary sensory nuclei in the brain stem. The axones of the ganglion cells constitute the nerve fiber layer of the retina lying between the ganglion cells and the internal limiting membrane of the retina; they are comparable to the ascending spinothalamic tracts in the cord. Although not myelinated within the eye, the axones of the ganglion cells acquire myelin immediately after leaving the eye and thereby form the optic nerves (Figure 4).

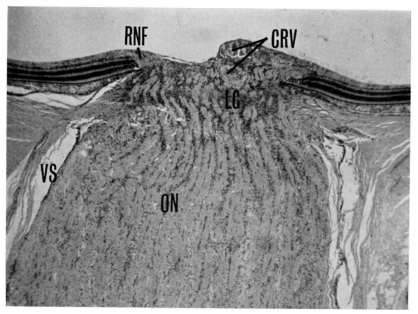

FIGURE 4. Cross section of the optic nerve head. H. & E. stain.
CRV, central retinal vessels; LC, lamina cribrosa; ON, optic nerve; RNF, retinal nerve fibers; VS, vaginal sheaths.

After traversing the optic nerve the fibers which arose in the ganglion cells of the retina pass by way of the optic chiasm and tracts to terminate in the lateral geniculate bodies. Thus, the optic nerves and tracts are the photoconductive counterparts of sensory tracts within the spinal cord and lemnisci of the brain stem. Despite their designation as nerves, the optic nerves are, therefore, more analogous to tracts of the central nervous system than they are to peripheral nerves. This becomes clinically apparent when we consider their lack of regenerative capacity and their susceptibility to certain demyelinative diseases.

The first neural relay of the visual system within the cranium is the lateral geniculate body. These paired bodies, one on each side of the brain, consist of laminated cell structures forming the posterior tips of the thalami. They are, in fact, the visual relays corresponding to the thalamic cells that relay other modalities of sensation. The cells of each lateral geniculate body then project their axonal fibers to the occipital cortex, forming the geniculostriate radiation, just as the sensory fibers from each thalamus project to the parietal cortex. The course of these visual fibers through the cerebral hemispheres is of the greatest neuro-ophthalmic importance (see p. 253).

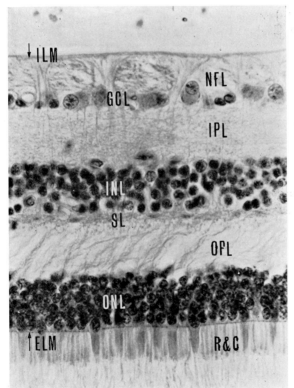

FIGURE 5. Cross section of the retina in the region between macula and equator H. & E. stain.

ILM, internal limiting membrane; NFL, nerve fiber layer; GCL, ganglion cell layer; IPL, inner plexiform layer; INL, inner nuclear layer; SL, synaptic layer; OPL, outer plexiform layer; ONL, outer nuclear layer; ELM, external limiting membrane; R&C, rods and cones.

(b) **Rods and cones.** The rods and cones lie just outside the external limiting membrane of the retina while their cell bodies lie just internal to it (Figure 5). Each outermost segment, about 15 μ in length, may be seen by electron microscopy to contain hundreds of protein plates separated by as many lipid membranes[1332] (Figure 6). Within this outermost segment is the photosensitive pigment, rhodopsin in the case of rods and iodopsin in the case of cones, which is responsible for the absorption of the light stimulus. The pigment portion of both rhodopsin and iodopsin is retinene,[1509] an oxidative derivative of vitamin A[62] supplied by the pigment epithelium, and a protein fraction called opsin.[1514, 1512] On exposure to light this photosensitive substance is bleached and in some way triggers off a neural discharge that is ultimately registered as a visual stimulus. Visibility curves determined in vivo thus correspond to the bleaching curves of the pigment in vitro.[822, 1515] The energy required to stimulate visual perception is only a few quanta of light; that is, the energy necessary to decompose only a few molecules of the pigment.[626, 158, 157, 1154] Nowhere else in the body has such a precise and sensitive correlation been found between excitation and neural response as in the case of vision.

The inner portions of the rods and cones, also measuring about 15 μ in length, contain no photosensitive substance but do contain an abundance of mitochondria packed into an area called an ellipsoid. The fact that the ellipsoids are larger in the cones than in the rods gives to these receptors their different and characteristic shapes. Since mitochondria are generally associated with energy production, the ellipsoids of the rods and cones are thought to be the power packs of the photoreceptive process; it is here that the oxidation of glucose and other fuels is believed to provide the energy for conversion of the photochemical stimulus into a neural discharge. Whereas the outer portions of the rods and cones contain the detectors, the inner portions provide the amplification for photic stimulation.

Connecting the outer and inner segments are several cilia. Although some investigators have interpreted these cilia as neuroconductive it would seem more likely that they were supportive; on cross section they have the ultrastructure (seven pairs of osmiophilic bodies) seen in non-motile cilia elsewhere. How the impulse is relayed from the outer to the inner segments is not clear but it may be simply by change in membrane potential such as occurs in neurones elsewhere.

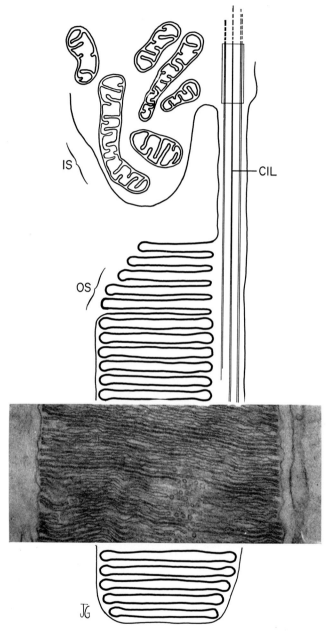

FIGURE 6. Representation of a single rod based on information obtained from electron microscopy.

IS, inner segment containing many mitochondria and collectively called the ellipsoid; OS, outer segment consisting of laminated plates believed to result from infolding of the cell wall. (An actual electron micrograph from an outer segment is superimposed on the diagram.) Cil, cilia connecting the outer and inner segments.

The cones, concentrated in the macula, function most effectively in conditions of daylight illumination whence they are said to mediate photopic vision. Their photosensitive pigment, iodopsin, has a peak absorption at 540 mμ (in contrast to the peak absorption of 500 for the rod pigment, rhodopsin)[1510, 1516]. While the threshold for cone stimulation is high, owing to the small amount of visual pigment present, the cones show little functional summation with other rods and cones, whence the visual discrimination (visual acuity) from cone stimulation is of a high order.

The rods, scattered widely throughout the retina but absent in the macula, function most effectively at low illumination; they are therefore said to mediate scotopic vision. The threshold for rod stimulation is low because they contain large amounts of the photosensitive pigment rhodopsin and also, according to some authorities, because many rods are summated in one bipolar cell and again in one ganglion cell.[1162] While thus gaining in sensitivity by summation the rods lose in visual discrimination.

The difference between rods and cones is analogous to that between coarse and fine grains of photographic film. The coarse-grain film has greater sensitivity but lacks the qualities of detail of the fine-grain film.

One further difference in rod and cone function is color perception. This appears to be a function of cones and preliminary evidence suggests specific pigments for each of the three primary colors.[1252]

(c) *External limiting membrane.* What appears by light microscopy (Figure 5) to be a fenestrated membrane, long known as the external limiting membrane, has been found by electron microscopy to be a series of cytoplasmic condensations connecting the rod and cone bases with extensions of glial cells.[441] In the language of electron microscopists these are desmosomes (terminal bars) and do not constitute a true membrane.

The extensions of the glial cells (Müller cells) outward beyond the external limiting membrane form knob-like processes, called the fiber baskets of Schwalbe, surrounding the bases of the rods and cones (Figure 7).

(d) *Bipolar cell layer.* Most of the cell bodies in this inner nuclear layer are the bipolar cells that relay impulses from the rod and cone cells to the ganglion cells within. The connecting synapses with their axones and dendrites form the outer and inner plexiform layers which bound the bipolar cell layer (Figure 5).

Aside from the internuncial bipolar cells, this layer contains on its outer regions horizontal cells which also synapse with the rod and cone cells but have certain of the metabolic functions of glia (such as abundant diaphorase activity).[839] These horizontal cells may well serve

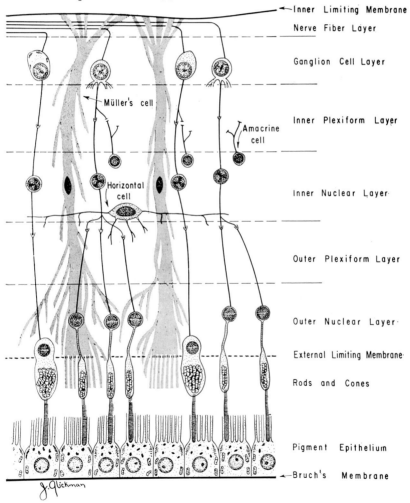

Inner Limiting Membrane

Nerve Fiber Layer

Ganglion Cell Layer

Müller's cell

Amacrine cell

Inner Plexiform Layer

Horizontal cell

Inner Nuclear Layer

Outer Plexiform Layer

Outer Nuclear Layer

External Limiting Membrane

Rods and Cones

Pigment Epithelium

Bruch's Membrane

FIGURE 7. Diagram of neurones and glia within the retina based on a drawing by T. Kuwabara.

for facilitation, inhibition (as in contour discrimination), and other neuronal associations within the retina (Figure 7).

Most of the bodies of Müller cells are situated in the bipolar cell layer. These glial cells course radially through the whole thickness of the retina sending processes externally to form the fiber baskets beyond the external limiting membrane and inward to form a dense plexus of fibers in the innermost layers of the retina (Figure 7). Müller cells have long been identified with mechanical support of the retina, serving to hold the retina together as an integral membrane; recently their metabolic and neuroregulatory roles have come to be stressed. They provide a reservoir of glycogen for the glucose requirements of the retina [850] and have the requisite enzymes for conversion of this glucose into useful energy.[849] These cell processes ramify widely throughout the retina serving, it would seem, as the route of supply from the blood vessels to the nerve cells in a tissue which has a notable lack of extracellular space for diffusion of nutritive substances. That they also provide a neuroregulatory function is suggested by their electrophysiologic responses to flashes of light.[1394] It would appear that Müller's cells (and the same is true of glia elsewhere) have much to do with conditioning the responses in the neurones; no longer are they considered merely passive supports of the retina.

Finally, the inner portion of the bipolar cell layer contains large cells which appear to have been misplaced from the ganglion cell layer. The bipolar cell layer also contains certain cells called amacrine cells because they have no large axone; their function is unknown.

(e) *Ganglion cell layer.* The cells of this layer are distinctive in having abundant cytoplasm to serve the long axones that extend back into the brain. The use of silver stains has permitted the differentiation of small and large ganglion cells. The small ganglion cells are believed to serve cone functions and it has been suggested that each cone is represented by a single ganglion cell on a one-to-one basis whereas the large ganglion cells serving rod functions have a wide representation, each ganglion cell representing as many as eighty rods.[1162]

The concentration of ganglion cells varies widely in different portions of the retina. It is maximal about the macula, where the nuclei form a layer eight to ten cells thick, and minimal in the periphery where the ganglion cells are sparse and situated far apart.

(f) *Nerve fiber layer.* Situated between the ganglion cells and the internal limiting membrane this layer consists of the axones from the ganglion cells, a dense plexus of fibers from Müller's cells, a sprinkling of glia with small round nuclei (lemmocytes), and occasional astrocytes.

The axones of the ganglion cells course horizontally toward the disc and exit from the eye to become myelinated and form the optic nerve. In the retina they radiate toward the disc everywhere except centrally where they form an upper and lower arch to circumvent the macula. The greatest bulk of the nerve fiber layer is immediately adjacent to and overlying the disc.

Occasionally the nerve fibres about the disc are myelinated. Only in such cases are oligodendrocytes found in the retina. This anomalous occurrence of myelin is infrequent in human retinas (Figure 8) but is a regular occurrence in the rabbit retina [112].

(g) *Internal limiting membrane.* By light microscopy the internal limiting membrane is a distinct structure staining most conspic-

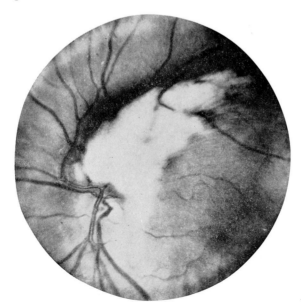

FIGURE 8. Myelinated nerve fibers contiguous with the optic disc. Characteristic is the dense white opacity obscuring the vessels and having fibrillary peripheral edges indicating the course of the nerve fibers.

uously by the periodic acid Schiff method. With the electron micro-scope it appears to be less robust but is nevertheless distinct from both the vitreous with which it has tenuous connections and from the Müller fibers which lie immediately beneath it.[441, 1126] With autolysis or trypsin digestion (and with many pathologic processes) the internal limiting membrane may be separated as a sheet bearing the "finger-prints" of Müller fibers.

This membrane covers the entire inner surface of the retina, merging with the epithelial cells of the pars plana at the ora serrata, but is absent over the nerve head. It is from this latter region, therefore, that fibrovascular tissue can grow into the vitreous under pathologic conditions.

The light reflexes seen with the ophthalmoscope come chiefly from the internal limiting membrane. These appear as a sheen or dotted highlights scattered throughout the fundi. A few clinical observations have been made on the aberrations of these reflexes in disease (thus, retinal edema is said to produce a loss of the sheen)[565, 446] but the field warrants further study.

(h) *Macula.* The macula lutea (yellow spot) is an ill-defined area at the posterior pole of the eye having approximately the same dimensions as the optic disc. The yellow color is not ordinarily visible during

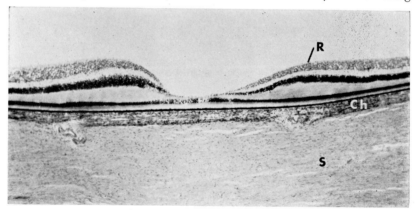

FIGURE 9. Cross section of posterior pole of eye through the macula. H. & E. stain. Characteristic of the macula is the central declivity or fovea (where the inner retinal layers are attenuated) and the abundance of ganglion cells in the parafoveal regions.

R, retina; Ch, choroid; S, sclera.

life against the orange background of the choroid but stands out in death or whenever the retina becomes opaque. The yellow color increases with age[1264, 1162] and corresponds to the "pigment" granules in the ganglion cells seen by electron microscopy.[442]

The fovea is the central declivity of the macula (about the size of the head of a pin) caused by local attenuation of the inner layers of the retina (Figure 9). Ophthalmoscopically it is identifiable by a central bright highlight reflected from its concave inner surface. Having the densest population of cones, the fovea is the portion of the retina on which objects of attention are focussed under photopic conditions but which, having no rods, is effectively blind under scotopic conditions. Covering approximately 2° of the central visual field it is the region of greatest acuity.

Subprimate mammals have only rudimentary maculas. They also have only slight motility of their eyes in comparison with man since the entire function of the ocular motor system is to focus objects of regard on the macula.

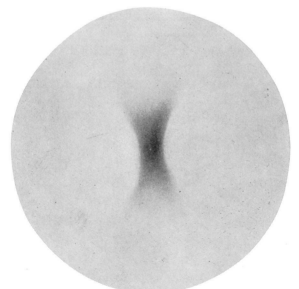

FIGURE 10. Haidinger's brushes. When one looks at a uniformly blue background (such as the sky) through a single polarizing filter one see yellowish brushes, here illustrated by the gray tone, alternating with light blue quadrants. This occupies only the center 2°-3° of the visual field and is therefore thought to correspond to the radiating fibers of Henle.

Since the ganglion and bipolar layers are absent in the center of the macula the axones of the rod and cone cells in the outer plexiform layer must reach their next higher layer by radiating obliquely rather than vertically. This locally skewed direction of the nerve fibers and glia is given the special name of Henle's layer and accounts for the star arrangement of light reflexes and deposits about the macula.

Haidinger's brushes are entoptic phenomena seen best when a uniformly blue background is visualized through a single polarizing lens[1373]. The brushes are two yellow sheaths extending out 2°-3° from the point of fixation and separated by bright blue quadrants (Fig. 10). They are related to the radiating pattern of Henle's layer and have been recommended as a clinical test for macular function[556, 466, 1285, 1338].

The reduction of the nerve fiber layer over the macula is attained by an arching arrangement of fibers about the fovea. This results in a pattern of nerve fibers as sketched in Figure 11 and permits lesions of the disc to produce field defects sharply demarcated by the horizontal meridian.

Although there is no anatomic landmark for the vertical meridian of the retina, an arbitrary line drawn vertically through the fovea will

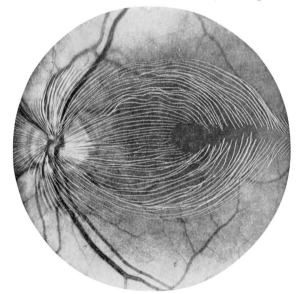

FIGURE 11. Sketch of nerve fibers superimposed on a fundus photograph to show the arching arrangement about the fovea.

divide the retina into approximate halves corresponding to separate representation on the two sides of the brain. This division is seen impressively in histologic preparations of optic atrophy following tract lesions: the ganglion cells have completely disappeared from one side of the fovea but are normally abundant on the opposite side (Figure 12).

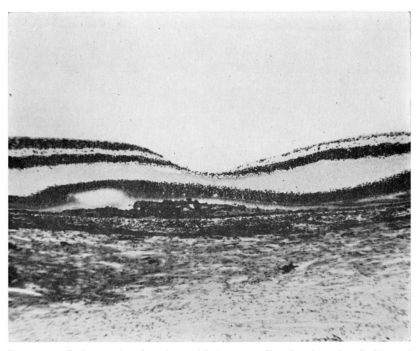

FIGURE 12. Left macula of patient with long standing hemianopia of chiasmal origin. The area on the temporal side of the fovea *(left in the photograph)* shows normally abundant ganglion cells whereas the corresponding area on the nasal side *(right in the photograph)* shows glial cells only. (The elevation of the macula by residual folded layers of pigment epithelium is an artifact.)

The sparing of the central portions of the visual field in an otherwise complete hemianopia has suggested a bilateral representation of the macula in the brain. An alternative suggestion has been an assumed spread of the stimulus within the retina[574]! The thesis of bilateral representation, however, seems unlikely (see p. 255) and the specific possibility of intraretinal cross-stimulation is disproved by the absence of sparing in cases of hemianopia from optic tract lesions.

(i) *Inversion of the retina and transparency.* The retina is re-markably transparent; yet the "inverse" orientation whereby light has to penetrate the full thickness of the retina before stimulating the photoreceptors must present some handicap to vision. This inversion is presumably necessary so that the rods and cones will be in immediate proximity to the pigment epithelium and the choriocapillaris from which their stores of photosensitive substances are derived. In the re-gion of the fovea the handicap is minimized by attenuation of the innermost layers.

A further limitation imposed on the nerve fibers of the retina by this necessity of maintaining transparency is their lack of insulation by myelin. In consequence, there is spread or leakage of stimulus by impulses traversing the nerve fiber layer. This adventitious spread pro-duces a glare that can be observed entoptically in the "blue arc" phenomenon wherein the impulse spreads from the fibers arching about the macula to underlying neurones[1363, 503] (Figure 13).

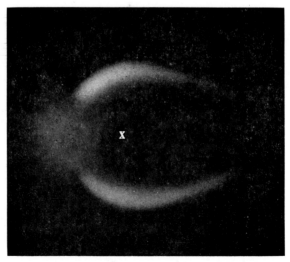

FIGURE 13. Blue arc phenomenon as seen when an observer in the dark gazes with his right eye to the right of a small red light. The point of fixation is rep-resented by the area marked X, the red light is represented by the blur to the left of this, and the two "horns" are the vividly blue entoptic arcs extending to the region of the blind spot on the right. The phenomenon is thought to be due to transneuronal spread of a stimulus within the retina and to indicate the nor-mal lack of complete insulation.

(j) *Blood supply.* The blood supply to the human retina accords with the division of the retina into outer and inner layers. The rods, cones, and outer nuclear layer are supplied through diffusion from the choriocapillaris (at least in the posterior portions of the eye). The rest of the retina, comprising the bipolar cell layer, the ganglion cell layer, the inner reticular and the nerve fiber layers, is supplied by branches of the central retinal artery.

The central artery has four branches, one for each quadrant of the eye, with little overlap in distribution between each branch—they are end-arteries. The superior and inferior temporal arteries thus show a sharp division in area of supply demarcated by a hypothetical horizontal line; an occlusion of either of these branches will cause an altitudinal hemianopia.

A common variant is a small artery derived from the choroid, emerging at the temporal edge of the disc, and supplying the cecocentral area of the retina (Figure 14). This is called a cilioretinal artery and may be the means of saving a small amount of sight when the main retinal artery is occluded. Or, conversely, it may be

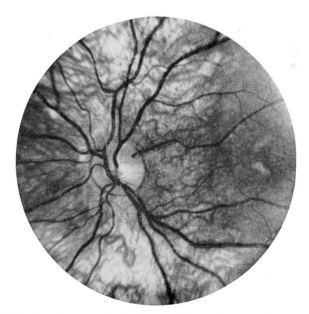

FIGURE 14. Fundus photograph showing a cilioretinal artery in upper temporal quadrant of the disc. This artery is derived from the choroidal circulation.

occluded and cause a cecocentral scotoma with a full peripheral field when the main retinal artery is patent[505].

The central retinal artery is usually the first branch of the ophthalmic artery as this latter vessel enters the orbit. The ophthalmic artery is in turn the first major intracranial branch of the internal carotid artery as the latter emerges from the cavernous sinus. Thus, the retinal artery arises close to the major cranial artery of the head and may accordingly be expected to have a high pressure.

A frequent variant in this arterial supply is the origin of the ophthalmic artery (and therefore of the retinal artery) from the middle meningeal artery. Since this latter is derived from the external carotid system, through the maxillary artery, the eye will be supplied in such cases by the external carotid rather than the internal system.

The retina has a rich meshwork of capillaries that can be isolated by trypsin digestion and studied in whole mounts[848] (Figure 15). In the posterior part of the eye the capillaries are supplied by small pre-capillary arterioles that come off the main artery as side-arm branches

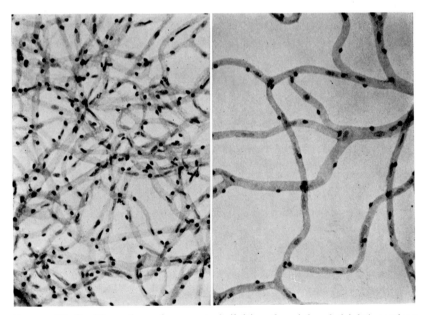

FIGURE 15. Capillary plexus from central *(left)* and peripheral *(right)* portions of the retina. The vessels were isolated by trypsin digestion, stained by the periodic acid Schiff method and hematoxylin, and mounted on the flat.

and undergo multiple subdivisions before rejoining into one or more venules. In the periphery where they are much more sparse the capillaries arise from repeated subdivision of the arteries and form simpler capillary plexuses.

This progressive dichotomy would lead one to expect a lower hydrostatic pressure in the peripheral capillaries as compared with the central capillaries which arise from larger arteriolar trunks. This effect is mitigated, however, by the greater capillary bed served by the precapillary arteriole in the central area.

The basement membrane of the retinal capillaries is, by comparison with that of capillaries elsewhere in the body, unusually thick. The capillary cells consist of endothelial cells lining the lumina and cells within the substance of the wall called by some pericytes but by others mural cells[851] (Figure 16). We prefer this latter name since it sets these cells apart from the heterogeneous cells that have been labelled pericytes and it more properly refers to their localization *within* the wall

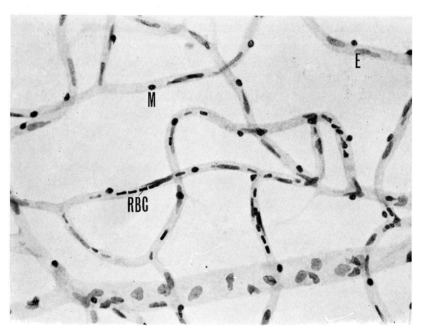

FIGURE 16. Enlarged view of retinal capillaries isolated by trypsin digestion, stained with hematoxylin and eosin, and mounted on the flat.

E, endothelial cell nucleus; M, mural cell nucleus; and RBC, red blood cells.

substance. Mural cells are readily demonstrable in flat mounts and are about as numerous as the endothelial cells. Their function is not known with certainty but they may be responsible for the uniform distribution of blood throughout the capillary meshwork; we know that, unlike capillaries which have no mural cells, the retinal capillaries show a continuous flow of blood all the time and are incapable of reversible congestion. The clinical importance of the mural cells is determined in part by their relative resistance (in comparison with endothelial cells) to ischemia but more especially by their specific vulnerability in diabetes (see p. 57f).

The retinal veins follow the same general pattern as the arteries and similarly form a central vein in the axis of the optic nerve (Figure 14). The occasional vein that leaves at the edge of the disc to connect with the choroidal circulation is called an opticociliary vein but these vessels are much less frequent than are their arterial counterparts, the cilioretinal arteries. Lymphatics are absent in the retina[882] and there is no extravascular space except immediately about the main vessels near the disc.

The presence or absence of pulsation in the large retinal vessels is determined by the relation of intraocular to intravascular pressure. Arterial pulsations are never present normally but will occur whenever the diastolic pressure is pathologically low (syncope, vasomotor collapse, aortic regurgitation ,or hyperthyroidism) or when the intraocular pressure is pathologically high (glaucoma). Indeed, retinal arterial pressures are measured by a process called ophthalmodynamometry whereby those points are determined in which increasing pressure on the eye first causes pulsation (diastole) and further pressure causes continued collapse of the arteries (systole) (see p. 36). The eye can thus be used as a sphygmomanometer.

In contrast to arterial pulsations, venous pulsations are present in about half of all normal persons and can be elicited by gentle pressure on the eye in most other persons. This is not, however, a primary venous pulsation but is a rhythmic collapse of the veins secondary to pulsatile oscillations of the intraocular pressure. The absolute level of the retinal venous pressure has no significance; it adjusts itself automatically to the mean intraocular pressure. When this latter is elevated the vein momentarily collapses at the site of lowest pressure, that is at the point of exit from the eye, and the intravascular pressure builds up until it again exceeds the intraocular pressure and allows blood to flow out of the eye.

(k) *Electroretinogram.* The function of some portions of the retina may be evaluated by recording the electric impulse resulting from flashing a light into the eye. One electrode is placed on the cornea by means of a contact glass and the other electrode is connected with some indifferent site such as the eyelids or mouth. A graph re-

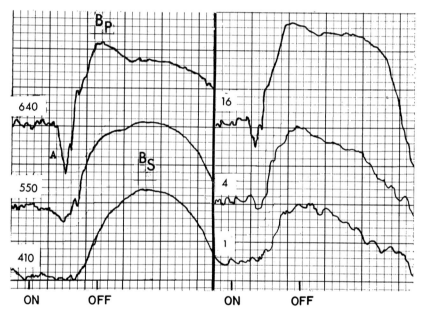

Figure 17. Typical electroetinograms from the eye of a twenty-one year old normal subject. The records were made with a CAT computer and represent the average response to a flash whose duration was 0.1 second. (The records and interpretation were provided by Prof. Lorrin A. Riggs, Brown University.)

The three records on the left illustrate differences in waveform due to changes in wavelength of stimulation. For the top record the grating monochromotor was set at 640 mu which strongly stimulated cone receptors; a deep *a*-wave and large photopic *b*-wave resulted. For the bottom record the monochromotor was set at 410 mu which caused scarcely any cone response but an effective rod response; a scotopic *b*-wave was the only prominent feature.

The three records on the right illustrate the effect of stimulus intensity. The wavelength for all of them was 640 mu and the relative intensities of the stimulus flash were 16, 4, and 1. The drop in intensity resulted in a loss of both photopic and scotopic portions of the wave.

cording the change in potential following exposure to the flash of light is called an electroretinogram.[1213, 575]

Although requiring equipment of a fairly elaborate nature (shielded room, electronic amplifiers, and recorders), electroretinography is a relatively simple test. A sample normal curve is shown in the accompanying Figure 17. The a wave is believed to arise from the outer layers of the retina (possibly from the rods and cones themselves[185]), the b wave from the intermediate layers of the retina and the c wave from the pigment epithelium.

Lesions of the outer retinal layers abolish the electroretinographic response whereas lesions of the inner retinal layers, however extensive, show a normal response[616]. Thus the electroretinogram is extinguished (or nearly so[38]) with retinitis pigmentosa but is normal in Tay-Sachs disease[295]. Although electroretinography is a valuable research tool it has only limited clinical usefulness because of its non-localizability to specific areas of the retina and because of the fact that other clinical evidence can usually provide all the practical information needed for diagnosis.

(1) ***Pigment Epithelium and Bruch's Membrane.*** Lying imme-

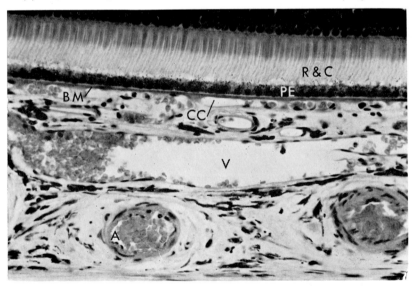

Figure 18. Cross section of choroid and outer layers of retina.
R&C, rods and cones; PE, pigment epithelium; BM, Bruch's membrane; CC, choriocapillaris; V, vein of choroid; A, artery of choroid.

diately external to the retina is the pigment epithelium and external to this a hyaloelastic layer, Bruch's membrane, intimately associated with the choriocapillaris (Figure 18). The pigment epithelium is a monocellular layer of hexagonal cells that send interdigitating processes between the photoreceptive elements of the retina. Some have likened the pigment epithelium, with its intimate relation to the outer layer of the retina, to the sheath of Schwann in the peripheral nerve.[1513] Aside from their function as bearers of pigment that absorbs the extraneous light, the pigment cells participate in the removal of vitamin A from the blood and conversion of the vitamin A into the photosensitive substance, retinene. The pigment epithelium comprises a highly active group of cells, as judged by their rich content of mitochondria, and can proliferate vigorously under pathologic conditions.

Bruchs' membrane is a modified basement membrane of the pigment epithelium that is hyaline on its inner portion and elastic on its outer portion. It commonly forms wart-like excrescenes, called drusen, and regularly undergoes lipid and calcific changes with age. Many of the lesions of the outer layers of the retina that occur with age are caused by ruptures of a calcified Bruchs' membrane with consequent hemorrhage from the choriocapillaris.

B. DEVELOPMENTAL ABNORMALTIES

Most common are the developmental abnormalities of the retina which occur in association with anencephaly[396] and other gross brain defects. The ophthalmoscope may reveal in such cases a large chorioretinal coloboma (Figure 19) occupying much of the lower fundus or simply a white disc and attenuated vessels extending onto the fundus. Such infants are effectively blind but they often show a surprising blepharospasm in response to light and at least a vestige of pupillary reactivity[646].

Aplastic retinas show an abortive development of the cellular layers, an absence of the rods and cones, and a gliosis of the inner layers of the retina. When the outer layers are distorted there is a characteristic rosette formation with abortive rod and cone elements facing inward toward the center of the rosette. Or there may be congenital folds in the retina with retention of portions of the vestigial hyaloid system and proliferation of blood vessels from the retina.

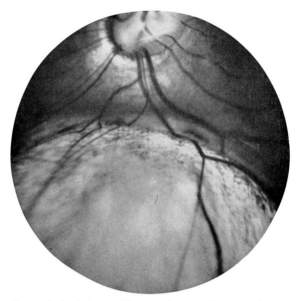

Figure 19. Congenital coloboma. Noteworthy are the anomalous vessels emerging from the disc and the large chorioretinal defect below the disc. This latter was depressed one to two diopters behind the level of the adjacent fundus.

Retrolental fibroplasia is a disease of premature infants (weighing less than four pounds) who have been exposed to high concentrations of oxygen in an incubator. The oxygen causes swelling and necrosis of the capillary endothelium (but only of the retina) with early occlusion of the vessels. Later vasoproliferation occurs when the infant is removed from the incubator. The name retrolental fibroplasia was adopted under the erroneous impression that the pathogenesis lay in a fibrous metaplasia of the fetal hyaloid system[1420].

Developmental abnormalities involving absence of rod function (congenital night blindness and Oguchi's disease) or of cone function (achromatopsia) will be discussed in association with degenerative lesions to which they are symptomatically related (see p. 88f).

Many other developmental anomalies involving the retina will be mentioned only in passing since they have limited neuro-ophthalmic significance. These include congenital folds of the retina[975] (often with other malformations of the eye[1554] or face[759]), massive retinal dysplasia with the 13-15 trisomy syndrome[276], curious tapetoretinal reflexes, colobomas beneath the disc, massive retinal gliosis[1184, 1256] (sometimes transmitted as a sex linked trait and then called Norrie's disease[1076, 28, 1533]), and abnormal tortuosity of the retinal arteries in association with coarctation of the aorta[432]. Some of these are determined as genetic errors of metabolism and some result from viral or other disturbances of the mother during gestation. In all these abnormalities the problem is to differentiate primarily aplastic defects from secondary reactions. This is often impossible.

SUMMARY

The retina is the seeing portion of the eye that transmutes a light stimulus into a neuronal excitation. Derived embryologically from an evagination of the central neural tube the human retina consists of a neuroectodermal layer of rods and cones, an intermediate layer of bipolar cells, horizontal cells, and Müller's cells, and the inner layers containing ganglion cells, glia, nerve fibers and internal limiting membrane.

The rods and cones are the photoreceptors and consist essentially of outer segments containing laminated plates with a photoreceptive pigment and inner segments with dense packing of mitochondria. The so-called external limiting membrane is seen by electron microscopy to consist of a series of terminal bars joining the rod and cone cells to the adjacent extensions of Müller's cells. The bipolar cells are the internuncial neurones corresponding to the dorsal-root ganglia in the peripheral nervous system. Within the bipolar layer are the cell bodies of those modified glia called Müller's fibers which extend through the full thickness of the retina. The ganglion cells in the inner layer correspond to neurones in the gray matter of the spinal cord, while the nerve fiber layer of the retina and the optic nerve itself correspond to the spinothalamic tracts within the brain stem and spinal cord that relay impulses to the basal ganglia. The lateral geniculate body and visual radiation correspond in turn to the thalamic nuclei and parietal radiation of the sensory system. The internal limiting membrane is a true basement membrane of the retina.

The macula in the human retina is a region where there is a condensation of special cones and a concentration of ganglion cells that permit high visual resolution. In its center the retina is thinned by attenuation of the inner layers forming a central declivity called the foveola which is the region of maximal visual acuity.

Nutrition to the inner layers of the human retina is supplied by branches of the central retinal artery and an elaborate capillary plexus. The outer retinal layers are supplied by diffusion from the choriocapillaris.

The pigment epithelium consists of a monocellular layer of hexagonal cells lying just external to the rods and cones. It provides the photoreceptors with a sheathing of melanin pigment and the vitamin A substrates for the photosensitive pigments.

External to the pigment epithelium and constituting the basement membrane is the hyaloelastic layer called Bruch's membrane. Just external to this and intimately associated with it is the plexus of venous sinuses called the choriocapillaris.

Developmental anomalies are manifest in the retina by aplasia, replacement of the inner layers by glial tissue, rosette formation in the outer layers, accessory folds of the entire retina, persistence of the fetal hyaloid system, proliferation of the retinal vessels into the vitreous (retrolental fibrophasia), massive retinal gliosis, and simple absence of either rod or cone function. Some of these anomalies are determined genetically. Others occur idiopathically either as isolated occurrences or in association with abnormalities of the brain and rest of the body. Some result from viral infections of the mother during pregnancy.

CHAPTER II

RETINA: Vascular Lesions

1. Occlusive Disease of Retinal Arteries

T HE CLINICAL PICTURE of occlusive arterial disease is characteristic. Sudden blindness occurs when the entire retinal artery is obstructed and altitudinal hemianopia when the superior or inferior branch is obstructed. The ophthalmoscope reveals a diffuse cloudiness of the retina (Figure 20) with a contrasting red center, the cherry red spot in the macula. This opacification, often erroneously attributed to edema, is actually due to cloudy swelling of the ganglion cells and is, consequently, most evident in those portions of the retina where the ganglion cells are concentrated. The cloudiness is followed after

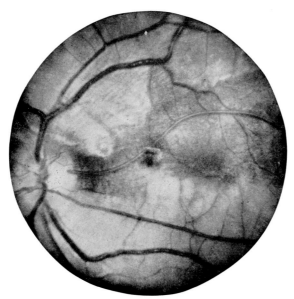

FIGURE 20. Occlusion of the central retinal artery. The opacification of the retina is shown particularly well in the present photograph because of the sparing of the retina in the region of the cilioretinal artery.

[31]

several days by pallor of the nerve head. A similar cloudiness and cherry red spot occur post-mortem and occasionally in otherwise normal eyes.

The actual obstruction is usually short-lived and has disappeared by the time the patient is seen by a physician. However, it may occasionally persist for several hours or even days and is then manifest by static or slowly moving segments of blood with an appearance that has been likened to "box-car" or "freight-car" trains.

The segmentation of the blood column indicates a slow movement of the red blood cells. When it does not occur spontaneously it may be induced by gentle pressure on the eye[752]. It is seen most commonly in veins but may be seen in the arteries when the obstruction is severe. Segmentation may be a manifestation of arterial obstruction, excessively viscous blood (so-called sludged blood) or a sequel of cardiac failure. It occurs regularly at the time of death and is said to be a useful sign in the detection of cardiac arrest and in evaluating the effectiveness of resuscitation[790, 788]. In addition to segmentation one occasionally sees an actual reversal of flow with blood coursing toward the disc in some arteries[1183].

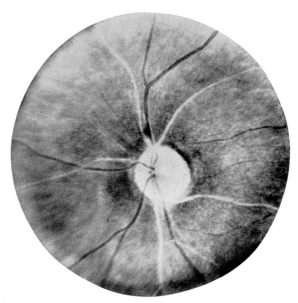

FIGURE 21. White disc (optic atrophy) and ensheathed arteries in a patient with long standing occlusion of the central retinal artery.

The late manifestations of retinal artery occlusion are pale nerve heads with narrowed, often ensheathed arteries (Figure 21). Hemorrhages are not a regular feature but they may occur as the circulation returns. They probably represent leaks through the vessels damaged during the period of obstruction. Occasionally they are massive.

(a) *Syndromes.* Arterial obstructions may be embolic, atherosclerotic, ischemic, or inflammatory.

Emboli occur precipitously without warning. They may occlude the main retinal artery and thus cause complete blindness or they may occlude a branch of the artery causing an altitudinal field defect. Calcific emboli can frequently be seen in branch occlusions and have the curious feature of being considerably larger than the apparent lumen of the vessel (Figure 22). With total occlusion the region immediately about the disc is often spared, due to collateral choroidal circulation, thus permitting retention of a vestige of vision.

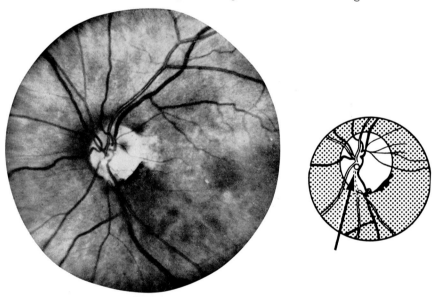

FIGURE 22. Calcific embolus lodged just below center of disc. The embolus appeared along with a corresponding field defect at the time of a mitral valvulotomy. The appearance of the embolus did not change over an observation period of four years. Collateral circulation (evident in the photograph) occurred within a few weeks but without improvement in vision. The arrow in the accompanying sketch points to the embolus and to the occluded portion of the inferior temporal artery.

A larger field often including central vision will be spared with the fortuitous presence of a cilo-retinal artery (Figure 14). Conversely the cilio-retinal artery may be occluded while the rest of the retinal circulation is intact; the visual field then shows a cecocentral scotoma[182].

Emboli usually occur in persons with cardiac or pulmonary sources for the emboli. Cardiac sources have been held to account for three-fourths of all emboli[638]. In young persons the embolus most frequently comes from post-rheumatic vegetations[664], especially following cardiac catheterization or mitral valvulotomies, while in older persons the source is more commonly atheromata in the carotid system. Less common causes are cardiac myxomas[981] and iatrogenic traumas of angiography[1034, 277, 340] (Figure 23).

The prognosis following embolization is poor. Rarely does one have an opportunity to do paracentesis within the few minutes that would be necessary to salvage vision and even then emboli can rarely be dislodged by such a maneuver. On the other hand, some success has

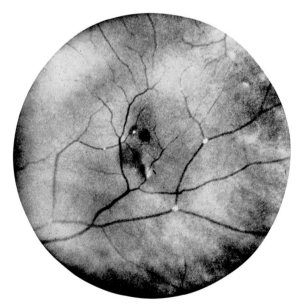

FIGURE 23. Multiple emboli in the retinal arteries. These occurred during a carotid endarterectomy and are presumed to be fat. They occur preferentially but not exclusively at bifurcation sites.

been obtained by prompt massage and use of carbon dioxide and oxygen[608, 1123].

Atheromatosis is probably a common cause of retinal artery occlusion in older persons although rarely is there an opportunity to prove this histologically. The ultimate occlusions, characterized by blindness and cherry red spot in the macula, are often preceded by several episodes of blackouts (amaurosis fugax) lasting a few minutes. Nevertheless black-outs do not necessarily all end up in occlusion even when they are due to atheroma. Some black-outs may occur repeatedly for years and then, presumably due to development of collateral circulation, cease permanently[265].

Atheromatous occlusion of the retinal arteries differs from embolic occlusion in several respects. Due to the anatomic difference in the main retinal arteries and their branches (see discussion on pathology, p. 43) atheromata cause occlusion of the retinal arteries within the eye less often than do emboli. But the reverse is true for occlusion of the central retinal artery behind the eye. There atheromatosis is more commonly the cause of occlusion than is embolus. Since atheromatous occlusion is gradual there is more chance for the development of collateral channels and the prognosis is better.

The wide variety of therapeutic procedures which have been reported to be successful in this type of occlusion probably reflects to a considerable degree the spontaneous reversibility of atheromatous ischemia. On the other hand the occlusion may persist beyond the recoverable stage and the result will be permanent blindness, optic atrophy and narrow vessels.

One might expect ophthalmodynamometry to be of great service in evaluating obstructions to the central retinal artery. This is not the case. Usually blood flow has been restored by the time a physician sees the patient and since the pressure in the retinal artery reflects that in the ophthalmic artery[395], even when it is narrowed, the pressure will not be appreciably lowered[1345]. As long as the retinal artery is sufficiently patent to permit some blood flow, however restricted, its pressure will be that of the artery from which it is derived.

The character of the arterial pulse, induced by pressure on the eye is, however, altered in partial arterial occlusion. For the first few days after a retinal occlusion a pulse may not be elicitable[920].

Later it will be present but lack the brisk, snapping quality of the normal pulse. While it fills and empties with each pulsation, it does so more sluggishly.

Atheromatous occlusion of the retinal arteries is often confused with atheromatous occlusion of small arteries to the optic nerve. These latter give rise to less complete blindness and less regular field defects, and do not show the cloudy swelling of the retina as do the retinal occlusions.

Ischemia of the retina is a comprehensive term covering all forms of inadequate blood supply to the retina sufficient to cause blackouts or blindness. Occasionally it follows massive hemorrhages[672] (hematemesis, bleeding from bowel, or surgery) and it is then associated with generalized shock. The blindness, which may be unilateral but is generally bilateral, does not usually come on until several days after the blood loss and is then followed by central retinal cloudiness and optic atrophy such as occurs after occlusive arterial disease. Rarely the ischemia results from heart failure or too rapid lowering of the blood pressure in the treatment of hypertension[807]. It has been the cause of black-outs in aviators subjected to more than 4.5 G acceleration[389].

More commonly, ischemia results from carotid occlusion and is part of a syndrome of black-outs or blindness in one eye and hemiplegia or hemisensory symptoms of the opposite side of the body. This syndrome has long been recognized[729,570] but recently re-emphasized[454, 666] as a cause of "small strokes." It can be readily diagnosed by ophthalmodynamometry when the retinal diastolic pressure on one side is significantly lower than on the other side.

Ophthalmodynamometry is usually performed by two persons, one who exerts an increasing pressure against the sclera while the other watches for the collapse of the artery on the nerve head. The point at which the retinal artery begins to pulsate corresponds to diastole while that where it just remains collapsed corresponds to systole. Usually the mean of several readings is taken and recordings are often made with the patient in supine and erect positions successively[1350]. Most ophthalmodynamometers are calibrated to record pressures in the range of 10-150 grams. This can be converted into mm Hg. pressure by re-exerting the diastolic and systolic pressures on the eye while a tonometer simultaneously records the intraocular pressure, but this is seldom necessary since one is ordinarily interested in the relative differences between the two eyes rather than in absolute values.

Variation between the two eyes is normally less than 15 per cent[1364] but allowances must be made for the experience of the observers and for the visibility of the vessels during the examination. Needless to say, dilatation of the pupil facilitates the measurements and indirect ophthalmoscopy is easier for both the examiner and the patient.

The diagnosis of carotid occlusion is fortified by hearing a bruit in the supraclavicular region on the affected side[448, 308] and occasionally by hearing a bruit over the ipsilateral[284] or contralateral[453] eye. Pressure on the patent carotid may produce an informative syncope but is a dangerous diagnostic maneuver[1398, 1347]. The common site[776] of the occlusion is either at the bifurcation of the common carotid or at the arch of the aorta (whence the name aortic arch syndrome[1238]). When the obstruction is in the internal carotid artery a collateral circulation may develop through the external carotid, angular and ophthalmic arteries so that the main blood supply to the eye on the affected side is by way of the external carotid system[413, 1331, 1529, 356, 749, 1260, 1463, 244, 539, 1410, 1595, 1489, 1531, 155] (Figure 24). In such patients there will be no significant difference in the ophthalmodynamometric readings despite the carotid occlusion.

As might be expected, a wide variation in symptoms results from carotid occlusion. Some of the variables resulting from anatomic structure are the different sites of the occlusion, the patency of collateral channels through the Circle of Willis and external carotid arteries[1017, 1051] (see p. 187) and the inconstancy of the vascular architecture[1212]. In general, symptoms will be more severe the lower the obstruction is in the carotid system, the more extensive the atheromatosis is in the collateral channels (opposite carotid artery and anterior communicating artery) and the older the patient[708].

Black-outs from carotid occlusion may occur over a long period before blindness results. They frequently cease when hemiplegia supervenes[455]. Yet they occur in only a minority of patients with carotid occlusion[666]. About as common as blindness are field defects which, as in other forms of retinal artery occlusion, show a predilection to involve the lower fields.

The black-outs and other symptoms of carotid occlusion are often dramatically relieved by anticoagulant treatment[1025]. This improvement occurs even when there is no measurable elevation in the retinal arterial pressure; it is as though anticoagulation improved blood flow by means other than pressure changes.

Bilateral occlusion of the carotid arteries occurs with wide-spread vascular occlusion in a syndrome known as pulseless disease or the aortic arch syndrome. One variety of this is caused by athero-sclerosis[1433], often with aortic aneurysms, and produces incapacitating black-outs and fainting whenever the patient stands up. The retinal arterial pressures are extremely low in such cases and the retinal vessels develop microaneurysms[1151, 381], often in great numbers. Ophthalmo-dynamometry may be especially useful in such cases not only for confirming the diagnosis[644, 673, 134, 1443] but the fundus may be the only place in the body where blood pressure readings can be obtained[1349]. Another form of the pulseless syndrome, Takayasu's disease, occurs chiefly (but not exclusively[43]), in Japanese young women and is due to widespread arteritis (see p. 42). The retinal pressures in these cases are also profoundly low and the vessels themselves develop arterio-venous shunts about the disc. A third cause for pulseless disease, more common in years past than at present, is syphilitic disease of the carotid and aortic arteries[1238, 823].

There are many reasons for amaurosis fugax other than carotid occlusion although most involve retinal ischemia. Such is the case with

---

FIGURE 24. Arteriogram illustrating obstruction of the internal carotid artery with collateral circulation to the brain by way of branches of the external carotid artery.

The site of obstruction is just below the point marked for the carotid artery (C.A.). In consequence the distal portion of the carotid siphon is filled by retrograde flow through the ophthalmic artery (Oph.A.) by the hypertrophied internal maxillary artery (I.M.A.) and superficial temporal artery (S.T.A.). These latter two arteries are branches of the external carotid artery (E.C.A.). The direction of flow is indicated by arrows.

Of incidental interest is the hypertrophied middle meningeal artery (M.M.A.) which is also a branch of the external carotid artery and supplies the parietal region along with the occipital artery (Occ.A.). This compensates for the inadequacy of the terminal branches of the middle cerebral artery which normally supply this area.

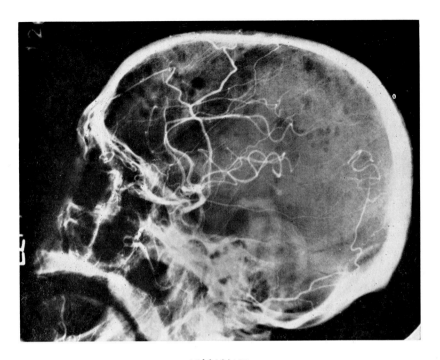

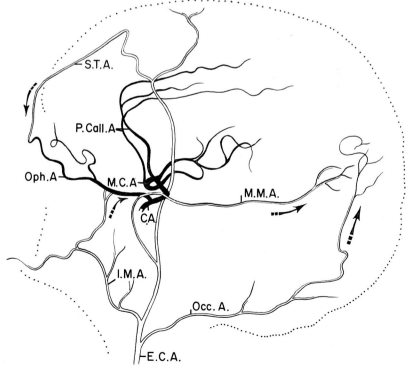

S.T.A.

P.Call.A.

Oph.A.

M.C.A.

C.A.

M.M.A.

I.M.A.

Occ. A.

E.C.A.

black-outs in papilledema and in the uniocular variety of ophthalmic migraine[823, 265] (if indeed such an entity exists). Several cases of black-outs have been reported with transient dilatation of the retinal veins and with abnormal tissue on the nerve head[928, 573]. There are still other cases, however, which do not reveal evidence for a vascular basis and must be assumed to be functional[265].

The term spasm has been widely used, and abused, to designate intermittent blackouts. It would be improper to deny that spasm may occur but to call every case of amaurosis fugax a spasm is also unwarranted; the majority, including those in which the retinal arteries are narrowed during an attack, are clearly the result of failure of the blood to get into the eye. This may be due to retinal artery obstruction or to hypotension in the ophthalmic artery and should not necessarily imply spasm.

Aside from the spontaneous variety, retinal ischemia is often induced artificially in ligations of the carotid artery for intracranial aneurysms or fistulas[1198]. In fact black-outs are one of the signs warning against surgery by ligation. Ophthalmodynamometry may be usefully employed to evaluate the effectiveness of ligation and to follow the course of events after surgery[1396]. Ligation of the common carotid artery results usually in a permanent lowering of the retinal arterial pressures whereas ligation of the internal carotid results in less effective lowering of the pressure. This decreased effectivity is due, presumably, to collateral circulation through the external carotid artery (see p. 37).

Inflammatory occlusion of the retinal arteries occurs in two distinct entities and probably in many non-specific entities. The two distinct syndromes with inflammatory retinal artery occlusion are temporal arteritis and Takayasu's disease. Temporal arteritis occurs in elderly persons as a manifestation of a systemic disease characterized by fever, elevated sedimentation rate, and a giant cell arteritis that is steroid sensitive[126, 1050]. While the etiology of this disease is obscure, the pathologic changes center about the elastica; and the serum of the affected patients is said to show a fall in elastase inhibitor substance[64]. The disease is identified in the literature as temporal arteritis because the symptoms of preauricular tenderness, headache, and painful jaw movements point to these arteries and biopsy permits ready confirmation. But arteries elsewhere in the body (including the coronaries) may be involved[1257] so that giant cell arteritis would have been a preferable name[1367] if usage had not established its present designation in the literature.

Temporal arteritis may cause blindness with no clinical symptoms pointing to the temporal arteries[1329, 1018, 1140]. This has been called occult temporal arteritis and definitive diagnosis can be established only by biopsy[1329]. Even biopsies may not be conclusive, for one portion of the temporal artery may be negative while another portion is positive[43] or the ophthalmic artery may show an inflammation while the temporal artery is negative[1395].

Although the inflammatory process has been localized in the retinal arteries in a few cases[294], most of the visual disturbances with temporal arteritis, especially those associated with swelling of the disc, have been due to involvement of the ophthalmic artery[210, 315, 1395] and of the ciliary branches to the optic nerve[210, 836, 1367, 315].

Approximately one-half of the patients with temporal arteritis

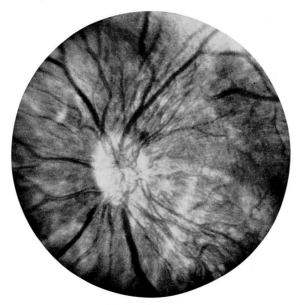

Figure 25. Takayasu's disease. The patient was a twenty-seven year old Chinese girl whose brachial and femoral blood pressures were not measurable and whose intracranial arterial pressure was so low she fainted whenever she stood up. Both fundi showed a plexus of proliferated vessels coming from the discs.

develop visual symptoms[1503, 186] and these symptoms come on generally three to four weeks after the symptoms of malaise and temporal arterial disease. The sedimentation rate is practically always elevated and is a most valuable aid for diagnosis and a guide to therapy. The blindness is generally irreversible but probably preventable by steroids[669].

The other specific type of inflammatory arterial occlusion affecting the retinal vessels is Takayasu's disease[1407] (Figure 25). This affects all the arteries of the body producing a syndrome of pulseless disease, with elevated sedimentation rate, leukocytosis, fever, and granulomatous arteritis[1317, 201]. Unlike the findings with the atherosclerotic type of pulseless disease the retinal changes in the inflammatory type consist of a proliferation of vessels and anomalous anastomoses about the disc in addition to the microaneurysms. Further ocular manifestations of this disease are cataracts and iris atrophy.

Other types of inflammatory disease of the retinal arteries are not so regularly associated with arterial occlusion, nor are they clearly distinct from inflammation of the veins. Hence discussion of these other

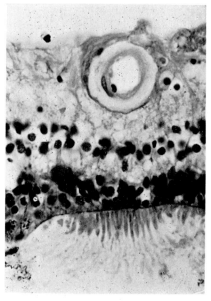

FIGURE 26. Hyaline thickening of the basement membrane in retinal arteriolar sclerosis. H. and E. stain.

types of arteritis will be reserved until a subsequent section on vasculitis (see p. 53).

(b) **Pathology.** Discussion of the pathology of retinal artery occlusion must first take into account the abrupt anatomic changes which occur as the artery enters the eye. While in the optic nerve, the central artery has an internal elastic lamina and a robust media and adventitia comparable to that of larger arteries, but after passing the lamina cribosa the artery loses its elastica, the media becomes much reduced, and all connective tissue of the adventitia disappears except immediately about the disc.

The pathologic changes in the extraocular and intraocular portions of the retinal artery show corresponding differences. Atherosclerotic occlusion of the arteries in the retina is manifest by mild proliferation of endothelial cells, thickening of the basement membrane (as visualized with periodic acid Schiff stains) and hyalinization of the wall (as seen in hematoxylin and eosin stains) (Figure 26). The lumina become narrowed and often multiple. By contrast, occlusion of the central artery in the optic nerve head shows a proliferation of

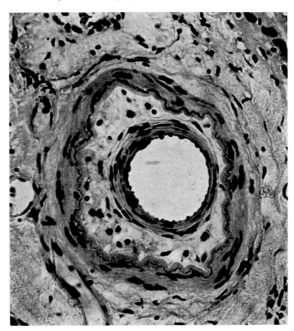

FIGURE 27. Atheroma of the central artery within the optic nerve. H. & S. stain.

the intima, transformation of intimal cells into foam cells, and deposition of sudanophilic, crystalline and calcific material in the wall entirely like that in the atheromatosis of the larger arteries (Figure 27).

Giant cell granuloma of arteries, such as occurs in temporal arteritis, is found in the central artery of the nerve head but not within the retina since this disease is associated with elastica. The retinal arteries *within* the eye show no arteritis, either clinically or pathologically. On the other hand, the central retinal artery within the optic nerve has shown the fragmentation of elastica, the giant cells localized in the lamina of the elastica, focal necroses in the media and round cell infiltration similar to that seen in the temporal and other arteries with this disease[294]. A similar process might be expected with Takayasu's form of pulseless disease but the one pathologic case reported in the literature[348] merely showed proliferation of vessels in front of the retina without definite evidence of vasculitis.

Infarction causes, as might be expected, loss of the inner retinal layers including nerve fibers, ganglion cells, inner reticular and part

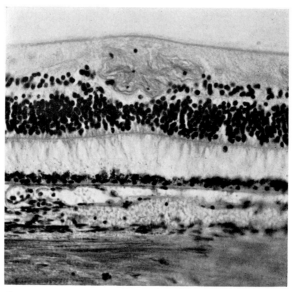

FIGURE 28. Completely occluded retinal artery (center of field) with loss of the inner retinal layers. H. & E. stain.

of the bipolar cell layers (Figure 28). The retina is thinned with remarkably little replacement by glial or fibrous tissue. With loss of the inner layers, the internal limiting membrane comes to be closely apposed to the bipolar cell layer. Yet the outer nuclear layer and rod and cone layer remain normal. Some exception to this gross disappearance of the inner retinal layers is seen in the region surrounding the disc and occasionally in the immediate vicinity of the larger arteries where the inner layers, including ganglion cells, may be partially preserved.

Glaucoma may follow occlusion of the central retinal artery[1138, 1582, 675, 592, 1502] but this occurs much less frequently than after occlusion of the central retinal vein.

SUMMARY

Occlusive disease of the retinal arteries is characterized chiefly by sudden blindness involving the entire visual field or by altitudinal hemianopia. The ophthalmoscopic appearance is that of perifoveal opacification of the retina (due to cloudy swelling of the ganglion cells) and segmentation of the blood column. Occasionally a portion of the retina is spared corresponding to the distribution of a cilio-retinal artery.

Embolic occlusion of the retinal artery occurs suddenly, without warning, and results commonly from a calcified plaque being released by cardiac vegetations. Atheromatosis is a common cause of occlusive arterial disease in older people with episodes of transient black-outs often preceding the definitive occlusion.

Ischemia of the retina may follow a general drop in blood pressure as from massive hemorrhage or heart failure. It may result from internal carotid artery occlusion and be associated with the "small strokes" syndrome. Ophthalmodynamometry is most useful in detecting such cases by revealing a significantly lower arterial pressure on the affected side. Bilateral retinal ischemia results from occlusion of both carotid arteries in the syndrome of pulseless disease. This is characterized subjectively by postural black-outs and objectively by the finding of a myriad of microaneurysms and anomalous vascular proliferations in the retina.

Inflammatory occlusion of the retinal arteries occurs in one form of pulseless disease, that which affects predominantly oriental young women (Takayasu's disease), and also in a giant cell process called temporal arteritis. This latter occurs in people of an older age group and affects predominantly the temporal and ophthalmic arteries.

CHAPTER III

RETINA: Vascular Lesions (Continued)

2. Occlusive Disease of the Retinal Vein

Occlusion of the central retinal vein or of its branches is a common and serious type of vascular accident. Perhaps nowhere else in the body has the occlusion of small veins the significance and importance that it has in the eye; certainly nowhere else can its course and sequela be as well followed during life.

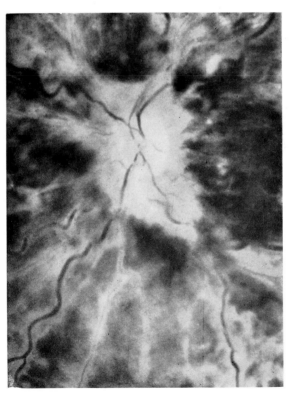

FIGURE 29. Recent occlusion of the central retinal vein showing massive hemorrhagic extravasations.

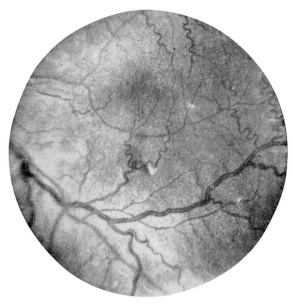

FIGURE 30. Distension and tortuosity of venules resulting from partial obstruction of the central retinal vein.

The typical ophthalmoscopic picture of central retinal vein occlusion is massive hemorrhage or hemorrhages into the retina obscuring all retinal details except for greatly distended loops of dark veins protruding through the hemorrhage (Figures 29 and 30). The disc may be covered with blood and its margins completely obliterated; usually the blood is oriented along the direction of nerve fibers radiating out from the disc. Variations from this typical picture include associated hemorrhage into the vitreous and lesser degrees of hemorrhage in the retina.

Occlusions of branches of the retinal vein (tributary occlusions) show similar hemorrhages and distension of the veins but the changes are confined to the distribution of one particular vein and the hemorrhages are distributed like a fan radiating out from the site of occlusion (Figures 31 and 32).

Obstruction of the central retinal vein or its branches occurs most commonly in middle or later life and is then generally attributed to arteriosclerosis. Yet it is not a valid index of either general or retinal arteriosclerosis. The most common site for obstruction of the central vein is at or just behind the lamina cribrosa while the most common site for tributary occlusion is at an arteriovenous crossing along the

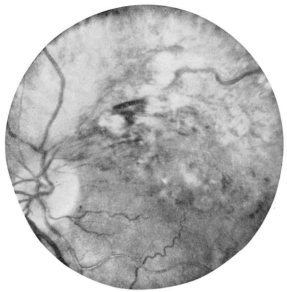

FIGURE 31. Occlusion of superior temporal vein (tributary occlusion) with much hemorrhage and exudate fanning out from an arteriovenous crossing just above the disc.

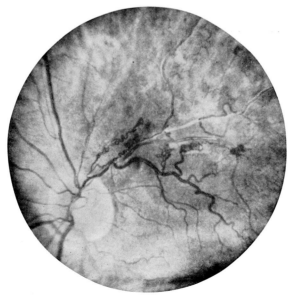

FIGURE 32. Residuum of a tributary occlusion. The area of venous obstruction, now represented by a white line, has been bypassed by collateral venules. As in the previous photograph the site of obstruction was an arteriovenous crossing.

superior temporal vessels. The lamina cribrosa imposes an anatomic constriction on the central retinal vein[87] and in a similar manner the retinal artery compresses the vein at arteriovenous crossings. Thus, although arteriosclerosis may be a precipitating factor in retinal vein occlusion, the basic cause must be an anatomic predisposition. In the presence of a vulnerable anatomic structure, occlusion of the central retinal vein may be a manifestation of some underlying disease that causes increased viscosity of the blood, such as polycythemia[23], multiple myeloma[1574, 1525h], other forms of hyperglobulinemia[1517, 334, 1363, 304, 1], and sickle cell disease[564, 908]. Probably the most common cause of diabetes[1234]. Less common causes are general infection, granuloma (interpreted as tuberculosis[1261, 1485]) contiguous inflammation in either the orbit or adjacent sinuses, gastric hemorrhage[1315] and trauma[598, 683]. A rare and unexplained entity is an intermittent dilatation of the retinal vein and blindness[928].

Occlusion of the central retinal vein is widely inferred to be thrombotic and, indeed, the term is commonly used synonymously with thrombosis of the central retinal vein. This was Coats' original contention[260] and is perhaps compatible with the finding of retinal venous occlusion with generalized thrombocythemia[803]. On the other hand Verhœff[1476] and others[1273, 1265, 804] failed to find histologic evidence of thrombosis, except in inflammatory cases, but did demonstrate endothelial proliferation. This intimal hyperplasia has not been frequently described in veins elsewhere in the body, whence the reservations to it on the part of general pathologists, but it is found in the retinal veins of eyes with either primary occlusion of the veins or occlusion secondary to glaucoma[1477, 571, 1389, 865, 84, 164, 416]. It is most akin to what is seen commonly in arteries and like the latter it shows recanalization by means of dissecting aneurysms[1476].

The immediate effect of central retinal vein occlusion is of course profound loss of vision but, contrary to what occurs with arterial occlusion, perception of light and hand movements is retained. The degree of visual loss with branch occlusion will depend on the involvement of the macula or vitreous. The later effects of venous occlusion depend on whether the entire central vein or just its branches were occluded. Central vein occlusion results frequently (probably in 5-10% of the cases[164]) in a particularly catastrophic type of glaucoma ("hemorrhagic glaucoma") after a matter of weeks or months. The obstruction to outflow of equeous humor follows a curious neovasculogenesis and fibrosis in the angle meshwork of the anterior chamber and on the surface of the iris. Tributary occlusion on the other hand rarely, if ever, causes secondary glaucoma and much of the vision lost may be regained as the hemorrhages clear.

Study of retinal venous occlusion has been handicapped for lack of a suitable experimental animal. Of the common laboratory animals the retinal veins in the rabbit are limited to the area overlying the myelinated portions of their retinas; the cat's veins derive entirely from the choroidal circulation; and the guinea pig has no retinal veins at all.

While the foregoing applies to acute occlusion of the veins, varying patterns of collateralization and symptom complexes are found in chronic obstruction. Anastomotic vessels are often conspicuous, forming a caput medusæ about the disc and establishing outflow by way of the choroidal vessels. With occlusion of a branch of the retinal vein some distance from the disc the collateral vessels form tortuous shunts circumventing the affected arteriovenous junction. With slow onset of the occlusion and adequate collateral circulation, the patient may develop few if any subjective symptoms.

3. Occlusive Disease of the Retinal Capillaries

Until recently knowledge of vascular lesions at the capillary level has been limited for lack of a suitable preparation by which the minute vessels and their cells could be examined in whole mounts. So long as we were dependent on injection techniques and periodic acid Schiff stains we could do no more than visualize the outlines of the lumina and walls. With the id of trypsin digestion the non-vascular components of the retina can now be eliminated so that appropriate cytologic stains can be applied to visualize the entire capillary panorama of the retina[848].

Occlusion of the capillaries is regularly accompanied by loss of the endothelial cells (or perhaps it is the loss of endothelium which determines the occlusion). This capillary occlusion is a normal occurrence in the periphery of the aging retina, beginning as early as the fifth decade of life, and is progressive[275]. It seems reasonable to assume that the development of cysts in the retinal periphery, which is also a regular function of age, and the tendency to develop retinal tears in the periphery and mid-periphery, are also functions of these capillary occlusions.

Spotty occlusions of capillaries involving either single capillaries or clusters of capillaries, are frequent findings in a variety of conditions such as arteriosclerosis, hypertension, diabetes, rheumatoid arthritis and lupus erythematosus (Figure 33). The actual occlusions cannot be seen ophthalmoscopically but they cause tiny infarcts in the nerve fiber layer that are called cotton wool exudates clinically and cytoid bodies pathologically.

Prior to complete occlusion, and probably responsible for it, the basement membrane of the arterioles and capillaries thickens. Following occlusion the wall frequently develops a sudanophilic stainability, but it does not develop the foam cells or other evidence of atheroma seen in the large vessels.

Petechial hemorrhages and sometimes microaneurysms are part of

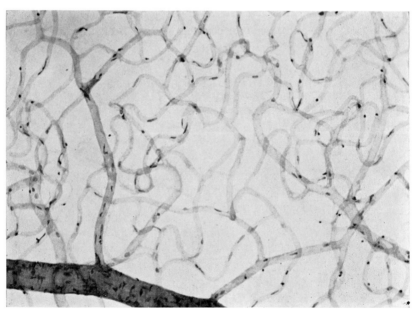

FIGURE 33. Acellularity and occlusion of a cluster of capillaries in the mid-periphery of the retina. This is a frequent finding in old age.

these capillary occlusions but their precise relation to the occluded vessels is not clear.

True neovasculogenesis within the retina probably does not occur in the adult retina. What appears as new vessel formation with the ophthalmoscope is either a dilatation of preformed channels to form shunt vessels or a proliferation of vessels on the surface of the retina internal to the inner limiting membrane. On the other hand, new vessel formation does occur in the developing retina of the fetus and of the newborn. In the fetus the proliferation of endothelial cells and formation of vessel spaces may be so lush as to simulate a hemangioma[275]. Neovasculogenesis also occurs with retinoblastomas. The vessels then consist of large interlacing spaces having walls rich in endothelial cells.

4. Vasculitis

Aside from the giant cell arteritides which were discussed in connection with arterial occlusion, many other inflammatory processes involve retinal arteries and veins. Unfortunately none of these has been satisfactorily defined on clinical or pathologic grounds and the etiology is at present little more than guess work. Indeed, it is by no means clear what should or should not be called vasculitis. While it is generally agreed that opacification of the vessel walls along with fine vitreous opacities and chorioretinitis represents inflammation of the vessels, can the same be said of the opacification that occurs, for instance, along the veins with Eale's disease[375] or with multiple sclerosis[1245, 1540]? Should inflammation of the walls secondary to obvious intraocular inflammation be called vasculitis (in which case some degree of vasculitis would be present in all cases of endophthalmitis)? Or should the term be confined to those cases where the inflammation appears to be primarily in the vessels? Compounding the confusion further, the clinician tends to infer a specific nosologic entity of an infectious or necrotic nature when he uses the term, whereas the pathologist infers an infiltration of the walls which may exist to varying degrees in non-inflammatory processes.

Granted these ambiguities in the term vasculitis, we will consider retinal vasculitis from the clinical point of view as referring to those conditions in which intraocular inflammation is highlighted by exudate along the vessels. This may be a retinal phlebitis or arteritis or both but, unless associated with a generalized vasculitis elsewhere, it is impossible to decide whether the primary lesion is in the vessels of the retina or in the optic nerve.

The absence of tissue spaces in the retina causes exudate to be confined, relatively, to the vessel walls. Thus white blood cells form heavy mantles or cuffs within the layers of the veins (Figures 34 and 35) whereas in other tissues, such as the choroid, the white blood cells diffuse widely in the adjacent tissue. This peculiar confinement in the retina results in the ensheathing of vessels that is commonly seen ophthalmoscopically with various forms of non-necrotizing vasculitis.

One form of vasculitis is that occurring especially in young adults, accompanied by profound visual loss and presenting as a papillitis[947] (Figures 36 and 37). It may be unilateral or bilateral, and is sometimes accompanied by increased sedimentation rate but little other

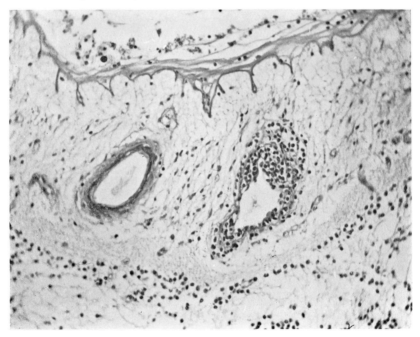

FIGURE 34. Inflammatory lesion of the retina showing considerable round cell infiltration in the vein wall but absence of infiltration in the arterial wall. PAS–hematoxylin stain.

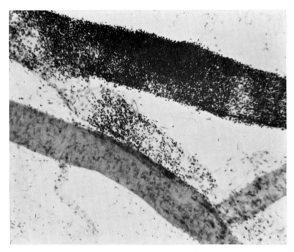

FIGURE 35. Flat mount of a retinal vein *(uppermost)* and a retinal artery *(lowermost)* in a trypsin-digested preparation showing round cell infiltration exclusively in the walls of the vein.

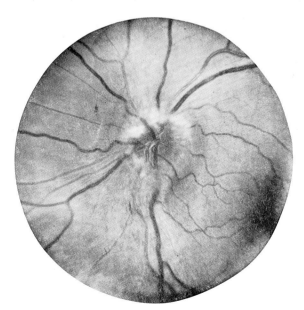

FIGURE 36. Incipient vasculitis in a thirty-six year old man. At this early stage the disc shows exudative inflammation (papillitis) with only mild ensheathing of the vessel walls.

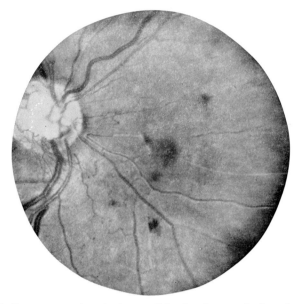

FIGURE 37. Late stage of retinal vasculitis showing marked ensheathing and occlusion of some arteries with optic atrophy and new vessel formation on disc.

evidence of systemic disease. The disc is usually edematous and the vessels show varying amounts of opacification of their walls. Later the vessels on the disc may proliferate to form a rete mirabile. The course is self limited and the disease becomes quiescent in several months time with a variable prognosis.

Perhaps related to the foregoing vasculitis limited to the eyes is the retinal vasculitis associated with generalized allergic angiitis. Here, too, there are woolly exudates along the vessels[391] and histologic evidence of florid inflammation in their walls[1052]. Also described is a unilateral, steroid-sensitive variety of undertermined etiology characterized by segmental infiltrates along the walls[853, 1056, 1432, 582].

Granulomatous disease may be manifest by deposits along the vessels. This is seen most characteristically in the perivascular white spots of the lower retinal periphery in sarcoid[1521, 900, 857, 568], likened to the drippings of candle wax[470]. Tuberculosis is also thought to induce a retinal vasculitis, and a granuloma, interpreted as tuberculous, has been identified within the central retinal vein[1261, 1485] or projecting into it[810]. Syphilis was a common cause in years past[647, 1241] but is infrequent now. Generalized periarteritis nodosa and lupus erythematosus which might be expected to induce arteritic involvement in the retina are more apt to show evidence of capillary lesions (see p. 69) than of arterial or venous lesions.

Retinal vasculitis has also been reported with infectious diseases (rheumatic fever[1385, 810] and pneumonia) and it is possible that the retinopathy following virus diseases is the result of a vasculitis.

5. Miscellaneous Vascular Retinopathies

Diabetes induces a retinopathy characterized by punctate hemorrhages, microaneurysms, and multiple white and yellowish spots that are often called "exudates" (Figures 38 and 39). These changes are most marked in the central area.

The hemorrhages are characteristic in that they are predominantly punctate, numerous and situated in the central retina. The aneurysms are round and when seen with the ophthalmoscope they do not appear to be connected with vessels. In no other condition do they occur as abundantly as in diabetes. Histologic preparations of these

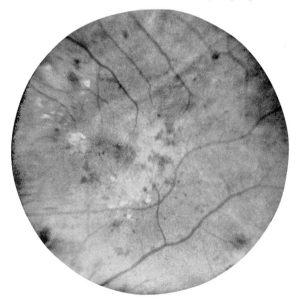

FIGURE 38. Moderately severe diabetic retinopathy showing white spots ("exudate") and red spots (hemorrhages and microaneurysms) about the central area of the fundus.

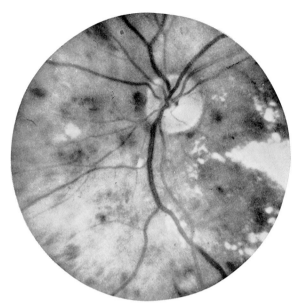

FIGURE 39. Severe diabetic retinopathy with "exudate" (cotton-wool and punctate types) and hemorrhages extending to the peripapillary region. The major retinal vessels appear normal.

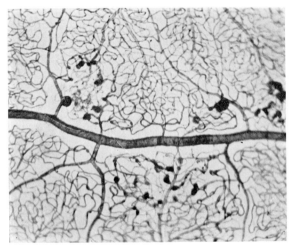

FIGURE 40. Flat mount of retinal vessels showing clusters of microaneurysms surrounding areas of occluded capillaries. These changes are characteristic of early diabetic retinopathy.

aneurysms, examined best in flat mounts, show them to be saccular outpouchings of capillary, arteriolar and venular walls (Figure 40).

In early diabetic retinopathy these microaneurysms are always arranged about and oriented toward a capillary infarct but are not themselves derived from the occluded vessels[282]. At first they consist of thin walled outpouchings (Figure 41) in which the endothelium proliferates. With this endothelial proliferation, more basement membrane is laid down and eventually as the endothelium dies the thickened walls of the microaneurysms undergo a succession of retrogressive and disintegrative changes similar to that which has been noted for occluded capillaries. First there is hyalinization of the wall, then accumulation of lipid, and eventual disruption and phagocytosis of the wall remnants. This sequence is evident ophthalmoscopically by sequential transformation of a red spot to a white spot and eventual disappearance of the spot.

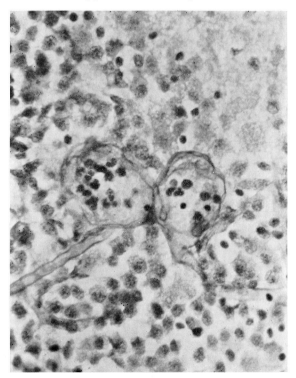

FIGURE 41. Cross section of a retinal capillary showing two microaneurysms. The relative thinness of the aneurysmal wall indicates an early stage of development.

Saccular microaneurysms occur, though rarely, unassociated with diabetes[930]. Those with pulseless disease are fusiform and always minute compared with the diabetic variety. Those with venous occlusion are also fusiform but large and always limited to the venous side of the vascular complex whereas in diabetes they are situated anywhere along the arteriolar-capillary-venular chain. No universally accepted explanation has been given for the predilection of microaneurysms for diabetes but it may be significant that this disease causes a highly selective loss of the mural cells of the capillaries and many of the microaneurysms appear to evolve from the sites of the former mural cells[282]. A characteristic finding in flat mounts of retinal vessels in diabetes is the presence of dilated vessels that by-pass occluded capillaries. It is from these distended vessels that the microaneurysms arise. The decreased vascular tone resulting from loss of the mural cells is assumed to allow distention and outpouching of some capillaries with consequent shunt formation[274]. The process occurs characteristically in the central retina where the hydrostatic

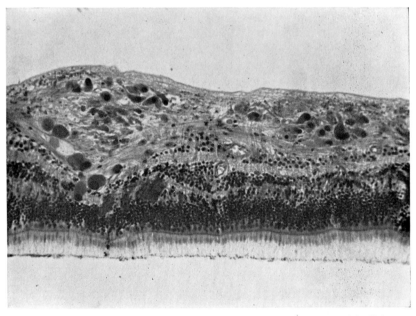

FIGURE 42. Cytoid bodies in inner layer of the retina in a patient with diabetes. These peculiar bodies, thought to represent microinfarcts, correspond to the cotton-wool spots that are seen with the ophthalmoscope.

pressure within the capillaries is greatest and is characteristic of diabetes inasmuch as this is the one condition in which mural cells are preferentially lost.

The white spots of diabetic retinopathy probably result from several pathologic processes. The blanket term exudates is a misnomer. The cotton wool spots are the cytoid bodies which, as stated previously, represent capillary infarcts in the inner layers of the retina (Figure 42). The deeper white or yellowish white spots correspond to the hyaline material in the outer layers of the retina; this material may be serum or it may be necrotic retina resulting from the infarcts (Figure 43). Fatty metamorphosis of this hyaline material contributes to the opacities seen ophthalmoscopically. Except for their predilection for the central regions of the retina, neither the cotton-wool nor deeper spots are specific for diabetes.

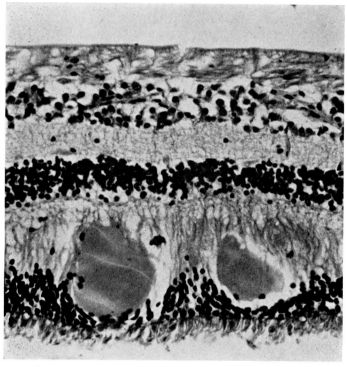

FIGURE 43. "Exudate" in diabetic retinopathy. An amorphous substance that stains like serum is found characteristically in the outer plexiform layer. These appear ophthalmoscopically as punctate white or yellowish white spots.

Retinitis proliferans, consisting of gliovascular tissue, extending into the vitreous, is a particularly serious complication of diabetes because of the associated separation of the retina (Figures 44 and 45). It usually follows in the wake of repeated vitreous hemorrhages with vessels growing out of the disc region, but a relatively benign type may develop spontaneously from portions of the retina away from the disc. Retinitis proliferans is not necessarily a late state of diabetic retinopathy (as is commonly stated)[447]; it appears to be an alternative type and may occur with little other evidence of retinopathy[56, 405]. It is commonly associated, however, with Kimmelstiel-Wilson changes in the kidney so that prognosis is poor not only for vision but for life as well.

Except for the pathologic and clinical evidence associating diabetic retinopathy and diabetic nephropathy there is unconvincing evidence of a correlation between the severity of diabetes, as indicated by insulin requirements, and the amount of retinopathy, or between the adequacy of control of the diabetes and control of the retinopathy.

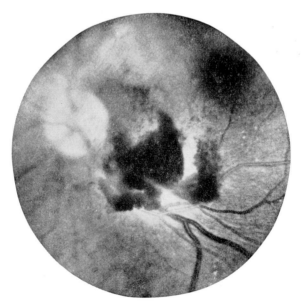

FIGURE 44. Pre-retinal hemorrhage occurring in a diabetic patient. Since the blood is in the vitreous it partially covers the retinal vessels and obscures the disc. Noteworthy is the absence of any marked diabetic retinopathy. Hemorrhages such as this commonly precede the formation of retinitis proliferans.

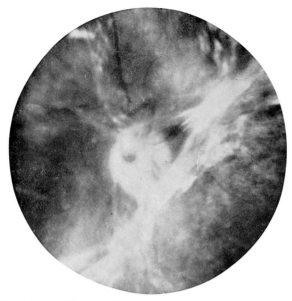

FIGURE 45. Retinitis proliferans. The patient was a twenty-eight year old woman with diabetes of many years duration. The photograph shows fibroglial tissue and vessels extending into the vitreous from the optic disc.

Nevertheless both the insulin requirements and the retinopathy are improved for a time at least by removal of the hypophysis[231, 940] and this procedure or a modification of it[1467, 293] is currently being advocated as a therapeutic procedure for severe cases[1404].

Finally, any discussion of diabetic retinopathy should mention the major retinal vessels. The retinal arteries are morphologically normal unless there is coincidental arteriosclerosis and hypertension. The retinal veins, however, are often distended and occasionally show sausage-shaped dilatation of their walls. This, however, is probably a reflection of viscosity changes in the blood and is not necessarily correlated with other manifestations of diabetic retinopathy.

Hypertension and arteriosclerosis produce characteristic changes in the retinal arteries, as seen by the ophthalmoscope, but it is not surprising that these changes fail to correlate well with those in other vessels generally used for comparison, for the retinal vessels are much smaller and lack the elastica, media, and adventitia of the larger vessels. It would be more appropriate to compare the retinal vessels with arteriolar manifestations elsewhere but this is rarely done and even then it is not apparent that the retinal arterioles are anatomically analogous to those elsewhere. For what it is worth, however, the hypertensive retinal arteriolar manifestations are said to stimulate those of the renal arterioles more closely than those of the cerebral arterioles[117].

Retinal manifestations of hypertension and arteriosclerosis are characteristic and important irrespective of their correlation with other vessels (Figures 46, 47 and 48). The prime hypertensive change in young persons is simply diffuse and focal narrowing of all the retinal arteries; in older persons it is more apt to be focal with irregularity of the lumina, or the changes may be absent altogether. Thus evaluation of hypertensive changes is less reliable the older the person. The hemorrhages and white spots in hypertensives do not parallel the morphologic changes in the arteries but usually do reflect the degree of encephalopathy present. The amount of papilledema is somewhat more significantly related to the degree of hypertension and is a fairly reliable index of the intracranial involvement.

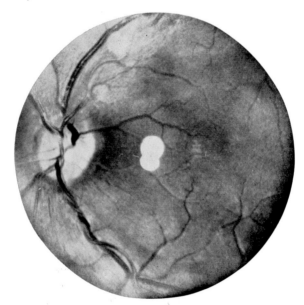

FIGURE 46. Mild hypertensive retinopathy characterized by slight narrowing with irregularity of lumen of superior temporal artery, and a single cotton-wool spot. (The double light reflex centrally is an artifact from the illuminating system.)

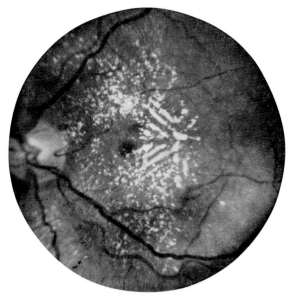

FIGURE 47. Moderate hypertensive retinopathy with considerable narrowing of retinal arteries and abundant exudate including a star figure in the macula.

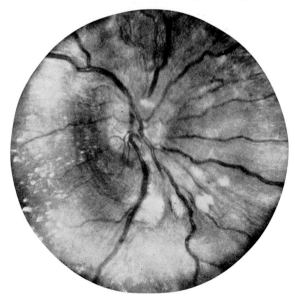

FIGURE 48. Severe hypertensive retinopathy. Both fundi showed narrowing and irregularity of the arterial lumina, multiple cotton-wool and punctate exudates, petechial hemorrhages, some edema of the discs and concentric folds of the retina temporal to the discs.

The degree of vascular change and extravascular retinopathy with hypertension and arteriosclerosis has been subjected to no less than eleven different classifications[899, 165]. These classifications serve for statistical studies and for abbreviating case findings but should not be made an end in themselves. There is no one sign or group of signs that can replace the over-all impression which one has from looking at the fundus and one should be guided by this impression quite as much as by an arbitrary number on a classification code.

Arteriosclerosis in the retina is characterized by broadening of the arterial light reflex, tortuosity of the vessels, spotty occurrence of "plaques" on the arterial walls, and most especially by venous nicking, banking, and obstruction at the arteriovenous junction (Figures 49 and 50). When acute, the latter shows massive hemorrhages peripheral to the point of obstruction; when chronic, it shows dilatation and proliferation of the small vessels circumventing the obstruction.

Retinopathy from *occlusion of the choroidal arteries* is less well characterized than that from occlusion of the retinal vessels. There is little reason to doubt, however, that the circumscribed ("punched-

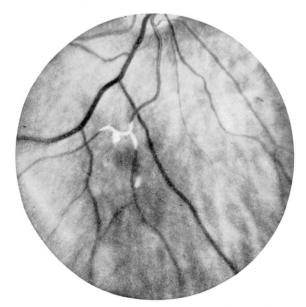

FIGURE 49. Plaque of the retinal artery. This type of abnormality occurring most frequently at the site of arterial branching is one of the manifestations of arteriosclerosis.

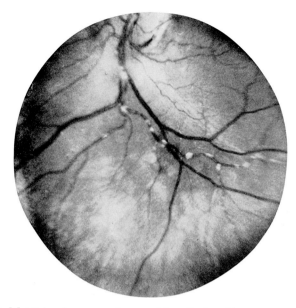

FIGURE 50. Multiple plaques on the arterial wall of a thirty-seven year old man with hypercholesterolemia.

out") patches of enhanced redness or loss of grayness that one sees frequently in the fundi of older people are the result of arteriolar occlusions in the choroid and in the choriocapillaris[1097] (Figure 51). The color change is due to loss of the pigment epithelium and the visual defect is due to the associated damage to the rods and cones. Some cases of widespread retinopathy simulating retinitis pigmentosa have been attributed to angiosclerosis of the choroid[1369, 1493, 953] but pathologic confirmation is lacking.

Then there is the *"retinopathy of abnormal proteins"*[1363] characterized by venous stasis, hemorrhages, and occasionally papilledema resulting from increased viscosity of the blood (macroglobulinemia of Waldenstrom[805, 203, 334, 828, 436, 606, 202, 1363, 917, 1293, 1437, 1429] (Figure 52), multiple myeloma[333, 258, 377], polycythemia[285, 23] (Figure 53), leukemia[152, 318, 19] (Figure 54), some cases of diabetes[1234], and cystic fibrosis of the pancreas[187]) and occasionally from arterial occlusion[29, 410]. These are manifestations of blood sludging that are often accompanied by visible movement of the blood through the vessels either spontaneously or induced by gentle pressure on the globe. One form of hyperglobulinemia, frequently associated with venous stasis and retinal hemorrhages, is called cryoglobulinemia because of the tendency of the blood proteins to gel in the cold. It may present as a combination of Raynaud's syndrome and vascular retinopathy[428, 376], although arterial occlusion may occur with Raynaud's syndrome without abnormal blood proteins being evident[1318, 399, 27].

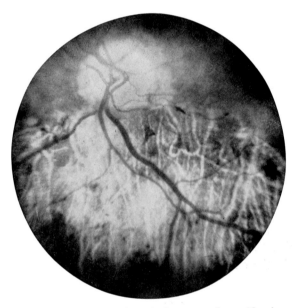

FIGURE 51. Circumscribed aggregation of pigment and opacification of choroidal vessels thought to be due to degeneration of the pigment epithelium and occlusion of the choroidal arteries. The optic disc and overlying retinal vessels are normal.

Some diseases cause arterial and venous obstruction preferentially in the peripheral arterioles and venules of the retina. Most frequent of these is Eale's disease[375, 1499] (Figure 55), an entity characterized by ensheathed and occluded vessels in the retinal periphery and sometimes by vitreous hemorrhage. Usually bilateral and occurring predominantly in males[371], Eale's disease is not regularly associated with systemic disease and its etiology is obscure[371]. Sickle cell anemia and trait produce a similar occlusion of the peripheral vessels and a fundus picture[630, 635, 784, 1058, 909] like that of Eale's disease.

Some diseases are manifest in the fundus by cotton wool spots (Figure 56). Histologically these are capillary infarcts and are not necessarily accompanied by changes in the larger retinal vessels. This type of fundus change has been termed in the French and German literature "dysoric retinopathy." The cotton wool spots are thought to be especially characteristic of lupus erythematosus[110, 798, 1002, 177, 259]

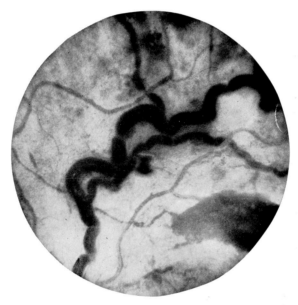

FIGURE 52. Severe distension of the retinal veins (with compression at the arteriolar crossings) and massive hemorrhage in a patient with hyperglobulinemia.

but they also occur in other diseases (Hodgkins[176]; periarteritis nodosa[502]; scleroderma[809, 1160]; dermatomyositis[355]; hypertension[809]; ischemia[667, 42]; rheumatoid arthritis; carotid ligation[938]; myeloma[491, 68]; leukemia[19]; etc.). On the other hand, megaloblastic (pernicious) anemia[300] and anoxic diseases are characterized by hemorrhages rather than by the cotton wool spots. One might venture the generalization that occlusive diseases cause cotton-wool spots whereas toxic and anoxic disturbances cause hemorrhages.

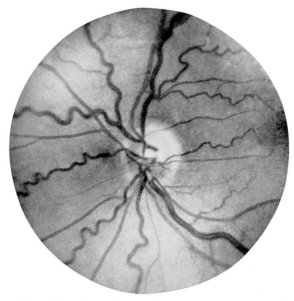

FIGURE 53. Mild, uniform distension and tortuosity of all the retinal veins in a patient with polycythemia.

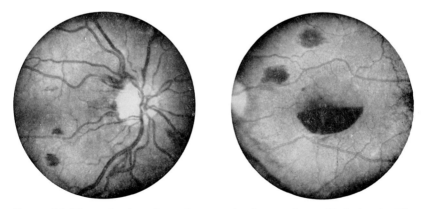

FIGURE 54. Hemorrhagic retinopathy occurring in a patient with leukemia. The right eye showed scattered flame-shaped hemorrhages throughout the fundus. The left eye showed, in addition, a preretinal hemorrhage in front of the macula.

Finally, occlusion of the arterial system in *both* retina and choroid produces a profound disintegration characterized ophthalmoscopically by splotchy pigmentation and pathologically by widespread necrosis and release of pigment. It results from extensive blood loss[815], from excessively high pressures of glaucoma and from the surgical procedure, opticociliary neurotomy, done formerly in blind eyes for intractable pain.

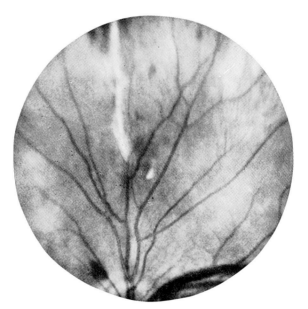

FIGURE 55. Ensheathing of vessels and hemorrhages in a twenty year old man with Eale's disease.

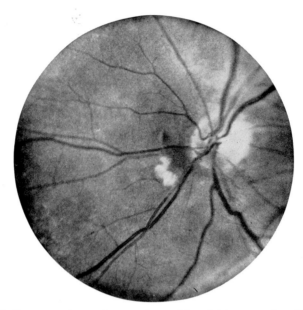

FIGURE 56. Cotton-wool spot in a patient with mild hypertension. These spots are thought to represent microinfarcts; they produce the pathologic entity known as cytoid bodies.

SUMMARY

Occlusion of the central retinal vein or of its superior temporal branch is a relatively frequent vascular accident. It is manifest by engorgement of the veins distal to the occlusion and by massive hemorrhages into the retina and occasionally into the vitreous. The occlusion occurs most commonly at the site of penetration of the vein through the lamina cribrosa or at an arteriovenous crossing. While arteriosclerosis may be an important contributing factor, the immediate cause of the occlusion is often some underlying disease that causes increased viscosity of the blood. Histologically, the occlusion is found to be an endothelial proliferation rather than thrombosis. Occlusion of the central vein, although not of its tributary branches, is followed by a particularly severe type of glaucoma (hemorrhagic glaucoma) in a significant number of cases. When the occlusion develops gradually, collateral circulation may be established that effectively by-passes the obstruction.

Occlusion of the retinal capillaries is a common occurrence in old age and in various disease states but it can be recognized in life only by the so-called "exudates" in the retina. Histologically the occluded vessels show preferential loss of endothelial cells, especially in the peripheral retina, with eventual loss of all cells and conversion of the capillaries into ragged cords. These capillary occlusions probably underlie the pseudocyst formation in the retina, the liability to hole formation, and the occurrence of white spots and hemorrhage in a miscellany of systemic diseases.

Vasculitis of the retinal vessels comprises some well defined and many ill-defined entities. The former include the inflammatory type of pulseless disease and temporal arteritis. The ill-defined entities include some cases of papillitis, Eale's disease, allergic angiitis, sarcoid vasculitis, Hodgkin's vasculitis, and probably many other poorly recognized types.

Diabetes produces an especially important variety of vascular retinopathy. Most characteristic are the abundant microaneurysms in the central area, the plethora of punctate hemorrhages, and the white spots that are called exudates. The histologic counterparts of these changes are capillary infarcts, preferential loss of the mural cells, outpouchings of the walls of the small vessels, and punctate necrosis and hyalinization of the retinal substance. The pathogenesis appears to be formation of shunt vessels consequent to loss of the mural cells and resultant alteration in the intracapillary pressure. A particularly serious form of diabetic retinopathy is that accompanied by pro-liferation of gliovascular tissue into the vitreous.

Hypertension produces a narrowing of the major branches of the retinal arterial lumina. This is evident especially in young persons and may involve focal portions of the artery or the entire artery. Sclerosis of the arteries in older people tends to prevent this narrow-ing and thereby masks the hypertensive narrowing that is evident in the young. The prime ophthalmoscopic changes of sclerosis of the retinal artery are broadening of the light reflex and arteriovenous nicking, angulation, and venous obstruction. Sclerosis and occlusion of the choroidal arteries is manifest ophthalmoscopically by loss of pigment epithelium (usually in discrete areas), accentuation of the choroidal tessellation, and often opacification of the choroidal vessel walls.

Various systemic diseases, especially those associated with elevated blood viscosity, may cause a vascular type of retinopathy. These include not only the various hyperglobulinemias but also the hemoglobinopathies, the neoplastic diseases of the blood, and the anemias. The characteristic fundus finding in all of these is hemorrhage and cotton wool spots. The larger arteries are morphologically normal but the veins are frequently distended and the terminal vessels show ensheathing and proliferation.

CHAPTER IV

RETINA: Degenerations

ASIDE from those due to vascular lesions, many specific types of retinal degeneration can be sorted out according to the layers of the retina which are primarily affected.

A. DEGENERATION OF THE
EXTERNAL LAYER OF THE RETINA

Selective loss of the rods and cones and of their cell bodies occurs in several disease entities: retinitis pigmentosa, choroideremia, some forms of macular degeneration, detachment of the retina, experimental vitamin A deficiency, and in association with deficiency of the choroidal blood supply. Related conditions are characterized by loss of *function* of the rods or cones, with only questionable morphologic changes: congenital stationary night blindness; Oguchi's disease; reversible night blindness (Uyemura's syndrome[511]); and congenital achromatopsia. The clinical symptom in the cases of faulty rod function is difficulty with dark adaptation ("night blindness") while with faulty cone function it is loss of central visual acuity and deficient color perception. In all cases with extensive loss of the outer retinal layer, the electroretinogram is characteristically negative[764] (i.e., gives no response).

Retinitis pigmentosa is an hereditary disease (usually recessive but occasionally dominant[1508]) coming on most commonly in the second decade of life and progressively constricting the visual field over the course of one or more decades. Occasionally it is associated with cerebral degeneration and epilepsy in a fulminant form called *Vogt-Spielmeyer and Bielschowsky's diseases*. The name retinitis pigmentosa is poorly chosen since the disease is neither inflammatory nor primarily a lesion of the pigment system. Historical precedent, however, establishes its use in preference to other terms such as nyctalopic retinosis[641] that might be more accurate.

Clinically, the disease first manifests visual difficulty at low levels of illumination (twilight); then the visual fields become constricted and the patient has poor peripheral vision even in broad daylight. He bumps into objects or stumbles over objects that are not directly in his line of vision. Yet central visual acuity remains normal for a long time. Ophthalmoscopically, the four typical findings are: conglomerations of pigment in bone-corpuscle or pepper-granule configuration (Figure 57); marked attenuation of the retinal arteries (the reason for which is not clear); increased visibility of the choroid through the attenuated pigment epithelium; and a posterior polar opacity of the lens. Occasionally one finds drusen of the nerve head. The fundus has a tessellated appearance, with unusual reflexes that vary according to the amount of lipid and calcific material in Bruch's membrane.

Whether pigment accumulates in bone-corpuscle clusters or in granular form probably depends on the rate with which the process develops. Slowly progressive processes enable the pigment cells to aggregate in clusters not only in the interstices of the retina but

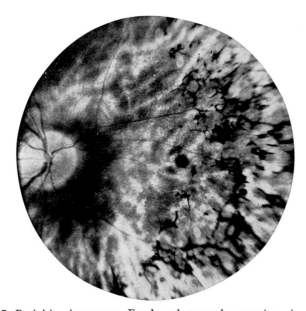

FIGURE 57. Retinitis pigmentosa. Fundus photograph centering about an area nasal to disc. Noteworthy are the severe narrowing of the arteries and the pigment clumping. The pigment is arranged like bone corpuscles in a circular area concentric with the macula.

about blood vessels, whereas more rapid processes cause a widespread scattering of the pigmentation in diffuse granular form.

Much of the pigment may eventually get into the blood stream and disappear. The extremes of such cases show little or no remaining pigment clumps and are therefore called retinitis pigmentosa sine pigmento.

Pathologically, retinitis pigmentosa consists of a primary loss of the rods and then of the cones with eventual replacement of the outer retinal layers by glial tissue[261]. As the rods and cones disappear the pigment epithelial cells insinuate through the sieve-like outer limiting membrane and "flow" into the retina much as white blood cells flow through small holes in capillary walls. The Vogt-Spielmeyer-Bielschowsky retinas show the same loss of the outer retinal elements with replacement by glia but, in contrast to retinitis pigmentosa, there is a more uniformly widespread invasion of pigment epithelial cells into the retina and involvement of the macula as well as of the rest of the retina (Figure 58). In some retinal dystrophies the entire retina is involved so that all layers are replaced by tenuous glial

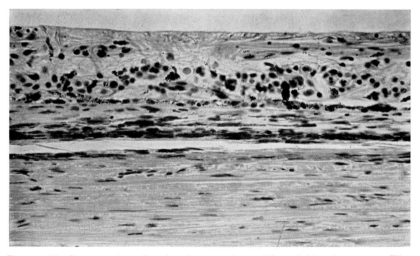

Figure 58. Cross section of retina from patient with retinitis pigmentosa. The rod and cone layer has completely disappeared. The bipolar layer, distorted by gliosis, is in direct contact with attenuated pigment epithelium. Pigment granules and some pigment cells are scattered throughout all layers of the retina. The ganglion cells are normally sparse in the mid-peripheral portions of the retina from which the present specimen was taken.

strands. These latter retinas show the same pathologic picture as is found in eyes which have been subjected to ischemia of both the arterial and choroidal circulation.

A congenital form of retinitis pigmentosa is known as Leber's congenital amaurosis[880] or heredoretinopathia congenitalis[22]. This causes blindness within the first few years of life with pigmentary clumping in the peripheral retina and equivocal changes in the optic nerve[1272]. It is transmitted as a recessive trait and is frequently associated with keratoglobus and keratoconus[1494].

The Laurence-Moon-Biedl syndrome is a variant in which retinitis pigmentosa is associated with obesity, polydactylism, hypogenitalism, and frequently mental deficiency[90]. Unlike typical retinitis pigmentosa the macula is sometimes involved early and differentiation from other forms of retinocerebral degeneration is then possible only by the progressive course of the latter disease.

Retinitis pigmentosa is associated with deafness in some ten percent of cases and less often with other congenital or hereditary syndromes (ophthalmoplegia externa[66, 1525d, 236, 16, 771], heart block[771], cerebellar degeneration[601], chronic polyneuritis in the syndrome of Refsum[1190] and acanthocytosis of the red blood cells in the Kornzweig-Bassen syndrome[825, 737, 388, 1020, 1297]) but these may be fortuitous associations of genetic defects closely situated on one chromosome rather than expressions of any common pathogenetic factor.

A genetically recessive disease analogous to retinitis pigmentosa occurs in rodents[777, 159, 1083, 380], dogs[657, 1288, 1115] and probably in other animals. It is characterized by progressive loss of dark adaptation (considerably more rapid loss than that in human beings), disappearance of the outer retinal layers, and extinction of the electroretinographic response.

Variants of retinitis pigmentosa comprise a diverse number of choroidoretinal degenerations. One of these is a sex linked trait in which an atypical retinitis occurs in males whereas the female carriers show a peculiar tapetal-like reflex (without subjective visual disturbances[976, 425, 1358, 1544, 254, 732]). Occasionally retinitis pigmentosa occurs in one eye only[88, 386, 483, 860] or it may be limited to sectors of eyes which show a normal electroretinographic response[841].

Certain retinal degenerations and inflammations may culminate in a clinical picture similar to that of retinitis pigmentosa and sometimes called pseudoretinitis pigmentosa[261]. This is encountered with syphilis, detachment of the retina, viral retinopathy and following injury—especially with injuries occurring early in life and accompanied by dislocation of the lens.

Retinitis punctata albescens refers to entities characterized by scattering of white dots throughout the fundi in persons with delayed or deficient dark-adaptation[1341, 838] (Figure 59). While there is one definite entity warranting the name, there are probably many others which are called by this name. The true retinitis punctata albescens is a congenital, non-progressive disease, with delayed dark-adaptation but full field and no definite abnormality of pigmentation, retinal vasculature, or nerve head.

Some other cases which have been called retinitis punctata albescens probably represent variants of retinitis pigmentosa since they occur in families with this disease and are accompanied by some bone

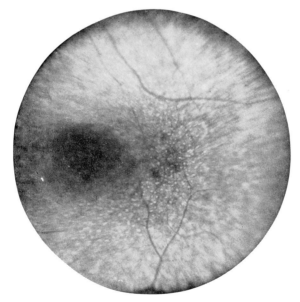

FIGURE 59. Retinitis punctata albescens. The patient was a thirty-one year old woman who had non-progressive night blindness all her life. Five other siblings from a sibship of fourteen were similarly affected. The fundi showed innumerable punctate white dots that were most abundant about the macula. The retinal vessels were minimally narrowed.

corpuscle pigmentation[1072, 633, 553]. These variant forms are progressive. The white spots are generally assumed to be drusen of Bruch's membrane or hyaline bodies within the retina derived from the pigment epithelium. Recently they have been described histopathologically as cysts in the inner layers of the retina[724] but it is questionable whether or not the case reported was one of true retinitis albescens.

Choroideremia is a less well defined and less common disease than retinitis pigmentosa but has in common with it an absence of the outer retinal elements. In addition there is an absence of most of the choroid so that the fundus presents a white reflex from the sclera rather than an orange color or tessellated pigmentation such as occurs with retinitis pigmentosa (Figure 60). Several types of choroideremia have been described but that which is most common and has been most thoroughly studied is a congenital, stationary variety affecting males and transmitted through heterozygous females who, while not showing choroideremia, do show abnormal pigmentary changes in their fundi[949]. The pathologic changes of choroideremia consist of

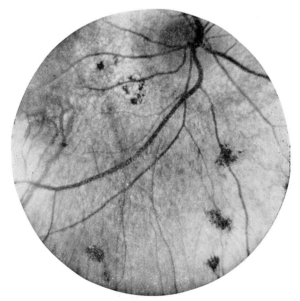

Figure 60. Choroideremia showing a white reflex from the fundus due to an absence of choroid. The patient was a forty-three year old man who had night blindness and severely constricted fields since childhood.

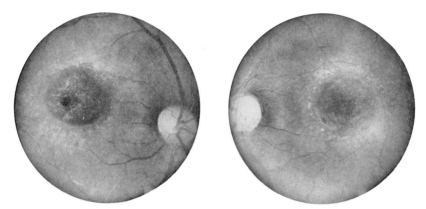

FIGURE 61. Macular degeneration with mottling of pigment about the maculas. The patient was an eighteen year old boy who had had slowly progressive decrease of vision over a two year period to the present level of 20/100 in each eye.

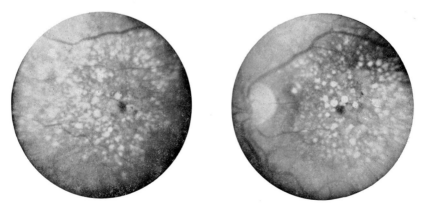

FIGURE 62. Macular degeneration with severe drusen formation in and about the maculas of the two eyes. The patient was a fifty-one year old man who had had progressive loss of vision for six to seven years. The present acuity was: O.D. 20/80; O.S. 20/400.

absence of most of the choroid and of the outer retinal layers so that the residual retinal tissue is apposed to the sclera directly.

Some forms of *macular degeneration* fall into the category of hereditary degeneration of the outer retinal layers[806, 475]. They are the reverse of retinitis pigmentosa in that the central areas are preferentially involved and they do not customarily extend to the periphery; they are sometimes called retinitis pigmentosa inversa (or Stargardt's disease[1374]) and are progressive[1466]. Central vision is lost so that the patients have what might be termed daylight blindness in contrast to the night blindness of retinitis pigmentosa. The occasional loss of color perception and of the photopic response on dark adaptation indicates a loss of cone function throughout the entire retina[1337]. The ophthalmoscopic picture varies. Some show merely mottled pigmentary changes about the macula (Figure 61) or massive drusen body formation (Figure 62). Others show a yellowish elevated mass likened to a fried egg and called vitelliform macular degeneration (Figure 63). Any one form may change with age[1197] and show variable expressivity in the same family[65, 584].

Of the many forms of macular degeneration the types of primary neuro-ophthalmic interest are those associated with cerebral degeneration in the entity of the Batten-Mayou type of amaurotic family idiocy[71, 72], those occurring abiotrophically in families[806, 475, 65], and

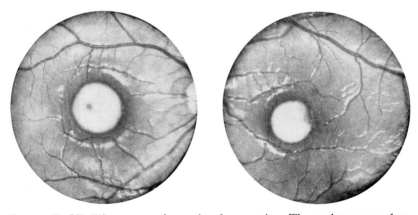

FIGURE 63. Vitelliform type of macular degeneration. The patient was a fourteen year old boy whose vision had deteriorated in the right eye to 20/40 and in the left eye to 20/200 over a two year period.

those occurring idiopathically in middle or old age. Retinal degeneration beginning in the macula may also occur occasionally with ophthalmoplegia, spinocerebellar ataxia, deafness and polyneuritis (Refsum's syndrome[1191, 736, 738]) or simply with central nervous system degeneration[467].

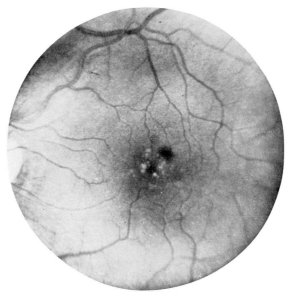

FIGURE 64. Forty-seven year old woman who has the typical pigmentary mottling in the macula such as is seen with senile macular degeneration. Yet the patient's vision was entirely normal, illustrating the discrepancy between what one sees in the fundus and what the patient is able to see.

Senile macular degeneration is a common but poorly understood process causing variable but often severe visual loss. The usual form is manifest by a granular pigmentation about the macula, loss of foveolar reflex, and sometimes increased visibility of the orange colored choroid in the central area. There is often a striking disparity between the ophthalmoscopic appearance and subjective loss of vision (Figure 64). Senile macular degeneration is not clearly distinguished from the abiotrophic variety previously referred to. The blood vessels appear to be normal ophthalmoscopically and the choroidal circulation shows no histologic abnormality[826] (although sclerosis of the choriocapillaris is often thought to be responsible for it[50]. Another variety of the senile form called disciform macular degeneration (Figure 65) is that associated with proliferation and metaplasia of the underlying pigment epithelium. This presents initially as a dark (occasionally black) mass centrally with red hemorrhage at its edge. Later the mass is elevated with a dark and white texture frequently simulating a melanoma.

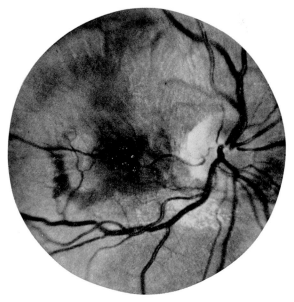

FIGURE 65. Disciform degeneration of the macula. Characteristic is the slightly elevated white mass near the macula partially surrounded by a corona of subretinal hemorrhage. The patient was an eighteen year old girl who gave a history of gradual blurring of vision in an eye for one year but sudden worsening recently. Visual acuity was 20/400.

Macular degeneration may take several pathologic forms corresponding to its various clinical types. Edema and multiple pseudocysts replacing Henle's layer are especially frequent, with circulatory disturbances of the retinal vessels (Figure 66). These cysts enlarge by confluence and may form large spaces bordered by the

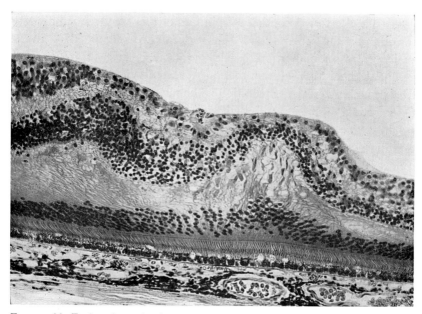

FIGURE 66. Early edema in the macular area characterized by fluid spaces in the outer plexiform layer and swelling of nerve fibers.

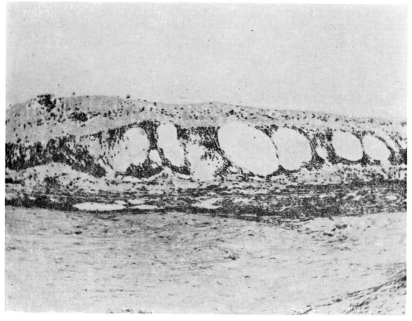

FIGURE 67. Ultimate pseudocysts near the macula with partial disorganization of retina and pigment epithelium.

internal and external limiting membranes or they may remain discrete forming a multilocular, honeycomb appearance (Figure 67). Eventually the cysts may rupture with consequent hole formation and potential separation of the retina. A second variety of pathologic change with macular degeneration is the selective disappearance of the outer retinal elements and ingrowth of pigment epithelial cells to produce the pigmentary macular degeneration (Figure 68). Like retinitis pigmentosa, but affecting the macula preferentially, it commonly occurs as a symmetric dystrophy in the two eyes but may occur as the result of idiopathic circulatory disturbances in the choroid. The third variety of macular degeneration, that which presents clinically as disciform degeneration, is characterized pathologically by ruptures of Bruch's membrane, hemorrhage from the choriocapillaris, proliferation of fibrous tissue about the pigment epithelium, and secondary changes in the overlying macula[1484] (Figure 69). In summary the pathology of macular degeneration is characterized by three major types of change according to whether the lesion was primarily in the retinal circulation, choroidal circulation, or in Bruch's membrane.

Other *degenerations of the outer retinal elements* are caused by *prolonged retinal detachment, experimental vitamin A deficiency,* and *insufficient choroidal blood supply.* These undoubtedly have a common pathogenesis in inadequate metabolic requirements for the rods and cones. That which occurs with prolonged retinal detachment has no great clinical significance. That which occurs with experimental vitamin A deficiency is of great theoretical interest in showing that lack of the photosensitive precursor will cause degeneration of the structure of the entire end organ[1411, 751, 383]. That it has not been reported to do so in human beings is due merely to the fact that sufficiently profound vitamin A deficiency in human beings is not compatible with life; in animals life may be maintained experimentally by supplements of vitamin A acid which is not metabolized by the eye[1043,382]. The degeneration secondary to insufficient choroidal blood supply undoubtedly accounts for many of the cases of senile visual loss but we have no means at present of differentiating clearly those

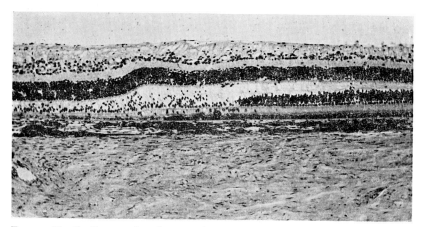

FIGURE 68. Senile macular degeneration in a seventy-five year old man. The area of the photomicrograph is just temporal to the macula. As one approaches the macula toward the left, the rods and cone cells gradually disappear and the pigment epithelium aggregates into clumped masses.

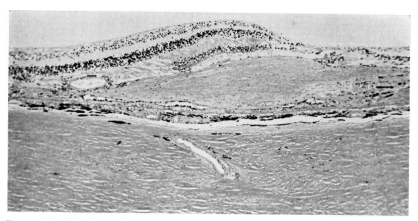

FIGURE 69. Disciform degeneration of the macula. Characteristic is the mass of tissue between the retina and Bruch's membrane, believed to be derived from the pigment epithelium. The reduced visual acuity is due largely to the destruction of the outer retinal layers.

due to circulatory disturbances and those due to other lesions (Figure 70). While of little practical importance it is of considerable theoretical interest that iodoacetate poisoning in animals[1081, 1082] and a phenothiazine derivative (N.P. 207)* in human beings[1486, 794, 1218, 196, 1539] have led to selective loss of the outer elements of the retina or of their functions.

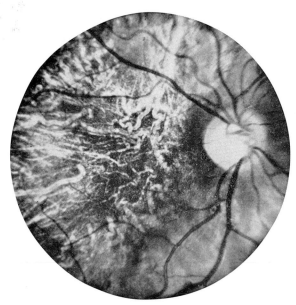

FIGURE 70. Chorioretinopathy thought to represent choroidal sclerosis and ischemia. Characteristic is the circumscribed nature of the lesion, the depigmentation (due to loss of pigment epithelium) and the apparent opacification of the choroidal arteries.

Congenital stationary night blindness. This is a well defined entity in which the patients have an hereditary lack of dark adaptability, as though the rods were congenitally lacking. It is stationary and not truly a degenerative condition but is included in the present category because of its obvious relationship to the progressive diseases with preferential involvement of the rods.

---

* This is an arbitrary designation for the chlorpromazine derivative 3-chloro-10 2-N-(methylpiperidyl) ethyl phenothiazine which was given a clinical trial as a tranquilizer.

Congenital stationary night blindness shows only the amount of dark adaptation which one would expect from cones[366]. Visual acuity is characteristically normal and the ophthalmoscope reveals no abnormalities[219]. No histologic study of the disease has been reported.

Congenital stationary night blindness has the distinction of comprising the most extensive pedigree of any human trait. The Nougaret family tree, showing the dominant variety of the disease, was first reported by Cunier (and Chauvet) in 1838[320], then brought up to date by Nettleship in 1907[1071], and finally completed by Dejean and Gassenc in 1949[351]. This covers ten generations and includes a total of 2,116 individuals.

Oguchi's disease. This disease reported in Japanese[1095, 1406] and rarely in other nationalities[1266, 122, 490] is also an hereditary night blindness transmitted as a recessive trait. The distinctive feature is a diffuse-white background color of the central fundus which disappears after several hours in the dark (Mizuo's phenomenon). The visual acuity, fields, and color perception are all normal. However, the absence of rod function is confirmed by the inadequate dark adaptation and by the negative electroretinogram.

Another form of degeneration of the outer layers has been called the *tapetal reflex type* because of a sheen that has been thought to simulate that from an animal's tapetum[254, 732]. This name has also been applied to a reflex from otherwise normal eyes[425, 976]. The degenerative type is a progressive disease, inducing an annular scotoma but surprisingly little abnormality of the electroretinogram. The peculiar reflex may well be due to lipid or calcific changes in Bruch's membrane which becomes unusually visible by reason of attenuation of the pigment epithelium.

Achromatopsia (monochromatism). This is also a well defined hereditary entity which, except for the fact that it is transmitted as a recessive instead of dominant trait, is the exact opposite of congenital stationary night blindness. These patients have poor visual acuity (usually), absence of color perception, and a form of photophobia. It is as though they had no cone function. We know that cones are present but they may be morphologically abnormal[863, 613] and they are functionally deficient[740]. The condition is stationary. With the poor vision there is nearly always a pendular nystagmus and a habitual blepharospasm in bright light. The absence of color perception which is so striking from an examiner's point of view may be so inconsequential to the patient that he may not complain of it unless directly questioned.

Albinism. Although not a degeneration, patients with albinism show, in addition to lack of pigment, an absence of macular function. The basis for this visual defect is not understood since the retina appears histologically normal but it results regularly in poor central vision and consequent pendular nystagmus. Color perception, dark adaptation and other retinal functions are, however, unaffected.

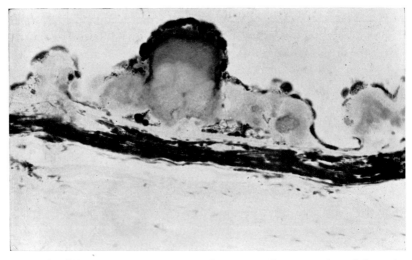

FIGURE 71. Massive drusen in an eye with long standing separation of the retina. The hyaline mounds are covered by attenuated pigment epithelium.

Drusen are hyaline excrescences of Bruch's membrane projecting forward beneath the pigment epithelium (Figure 71). They present ophthalmoscopically as discrete yellow dots scattered about the fundus. They are frequent concomitants of aging or of degeneration and are sometimes considered the primary abnormality. Thus, they are so conspicuous in one familial form of central retinal degeneration as to have been called Doyne's honeycomb degeneration. Ordinarily, however, they are undoubtedly secondary to aberrant activity of the pigment epithelium and are particularly prominent histopathologically in eyes with long standing separation of the retina.

B. DEGENERATION OF THE INTERMEDIATE LAYERS OF THE RETINA

Although the intermediate layers may be coincidentally affected by processes occurring elsewhere in the retina, no degenerative entity has been recognized which involves either the bipolar or reticular layers preferentially.

C. DEGENERATION OF THE INTERNAL LAYERS OF THE RETINA

The ganglion cells and their axones comprising the nerve fiber layer, disappear characteristically in several conditions. Aside from the arterial occlusion which has already been described, preferential loss of the ganglion cells occurs in glaucoma, Tay-Sachs form of amaurotic idiocy, and with certain poisons or trauma affecting the retina or optic nerve.

The loss of ganglion cells with glaucoma is explained by the strangulation of the nerve fibers at the cupped optic disc. The fibers become stretched on the relatively rigid edge of the sclera and when the cup is sufficiently deep the retina may be actually dragged into it. Although this would seem to be an adequate explanation, some have felt constrained to suggest that interference with the blood supply at the disc margin was the responsible modus operandi.

Tay-Sachs disease is an abiotrophy affecting particularly Jewish infants during the first two to three years of life. The ganglion cells of the retina[332, 273] and certain cells in the brain[125] become distended with a myelin-like substance that gives the ophthalmoscopic appearance of a white opacity in the central area (Figure 72). The absence of ganglion cells and therefore absence of opacification in the fovea leaves a zone of transparency in the center called a cherry-red spot.

The affected children, becoming progressively blind and apathetic, die within the first few years of life. The retinas of such patients show distension of some ganglion cells with abnormal lipid material (that stains like myelin and is vividly birefringent), loss of other ganglion

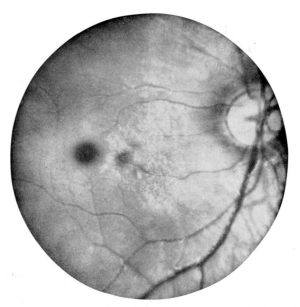

FIGURE 72. Tay-Sachs disease. The fundus shows an opacification of the central retina with sparing of the fovea (cherry-red spot) and an optic atrophy but normal retinal vessels.

cells and an extracellular deposition of the lipid material (Figure 73). Noteworthy is the absence of phagocytosis or other reaction.

The term infantile amaurotic family idiocy is often used synonymously with Tay-Sachs disease while the terms juvenile and adult amaurotic idiocy are used for other forms of degeneration of the retina associated with cerebral degeneration. This is confusing and should be avoided since it implies that the retinal degenerations are similar except for the variation with age. Actually Tay-Sachs disease is an exclusive degeneration of the inner retinal layer (the ganglion cells) while most other types involve either the outer layers exclusively (Vogt-Spielmeyer type) or all the layers of the retina (Bielschowsky type). The adult variety of amaurotic family idiocy, called Kuf's type, actually has no visual impairment[579]. One should thus avoid the ambiguous term amaurotic family idiocy or always qualify it as to the type by the appropriate eponym[264].

Less common than Tay-Sachs disease is a neurologic disorder that is called *metachromatic leucoencephalopathy* because of the staining characteristics of some of the white matter in the brain. Optic atrophy has been described in this entity and the retinal ganglion cells show a characteristic metachromasia with the cresyl violet stain[278]. Retinal ganglion cells also disappear selectively in the diffuse sclerosis of Schilder's disease[1409] but it is impossible to state whether the primary defect is in the retina or optic nerve.

With *poisons,* of which methyl alcohol is a prime example, it is

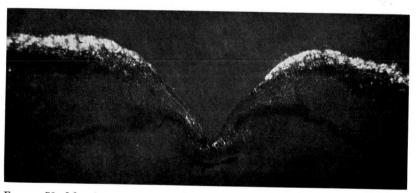

FIGURE 73. Macular area of patient with Tay-Sachs disease. The section was photographed between crossed polaroids to show the vividly birefringent material in what is normally the ganglion cell layer.

impossible to decide whether the point of attack is the ganglion cells or the optic nerve. The end result characterized by disappearance of the ganglion cells and optic atrophy would be the same wherever the process began.

The clinical manifestation of poisons appears to vary with the individual, and with the dose, and of course with the particular poison. Methyl alcohol causes preferential loss of central vision and does so in the wake of a debauch[107]. Quinine tends to cause peripheral constriction but may also involve central vision[1453].

Trauma causes loss of ganglion cells but this is clearly the result of nerve injury and the disappearance of the ganglion cells is a manifestation of retrograde degeneration such as occurs elsewhere in the central nervous system.

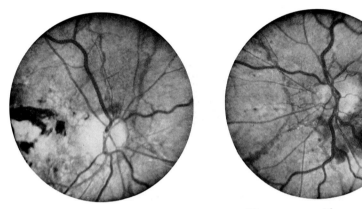

FIGURE 74. Angioid streaks. The patient was a fifty-two year old man who complained of failing vision for the previous several weeks. Aside from the streaks which surrounded and radiated outward from the discs of both eyes, the right eye showed a disciform degeneration of the macula and the left eye showed fresh subretinal hemorrhage in the peripapillary region.

D. MISCELLANEOUS DEGENERATIVE LESIONS

Aside from the vascular and specific degenerative changes in the retina there are correlates of aging which could not be included in the foregoing. Thus with aging a halo of chorioretinal degeneration frequently appears about the disc, the highlights reflected from the retina so brilliantly in youth disappear, and the diffuse redness of the youthful macula comes to be more like that of the rest of the retina[1150]. Pathologically pseudocysts develop in the periphery of the retina and the retina may show spotty loss of its outer elements (especially in the retinal periphery[1096]), hyaline excrescences (drusen) in Bruch's membrane, and occasional fusion to the choroid. Neverthe-less the retina is not known to show the gradual loss of its cells with age such as is said to occur in the gray matter of the cerebrum nor is there any ocular anatomic reason to suppose that the visual functions of an old person would be inferior to those of a young person.

In the entity *angioid streaks,* the retina undergoes secondary de-generative changes. This condition, often associated with pseudo-xanthoma elasticum in the skin[587, 1290] occasionally with Paget's disease of bone[1479, 1244, 1419] and systemic vascular disease[212, 1276, 458], sometimes with sickle cell disease[1120, 525, 526], acromegaly[674, 689, 1121] and hyperphosphatemia[960] is characterized ophthalmoscopically by brown-ish lines surrounding the disc and lines radiating toward the periphery of the fundus (Figure 74). The streaks actually represent proliferative changes in association with ruptures of Bruch's membrane and are called angioid because of their branched appearance simulating vessels. They eventually cause spotty destruction of the outer elements of the retina especially centrally where they produce the picture of disciform degeneration of the macula.

SUMMARY

Degeneration of the external layer of the retina results in loss of the rods and cones and of their cell bodies. Selective loss of rod function is characterized by night blindness whereas selective loss of cone function is characterized chiefly by lowering of visual acuity and loss of color discrimination.

Retinitis pigmentosa is the most common of the serious degenera-tions of the external retinal layers. It is an hereditary disease that begins usually within the first two decades of life with night blindness and progresses by unrelenting constriction of the visual fields. Follow-ing loss of the percipient elements the pigment epithelial cells migrate forward into the retina and produce the clusters of melanin, often in a bone corpuscular configuration, that give the name pigmentosa to the disease. The retinal arteries are also narrowed, the electrorentino-gram yields no response, and, curiously, the lens shows a posterior polar opacity. Variants of retinitis pigmentosa are about as common as the typical disease. These variants include a form associated with adiposogenital symptoms in an entity known as the Lawrence-Moon-Biedl syndrome, and a rapidly progressive retinopathy associated with cerebral degeneration in an entity known as the Vogt-Spielmeyer syndrome. There are many other variants which have no specific name. Indeed retinitis pigmentosa may be regarded as a generic diagnosis.

Retinitis punctata albescens includes a non-progressive fault of dark adaptation in persons whose fundi show a characteristic scattering of tiny white dots of undetermined origin; it also includes a progressive type in which fundal white dots, presumably drusen, accompany retinitis pigmentosa. Choroideremia is a loss of the choroid and may present in several forms; best documented is that which presents as progressive difficulty in dark adaptation and loss of the fundal orange color in males; the females show abnormal pigmentation but no subjective symptoms. Other degenerations with loss of the outer retinal elements are macular degeneration, prolonged detachment of the retina, experimental vitamin A deficiency and sclerosis of the choriocapillaris. Further clinical syndromes with either functional or organic defects in the percipient elements are congenital stationary night blindness, Oguchi's disease (night blindness with an anomalous white reflex from the fundus), progressive night blindness with a polychromatic luster from the fundus that has been likened to the tapetal reflex of animal eyes, achromatopsia that is characterized by nystagmus, poor central vision and absence of color perception as though the cones were functionally inactive, and, finally, albinism in which failure of pigmentation is accompanied by absence of macular function.

Degeneration of the bipolar layer has not been recognized as a distinct entity.

Degeneration of the inner layers of the retina may result secondarily from lesions of the optic nerve or nerve head; or the inner layers may be involved primarily in the dystrophies of the Tay-Sachs form of amaurotic family idiocy or in metachromatic leucoencephalopathy and possibly with certain systemic poisons. Tay-Sach's disease is a dystrophy affecting the ganglion cells of the retina and various neurones of the brain. It affects preferentially Jewish infants and is especially characterized by optic atrophy with a cherry-red spot in the macula. Metachromatic leucoencephalopathy causes a distention of some of the ganglion cells of the retina and of the brain cells with a metachromatic substance; it may or may not cause optic atrophy.

Miscellaneous degenerations of the retina include pseudocyst formation, spotty loss of the outer retinal layers, and occasional chorioretinal fusions. Angioid streaks result from a lesion that begins in the choroid and causes secondary retinal degeneration.

CHAPTER V

RETINA: Inflammatory, Toxic and Traumatic Lesions

A. INFLAMMATORY AND EXUDATIVE LESIONS OF THE RETINA

INFLAMMATORY processes occurring in both the retina and brain include the chorioretinitis of toxoplasmosis, cytomegalic inclusion disease, congenital syphilis, the retinitis of sarcoid and some virus diseases, and the curious retinopathy of Harada's disease and the allied Vogt-Koyanagi syndrome.

Toxoplasmosis is a frequent cause for focal inflammatory lesions

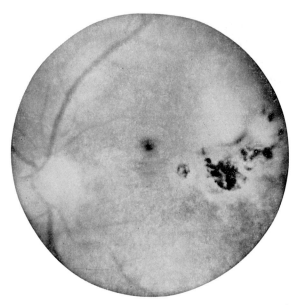

FIGURE 75. Active, recurrent chorioretinitis due to toxoplasmosis. An active exudative lesion is present on the edge of a previous, now-inactive lesion. The patient was a thirty-three year old woman with a serum titer for toxoplasmosis of 1:1024. The blurring of the fundus is due to vitreous opacities.

[98]

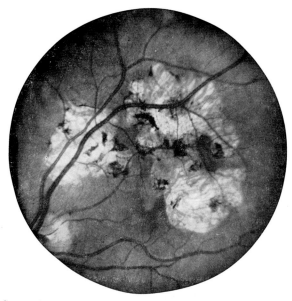

FIGURE 76. Scars of previous chorioretinitis. The patient gave a history of inflammation in the eye seven years previously. While not proved to be toxoplasmosis in origin the multilobate scars in this case are what one commonly associates with this disease.

of the fundus (Figure 75). During the acute stage these lesions present diffuse yellowish patches of varying size with much exudate in the vitreous. In the quiescent stage they present punched-out areas or chorioretinal scars, pigment mottling, baring of the sclera, and loss of most of the choroidal pattern but the media are usually clear (Figure 76). Recurrences are common and the reactivation almost always occurs in the manner of a satellite at the edge of a former lesion.

Although toxoplasmic retinitis may occur and may recur throughout one's adult life[1567, 731], the variety of chief neuro-ophthalmic interest occurs in the fetus. This results from subclinical infection in the mother during gestation[819]. The retinal lesions are commonly in the maculas of both eyes and result in great visual impairment. Concomitant foci are most always present in the brain and are manifest clinically by convulsions, hydrocephalus, various focal defects in the nervous system, and roentgenographic evidence of calcification[1522].

The organism of toxoplasmosis is a protozoan widespread in animals and in man. Human infection is common, as evidenced by positive skin test and serum agglutination, but rarely does it produce any marked clinical symptoms. In the case of the eye and brain, however, the toxoplasma (perhaps some strains particularly) become encysted in the nervous tissue and remain dormant over many years. Recurrences are presumably associated with periodic rupture of these cysts and release of the organisms into the adjacent tissue.

Pathologically, toxoplasmic chorioretinitis is characterized in the active phase by an intensely necrotic focus in which the retina and choroid are fused together and converted into a dense mass of inflammatory cells[665]. Organisms can be found in sections only after laborious search[1567] but may be demonstrated, even long after subsidence of active inflammation, by inoculation into mice.

Cytomegalic inclusion disease produces a syndrome in the newborn that is almost identical with that of toxoplasmosis[250, 595]. The focal chorioretinal necroses[1425] and the intracranial calcifications are both present. The differentiation is made histologically after death or by finding the characteristic cytomegaly in the saliva, gastric washings or urine of infected infants[1550, 595, 197, 982]. One case was confirmed by inoculation of aqueous humor onto tissue culture[197].

Congenital syphilis causes a disseminated type of chorioretinitis with diverse forms of central nervous system disease. The chorioretinitis presents spots of punched-out atrophic areas that are usually numerous and distributed randomly[712] (Figure 77). They are particularly common in patients with interstitial keratitis[799]. Active evidence of inflammation is only occasionally seen clinically but is common pathologically[500]. The inflammatory lesions and scars are often associated with other congenital anomalies of the eye (persistent hyaloid systems, microphthalmos, etc.). A bilateral and diffuse type of chorioretinitis producing a salt and pepper pigmentation of the fundus, has also been described as typical of congenital syphilis[1321].

Tuberculosis of the retina may be manifest as acute inflammatory foci with the military form of the disease or as an isolated granuloma. A more benign form characterized by an indolent chorioretinitis may occur, but it is rarely possible to prove the diagnosis histologically

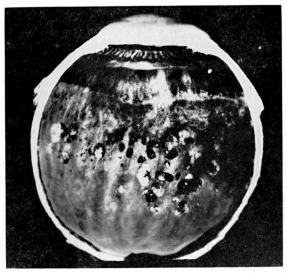

FIGURE 77. Disseminated chorioretinal scars due to congenital syphillis. The patient was a seventy year old woman who had had interstitial keratitis, perforated nasal septum and deafness in childhood. The eyes were removed post mortem and the picture taken of the opened eye.

and it is certain that many of the cases called tuberculous retinitis in former times were toxoplasmic or other infections by modern criteria.

Tuberculous chorioretinitis, if it exists, probably begins in the choroid rather than in the retina; granulomas, interpreted as tuberculous, have been described within the choroidal blood vessels[648].

Sarcoid involvement of the eye usually takes the form of a diffuse uveitis or nodular iritis but occasionally it produces a perivasculitis with highly characteristic white dots in the lower periphery[1521, 568, 309, 527]. These are collections of epithelioid cells situated in the superficial layers of the retina[876].

Some *virus diseases*, notably measles, may produce a severe retinopathy[621, 1319, 472, 734]. This comes on several days or weeks after the exanthem and may be associated with involvement of the central nervous system (encephalomyelitis). It is thought to result from an allergic vasculitis and not from a direct viral infection. A similar process may occur in the optic nerve (see p. 172); in fact, the resultant visual disturbance probably reflects both a retinitis and an optic neuritis. The presenting ocular symptom is blindness although this may not be appreciated at first because of the concomitant stupor and coma. Visual functions return in the course of several weeks but some defect usually persists, especially a deficiency in color perception. The fundus shows narrowed arteries and varying degrees of splotchy pigmentation suggestive of retinitis pigmentosa[472]. Viral infection of the mother during the first trimester of pregnancy is also said to produce a clinical picture similar to that of retinitis pigmentosa[414].

A necrotizing retinopathy due to herpes simplex has been seen in one patient with a fatal encephalitis[279, 1597]. The patient was an infant who at the age of three weeks became listless and progressed rapidly to profound mental deterioration. On the tenth day of illness the patient was noted to be unresponsive. Examination of the eyes which had been normal on the second day now showed areflexic pupils and a severe hemorrhagic retinopathy with obliteration of vessels; all landmarks, except the discs were obscured. The patient died at the age of fifteen weeks. Autopsy revealed loss of practically all cerebral tissue but fair preservation of brain stem and cerebellum. The eyes showed disappearance of all retinal tissue except for a thin glial membrane that was conspicuous only about the discs. The choroids appeared relatively intact. The optic nerves were completely atrophic. Etiologic tests, including those for toxoplasma and cytomegalic inclusion disease, were all negative except those for herpes simplex; the herpes titer rose 35-fold during the course of the illness.

Harada's disease is a poorly understood syndrome in which exudative detachment of the retina is associated with pleocytosis in the spinal fluid[1178, 541]. It appears allied to another entity, called *Vogt-Koyanagi disease,* in which a uveitis is associated with deafness, whitening of the eyelashes (poliosis ciliaris) and of the skin (vitiligo), with inflammatory cells in the spinal fluid[1112, 600, 936] (Figure 78). The etiology of these diseases is totally obscure but they are self-limited and much of the vision may return in the course of several months.

A common form of exudative retinopathy is that which is called *central serous retinopathy* (often miscalled angiospastic retinopathy). It is characterized by fairly rapid loss of central vision in one eye

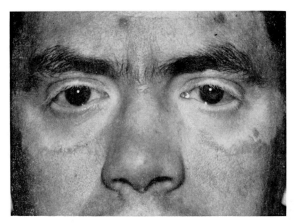

FIGURE 78. Vogt-Koyanagi syndrome. The patient was a twenty-four year old man who developed bilateral uveitis, vitiligo about the eyes, and 100-500 lymphocytes/mm³ in his spinal fluid.

with the frequent subjective observation of a red, orange or other colored ball[1303] in the line of sight and abnormal persistence of after-images. A subjective smallness of the image (micropsia[24]) or sensation of objects being far away (teleopsia) and difficulty in dark adaptation[735, 1498, 1474] are also frequent complaints. Ophthalmoscopically the entire central area of the retina is elevated by serum; a light reflex forms a circular line about the macula; and the macula itself may show a star figure. After a few weeks or months the retina recedes and the prognosis for recovery of most, if not all, the vision is good. There is no positive evidence to indicate what the etiology of this disease is but it occurs preferentially in young men, often of an apprehensive or obsessional personality[296, 609, 105], whence it is frequently believed to be an angioneurotic manifestation. It has also been reported to be associated with pits of the optic nerve[830]. Rarely is it bilateral or recurrent. Some evidence suggests increased pressure in the choroidal veins[808].

The persistence of after images together with prolongation of dark adaptation may be useful tests for the diagnosis of central serous retinopathy. A bright light as from the ophthalmoscope is shone on the macula for a minute or so. Patients with serous retinopathy, in contrast to those with degenerative macular disease, will recover visual acuity abnormally slowly[966].

Another almost specific sign for central serous retinopathy is the acquired hyperopia of 1-2 diopters which the patient is unable to overcome by accommodation. Thus patients with this disease may show considerable improvement of their vision when plus spheres are used over their normal correction. There is no obvious explanation why they cannot accommodate to overcome their small degree of acquired hyperopia.

Coats' disease is an exudative syndrome of obscure etiology occurring predominantly in boys and running a chronic course. It is characterized clinically by yellowish and sometimes glittering masses beneath the retina of one eye (Figure 79), and often by saccular dilatations of the retinal vessels. When the central area is involved vision will be greatly reduced and many eyes have been removed as retinoblastoma suspects.

Pathologically Coats' disease is characterized by masses of fat-

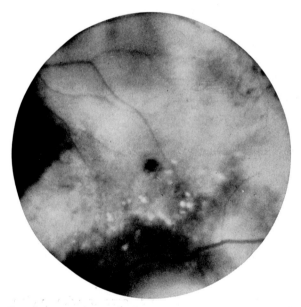

Figure 79. Coats' disease showing subretinal masses of yellowish white material in the central area of the fundus. The patient was an eight year old boy who incidentally discovered poor vision in one eye. At the time the photograph was taken his acuity was 1/200. Six months later the masses had increased with ballooning separation of the retina and the vision was nil. The temporal periphery of the fundus showed telangiectatic dilation of the veins.

laden histiocytes and cholesterol crystals in the outer portions of the retina and beneath the retina. It is generally an isolated occurrence without systemic disease but the pathologic abnormalities are similar to xanthomas elsewhere in the body (see p. 119).

One form of retinitis that has come to be recognized recently is that caused by *worms*[1566] (larval choroidoretinal granulomatosis). The worm may be seen to move actively during life[1019, 1291] (an observation noted by von Græfe in 1855[572]). After the worm dies, however, it causes either a massive intraocular inflammation with detachment of the retina and loss of all useful vision or a localized retinal lesion simulating a tumor or degenerative lesion[725, 41]. Since the reaction occurs only after the worm is dead and the eyes are removed late in the course of the disease it is usually impossible to identify the worm. The evidence available, however, has indicted the dog tape worm (toxocara canis)[41, 392, 82, 725], cysticercus[1019, 60] and common round worm (ascaris lumbricoides).

Fungus infections are occasional causes of retinitis and may begin in the retina. But by the time the patient is seen clinically, and certainly by the time the eye is enucleated, there is such a widespread endophthalmitis that it is impossible to determine the primary site of the infection.

B. POISONS AND INJURIES

Many poisons acting on the retina induce optic atrophy and it is often impossible to decide whether the initial site of injury is in the retina or optic nerve. Pathologic narrowing of the retinal artery, however, suggests a retinal site of action since simple loss of ganglion cells, such as might occur with optic nerve disease, is not known to cause arterial narrowing. Those poisons which induce degeneration of the macula, with little or no optic atrophy, may also be considered to have a focus of activity in the retina or in the subadjacent choroid.

Thus poisons affecting retinal function may be categorized into those producing simple optic atrophy, those with optic atrophy and arterial constriction, and those with evident macular changes. In addition some poisons cause retinal damage by obstructing the venous blood flow, and still other poisons produce an exudate in the retina. Recently a few poisons have been identified that act on the outermost layers of the retina and cause a clinical syndrome similar to that occurring with retinitis pigmentosa.

Methyl alcohol is perhaps the toxic substance that most notoriously produces simple optic atrophy and presents the quandary as to whether the site of intoxication is in the retina or optic nerve. Ingestion of methyl alcohol causes acute gastrointestinal symptoms, meningismus and visual symptoms that vary according to the amount absorbed. With a mild debauch the patient may develop simple and reversible blurring of vision but after a sufficiently intense debauch he can be completely blind on recovering consciousness. Some improvement in vision in the following few days is the rule but this recovery may in turn be followed by further loss of vision. The visual fields show central scotomas and irregular peripheral defects. The optic nerves become pale and the retinal arteries may or may not be constricted.

Methyl alcohol blindness is a peculiarly human (and primate) affection. Rarely has it been induced in lower animals. The toxic efflect is thought to be due to the oxidation of the methyl alcohol to formic acid and consequent acidosis[1159, 536, 578].

Ethyl alcohol may also cause an acute amaurosis but recovery is then usually prompt and complete[218]. More commonly, ethyl alcohol, along with tobacco, causes a chronic visual disturbance characterized by central or cecocentral scotoma and a particular impairment of color perception. Patients developing this chronic form of toxic amblyopia usually have an inadequate dietary intake and show other evidence of nutritional deficiency (such as polyneuritis)[1487]. Withdrawal of alcohol and restoration of an adequate diet will relieve the visual symptoms if done early in the course of the disease; otherwise central scotomas and optic atrophy will be permanent. The common histologic finding in the retinas of all these eyes is loss of ganglion cells.

Damage to the ganglion cells and inner retinal layers has also been induced experimentally in mice by levo glutamate or its precursor levo aspartate[939, 1170]. Yet no such effect has been observed in human beings despite widespread use of these compounds for epilepsy.

The prime example of retinal poisoning that culminates in optic atrophy with arterial constriction is that resulting from quinine (cinchonism). When taken in excessive amounts or, it is said, by patients who have a special susceptibility, quinine causes an acute blindness and prompt narrowing of the retinal arteries[884] (Figure 80). The visual symptoms are regularly accompanied by tinnitus and deafness[70]. Considerable recovery occurs after the acute episode but the patient is frequently left with constricted fields, thread-like retinal arteries, and pale discs. Other substances causing ophthalmologic signs and symptoms similar to those induced by quinine are organic arsenicals (especially atoxyl and tryparsamides), optochin, felix mas, ergot, salicylates, and methyl mercurial salts[578].

Hemorrhagic retinopathy results from a group of poisons that act on the blood vascular system. Most notable is the chronic poisoning with benzol and benzol derivatives (napthalenes and anilines). The fundi show characteristic distension of the veins and multiple flame-shaped hemorrhages. Such occurrences are presumably due to decreased platelets and increased viscosity of the blood rather than to any special vulnerability on the part of the retina.

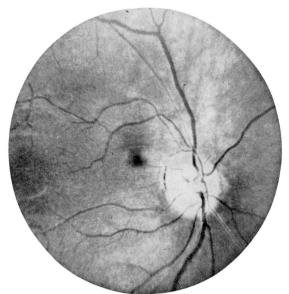

FIGURE 80. Optic atrophy and narrow arteries due to cinchonism. The patient was a forty year old woman who had ingested 100 grains of quinine over a three day period.

The whole retina, but most particularly the ganglion cells, is involved in siderosis. Apparently iron, whether it be from an intraocular foreign body or of hematogenous origin can cause blindness through a direct toxic effect on the retinal cells. The damage from repeated hemorrhages may be due in part to this siderosis and it is possible to cause blindness experimentally in dogs by repeated injections of blood[251].

Of practical significance are the retinotoxic effects of some of the phenothiazine drugs[1539, 230, 33]. This is a family of drugs having in common the molecular configuration of two phenyl rings joined by a sulphur and a nitrogen atom. Because of their different substituent groups they have variable effects as tranquilizers, antihelminthics, and insecticides. Two of the phenothiazine drugs which were found to be especially effective as sedatives have produced pigmentary degeneration of the retina and occasionally blindness in human beings[1486, 1218, 549, 196]. They are thioridazine (Mellaril) in exceptionally high dosage and NP207 [3-chloro-10,2'-(N-methylpiperidyl-2'')-ethyl-phenothiazine]. The retinal effects bear a superficial resemblance to retinitis pigmentosa in that night blindness occurs early and the retinal arteries show diffuse narrowing. Unlike the changes of typical retinitis pigmentosa, however, central vision is affected early, the electroretinogram is not completely extinguished[196], and the pigmentation occurs in large clumps rather than in bone corpuscle aggregates. The symptoms are partially reversible on discontinuance of the drugs. The pathologic changes remain to be ascertained since none of the eyes has been examined histologically and animal experimentation has been inconclusive[1486, 549]. The mechanism of toxicity is also unknown, but the phenothiazines have been found to concentrate in the uvea, most especially in the melanin fraction, suggesting that the vulnerability of the eye to these drugs is related to its pigmentation[1168]. Damage to the eye with these phenothiazines is not observed unless certain dosages are exceeded[32]. Thioridazine is not known to be harmful in doses less than 0.6 grams per day (continued for several months) and most of the patients who have had ocular damage had been taking as much as 2 grams per day. In the case of NP 207, the margin of safety between therapeutic and toxic amounts is narrower; pigmentary retinal degeneration occurs with doses of 0.8 grams per day but not with 0.3-0.4 grams per day which is the therapeutic range. Also toxic to the retina and optic nerve are certain of the quinoline drugs, sometimes used for treatment of malaria and other infections, but currently most widely used for treatment of rheumatoid arthritis and lupus erythematosus. In years past, one of this group of drugs, known as Optochin*, was used for pneumococcus infections but was discontinued when it was found to cause optic atrophy. Plasmocid†, another quinoline derivative used against malaria, was also discontinued because of resultant optic atrophy. In recent years other quinoline derivatives, chloroquine (Aralen) and hydroxychloroquine (Plaquenil), have been widely used, and a few patients have developed pigmentary degeneration of the retina as a consequence[656, 412, 655]. This retinal involvement has occurred with doses not exceeding the recommended therapeutic amounts (that is, not over 300 mg. per day) but only after the drug had been used for many months. The basis for the toxicity of chloroquine and of its analogs is incompletely understood, but the clinical manifestations are loss of central vision, granular pigmentation of the macula and sometimes of the rest of the retina, constriction of the arteries, and ring scotomas that may extend to the periphery producing a sort of altitudinal hemianopia. The visual loss is not necessarily progressive if the drug is discontinued, but, unlike the effects of the phenothiazines, it is irreversible.

An interesting form of blindness also occurs in dogs following a single injection of dithizone, a zinc chelating agent. Within a matter of hours the eyes of these dogs show an intense intraocular inflammation and become blinded with detachment of the retina. Histologic sections reveal severe necrosis of the tapetum lucidum and of all layers of the retina overlying the tapetum. The tapetum of dogs is made up largely of crystals of zinc cysteinate (18% of the dry weight is zinc). The significant conclusion is that an agent which binds the metal in the tapetum will cause degeneration of the overlying retina.

Dithizone has also been reported to damage the retina[1176] (and choroid) in rabbits which have no tapetum. The damage is due

---

* Ethylhydrocupreine

† (3-diethylaminopropylamino)-6-methoxyquinolone.

presumably to the high zinc content of the pigment epithelium[51]. One wonders whether other chelating substances which are normally consumed (as water softeners, etc.) in the human diet might not contribute to unexplained degenerations of the human retina.

A selective degeneration of the outer layers of the retina occurs in animals (rabbits and mice) given iodoacetic acid[1080] or bromacetate. This is a highly toxic substance but animals that survive intraperitoneal injections seem well except that they are blind; histologic sections of the eyes show within a few days a selective disappearance of the photoreceptors and eventual replacement by glial tissue[252]. The electroretinographic response disappears within a matter of seconds after the injection. From a biochemical point of view this selective effect on the rods and cones is significant in showing their especial vulnerability to at least one glycolytic inhibitor though apparently not to other sulfhydrl inhibitors[1359]. Another substance experimentally causing damage (in cats) to the outer retinal layers is 1,5-bis (p-aminophenoxy) pentane[40].

Ionizing radiation may damage the retina but only with doses of several thousand roentgens, that is with doses that are sufficient to cause cataracts and keratitis. These latter mask whatever retinopathy is present. Moreover the retinal damage results chiefly from occlusive vascular disease rather than from any direct effect of radiation on the retina. On the other hand, radiation from light or infrared sources may produce thermal burns on the retina by the focusing action of the ocular media. Such burns have long been associated with gazing at an eclipse[460] and have more recently come into prominence with gazing at the fire-ball of atomic explosions[260]. Unlike the case of the ionizing radiations, those due to light or infrared radiation are critically influenced by the size of the pupil and the direction of gaze at the time of the exposure.

Perforating *injuries* lacerate the retina but the prognosis depends on the amount of hemorrhage and associated injury to the lens and other ocular structures. Organization of hemorrhage in the vitreous and cicatricial detachment of the retina lead to loss of useful vision.

Blunt blows to the eye are usually tolerated remarkably well and tears of the retina do not necessarily cause serious impairment of the normal eye. If, however, the vitreous is liquefied as it is in middle age or in myopia, blunt blows may cause a tear that permits the fluid vitreous to insinuate beneath the retina and cause it to separate.

A traumatic type of retinopathy, called *Purtscher's disease,* results from crushing blows to the chest or to other remote parts of the body. This is manifest by hemorrhage, white spots, and edema. Suggested as causes have been fat emboli[768, 859], anoxia[1496] and extension of cerebrospinal fluid into the optic canal[362]. A similar ophthalmoscopic picture is said to have resulted from ligation of the common carotid artery[1279].

Hemorrhages in the retina, and into the vitreous, result also from traumatic *bleeding in the subdural and subarachnoid spaces.* This is believed to represent direct extension of blood about the optic nerve and thence into the eye (see p. 183). Retinal hemorrhages are also common in the newborn[534], presumably due to the trauma of birth, but they are benign and usually clear up without sequela in a matter of a few days.

Choroidal ruptures temporal to the disc are particularly frequent after blunt injuries to the globe. These tears are concentric with the disc, and separated from it by one or more millimeters. Immediately after the injury, eyes with choroidal tears show simply choroidal hemorrhage; later the tears are manifest by one or more white or pigmented lines concentric with the disc. They are usually associated with marked reduction in visual acuity.

SUMMARY

Toxoplasmic infection of the eye is characterized in the adult by a recurrent chorioretinitis and in the infant or fetus by a central chorioretinal scar and by intracranial calcification. Cytomegalic inclusion disease produces a nearly identical syndrome in the newborn. Congenital syphilis produces a disseminated variety of chorioretinitis. Tuberculosis has been alleged to be a frequent cause of retinitis but proved cases are rare. Sarcoid produces a characteristic vasculitis with white spots consisting of epithelioid cells scattered throughout the lower fundus. A particularly severe form of retinitis may follow various viral diseases.

Less well understood are the chorioretinopathies associated with pleocytosis in the spinal fluid and exudative separation of the retina (Harada's disease) or with vitiligo and deafness (Vogt-Koyanagi disease). Central serous retinopathy is also an exudative process of obscure eitology affecting the central area.

Worms and fungi cause retinopathy with more or less severe endophthalmitis. While the diagnosis may be suspected clinically, proof is usually possible only by histologic demonstration of the organisms.

Poisons may act directly on the retina and retinal blood supply or they may act on the optic nerve and cause secondary loss of the ganglion cells and nerve fibers in the retina. It is not always possible to distinguish which is primary and which is secondary. Methyl and ethyl alcohol fall into this category of indefinite localization. Quinine may be inferred to cause a direct retinal effect because of the characteristic narrowing of the retinal arteries, Chloroquine appears to cause predominantly macular degeneration while various agents (napthalenes and anilines) that act on the blood may manifest a vascular retinopathy in the eyes. Of particular interest is the selective degeneration of the outer retinal layers with iodoacetate poisoning in animals (or phenothiazine derivatives in man) and of the selective necrosis of that portion of the retina overlying the tapetum in dogs from dithizone.

Mechanical injury to the eye produces various retinopathies. Purtscher's disease consists of a hemorrhagic and exudative process resulting from crushing blows to the chest and long bones. Subarachnoid hemorrhages may extend into the eye by way of the optic nerve. Irradiation of the eye with ionizing rays produces primarily vascular occlusions while light or infrared rays produce a thermal and highly focal burn of the retina.

CHAPTER VI

RETINA: Tumors

RETINOBLASTOMA

THE MOST FREQUENT and most characteristic tumor of the retina is the retinoblastoma. With rare exception[1480, 948, 39, 1473, 970] this comes on in the first decade, usually in the first few years of life. It presents as a white mass behind the pupil of an eye that is found to be blind (Figure 81). Less frequently the tumor presents as daughter masses on the surface of the iris or even as a hypopyon. It is a tumor of moderate malignancy that may spread by way of the optic nerve through the cerebrospinal fluid into the brain or through the choroid into the orbit, or by way of the lymphatics into the lymph glands of the neck[209]. Less than half of all patients with retinoblastoma survive[353].

Retinoblastomas are tumors of unusual interest from many points

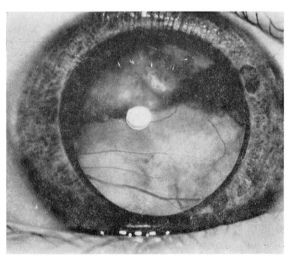

FIGURE 81. Retinoblastoma filling the vitreous space and visible through the pupil. The patient was a three year old girl whose mother had noted a white reflex from the pupil.

[113]

of view. Genetically they are the malignant tumors with the most impressive evidence for an hereditary transmission. In approximately one third of the cases the tumors are present in both eyes[1114]. Patho-

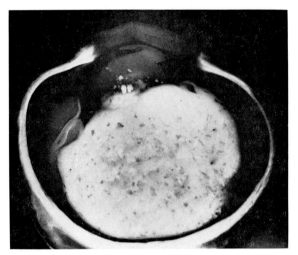

FIGURE 82. Retinoblastoma filling the interior of an opened eye. Portions of the detached retina are evident on either side of the anterior surface of the tumor.

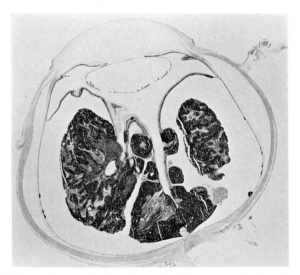

FIGURE 83. Photomicrograph showing retinoblastoma and detachment of the retina. The mottled appearance of the tumor is due to varying amounts of viable tissue, necrotic tissue, and calcification.

logically, retinoblastomas appear to arise from either the outer nuclear or bipolar cell layers of the retina (Figure 82) and have a characteristic and often marked rosette formation. They undergo necrosis readily (even to the extent of complete regression[1383]) and show abundant calcification (Figures 83 and 84).

The formation of rosettes is akin to what is seen occasionally with benign malformations of the outer portions of the retina; rosettes may be produced experimentally by interference with growth of the eye[1412, 548]. They are interpreted as neoplastic attempts to duplicate the rod and cone layer and are therefore most conspicuous with tumors arising from this layer[1581]; tumors arising from the bipolar layer have a similar cytology but are said to have no rosettes[243]. Rosette formation is also seen in medulloblastomas of the cerebellum but never as much as with retinoblastomas. Metastatic retinoblastomas ordinarily show few, if any, rosettes.

The clinical diagnosis of retinoblastoma is not always easy. Those entities which are most commonly confused with it are: persistent

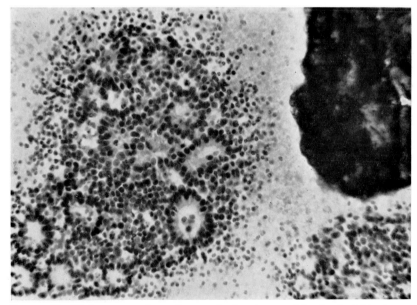

FIGURE 84. High power photomicrograph showing an island of viable tumor *(left center)* with characteristic rosettes, and a plaque of calcium *(upper right)* in necrotic tissue.

remnants of the lenticular vascular tissue, the exudative retinopathy of Coats' disease, massive retinal gliosis of infants, retrolental fibroplasia, metastatic endophthalmitis, and intraocular hemorrhage[643]. The presence of a solid mass in the fundus with satellite tumors in the vitreous is highly suggestive of retinoblastoma but perhaps the most indicative sign of retinoblastoma is the presence of a normal sized eye with normal or elevated tension. In most conditions simulating retinoblastoma the eyes are small and the tension is low. Only exceptionally are retinoblastomas found in phthisical eyes[1314].

The obvious treatment for retinoblastoma is enucleation but radiation also has its advocates[1368]. Antimetabolites are indicated when there is a likelihood of extrabulbar extension. The tragic circumstance of bilateral involvement requires the philosophic decision as to whether it is better to remove both eyes in the hope of saving life at the expense of total blindness or to maintain some vision as long as possible with the almost certain probability of death within a year or two.

Diktyomas (medullo-epitheliomas; teratoneuromas[1475]) arise from that non-pigmented portion of the retina which continues over the ciliary body. Rarely found elsewhere in the eye[1187], they usually present as white masses in the ciliary body region simulating organized glial tissue. Like retinoblastomas they occur most commonly in children and may be congenital but unlike retinoblastomas they are usually benign. They may, however, be locally invasive and a case has been reported in which the tumor invaded the orbit and brain[192].

Pathologically diktyomas have characteristic sheet-like laminæ of cells (resembling malformations of the pars plana of the ciliary body) and other teratoid aberrations[114]. Occasionally they contain rosettes and one can find all variations between true diktyomas and retinoblastomas.

Gliomas occasionally occur in the retina. These are benign tumors, simulating astrocytomas (although a few are said to simulate oligodendrocytomas[701]) and present as isolated white masses in the retina[349, 957, 990, 1102, 1465, 958]. They may be isolated occurences or occur, along with tumors of the nerve head and brain, in the entity of tuberous sclerosis[1012, 664].

Vascular tumors of several types occur in the retina. Typical cavernous or capillary hemangiomas may occur in the retina, as elsewhere in the body[1152], but are rare. A more frequent vascular tumor of the retina is that seen with the hemangiomatosis called von Hippel's disease (when it is limited to the eye) or Lindau's disease (when it is associated with lesions in the cerebellum and elsewhere). This hemangiomatosis retinæ is an hereditary process involving both eyes and coming on in childhood or early adult life. It is characterized ophthalmoscopically by aneurysmal tumors that are supplied by large arteries and veins (Figures 85 and 86). Later it is associated with extensive gliosis, local histiocytosis, detachment of the retina, and blindness. Hemangiomas and cysts in the kidneys and viscera are often found at autopsy or by roentgenography (Figure 87).

In addition to the frank angiomatosis retinæ, one occasionally encounters varices in the retina characterized by gross arteriovenous anastomoses and severe distension of the arteries and veins. These

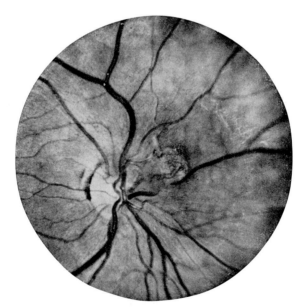

FIGURE 85. Retinal hemangioma (von Hippel-Lindau disease). The patient was a thirty-nine year old woman who had had headaches and difficulty in walking of several months duration. The patient's father, sister, and nephew had all died of brain tumors. Examination of the patient showed cerebellar ataxia and the hemangioma of the retina (which had produced no symptoms). Craniotomy revealed a cerebeller hemangioma.

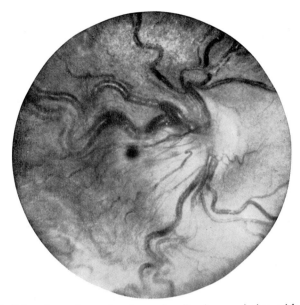

FIGURE 86. Dilated vessels coming from the disc in association with hemangiomatosis retinae. The patient was a sixteen year old girl with a discrete hemangiomatous mass in the temporal periphery. This was fed and drained by the large vessels seen in the region of the disc.

have been variously called cirsoid aneurysms, racemose aneurysms, and aneurysmal varices. Unlike the true angiomatosis retinæ, they are usually unilateral, congenital (but non-hereditary), stationary, not productive of visual symptoms, and discovered fortuitously during a routine eye examination. One syndrome has been described in which varices of the retina are associated with similar vascular anomalies in the mid brain and with dementia[1591].

The cavernous hemangiomas (nævus flammeus) of the face which commonly follow the distribution of the trigeminal nerve are characteristically associated with choroidal hemangiomas but not with retinal changes.

The *reticuloendothelioses* which produce tumorous enlargement of organs elsewhere, rarely result in infiltration of the retina. An infiltration of the maculæ has been reported, however, in both eyes of a patient with hepatosplenomegaly akin to Gaucher's disease[269] and a purely local reticuloendotheliosis occurs unilaterally in an eye with the entity known as Coats' disease (sometimes with hyperlipemia[135]).

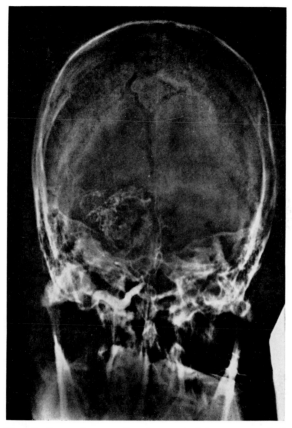

FIGURE 87. Vertebral arteriogram showing a vascular tumor of the cerebellar hemisphere. The patient had been blind since the age of twenty with vascular tumors of both retinas (von Hippel's disease). The present investigation was prompted by the recent development of suboccipital pain and hemianesthesia of face. Suboccipital exploration revealed a hemangioma overlying the left cerebellar hemisphere.

Coats' disease occurs predominantly in young males and presents at first as a white mass beneath the retina (see p. 104). Impressed by the abundance of fat-laden histiocytes in and beneath the retina, some have considered Coats' disease a form of xanthomatosis[988] (with phagocytes possibly derived from the pigment epithelium[347]); others, impressed by the aneurysmal dilatation of some of the retinal vessels consider it a telangiectasis[1186, 1442]; still others consider it toxo-plasmic[487, 75] or larval[392] infection.

Melanomas arising in the choroid may involve the retina second-arily. Usually they simply raise the retina by serous exudate and destroy the outer layers of the retina at the sites of contact. Occasion-ally the melanoma will penetrate into the retina and grow through it to present within the vitreous. In this way melanomas of the choroid may present with hemorrhage into the vitreous.

A benign type of melanoma, believed to arise from the pigment epithelium[1193], presents as a mass on the disc[299, 1119, 1011, 1604, 1472]. This occurs predominantly in Negroes and is compatible with normal visual functions (see p.   ).

Metastases to the retina occur[1472, 394, 1210] but they are rare in comparison to those in the choroid.

SUMMARY

The most frequent tumor of the retina is the retinoblastoma. With rare exception this occurs during the first decade of life, is moderately malignant, and frequently bilateral. It occurs as a sporadic mutation and is transmitted as a dominant hereditary trait. Pathologically these tumors are characterized by rosette formation, necrosis, and tendency to calcification.

Diktyomas are benign tumors usually arising from the ciliary epithelium and producing sheet-like laminæ of cells. They may simu-late retinoblastomas.

Less common tumors of the retina are the gliomas, hemangiomas, reticuloendothelioses (including Coats' disease), melanomas (from the choroid), and metastatic tumors. Most of these are sufficiently rare as to be considered curiosities.

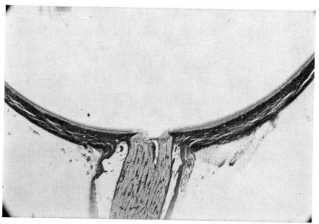

Cross section in region of nerve head, stained by van Gieson's method. Enlarged 5 times.

CHAPTER VII

OPTIC NERVE: Anatomy

THE OPTIC NERVE is a tract, consisting of myelinated nerve fibers and meningeal sheaths, that extends from the globe anteriorly to the chiasm posteriorly (Frontispiece). For convenience, it is arbitrarily divided into: (1) an ocular part traversing the sclera; (2) an orbital part having a sinuous course in the orbit about 40 mm in length; (3) an intracanalicular part within the foramen of the sphenoid bone; and (4) an intracranial part extending from the foramen to the chiasm. At the chiasm the nerve fibers separate, according to the rule for intracranial lateralization of sensorimotor representation; the fibers from the medial portions of the optic nerve (representing lateral visual fields) cross over in the chiasm to terminate in the contralateral geniculate body and midbrain while the fibers from the lateral portions of the optic nerve (representing medial visual fields) remain uncrossed to terminate in the homolateral geniculate body and midbrain.

1. Sheaths

The sheaths of the optic nerve are continuous with the meninges of the brain and are accordingly called the dura, arachnoid and pia respectively, or the vaginal sheaths collectively (Figures 89 and 90). The dura is the outermost and toughest of the three. It is composed of compact connective tissue with a considerable component of elastic fibers. The collagenous fibers of the outer portion of the dura are arranged along the axis of the nerve while those in the inner portions of the dura are arranged concentric to it.

On approaching the eye the dura frays out to insert along with the ciliary arteries and nerves in the sclera. In the posterior portion of the orbit the dura is continuous with the periorbita and passes through the foramen to be continuous with the dura in the skull.

The arachnoid of the optic nerve consists of a trabeculum of collagenous and elastic fibers lined by endothelium. It contains cerebrospinal fluid and is continuous with the corresponding intra-

[123]

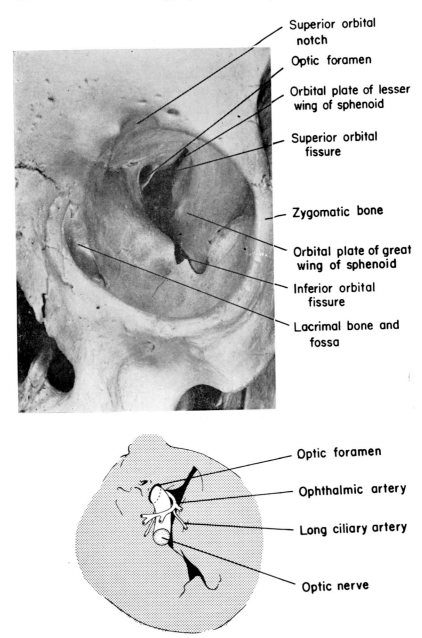

Superior orbital notch

Optic foramen

Orbital plate of lesser wing of sphenoid

Superior orbital fissure

Zygomatic bone

Orbital plate of great wing of sphenoid

Inferior orbital fissure

Lacrimal bone and fossa

Optic foramen

Ophthalmic artery

Long ciliary artery

Optic nerve

FIGURE 88. Photograph of orbit and sketch showing entrance of optic nerve and ophthalmic artery and adjacent orbital fissures.

cranial space[1577, 291, 583, 437]. As the optic nerve enters the globe the arachnoid ends in the sclera; at the apex of the orbit the arachnoid is continuous with the corresponding membrane of the intracranial meninges.

The pia, also consisting of collagenous fibers, elastic fibers, and endothelium, invests the nerve and sends fibers into it to form the characteristic septa. Anteriorly the pia is continuous with the sclera and choroid while posteriorly it continues through the optic foramen to form the only covering of the intracranial portion of the optic nerve.

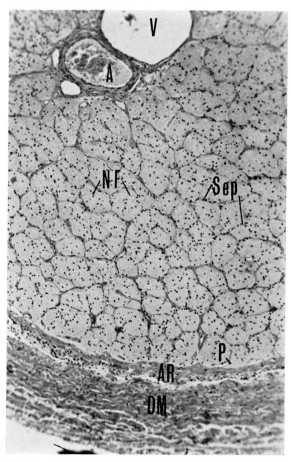

FIGURE 89. Cross section of a portion of the optic nerve just behind the eye. V, vein; A, artery; NF, nerve fibers; Sep, septa; P, pia; AR, arachnoid; DM, dura mater.

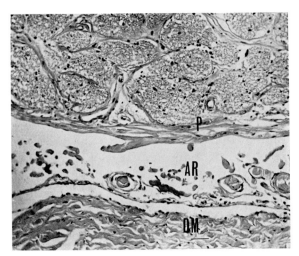

FIGURE 90. Sheaths of optic nerve. DM, dura mater; AR, arachnoid; P, pia.

As meninges elsewhere, those of the optic nerve contain characteristic clusters of cells, called meningoblasts, and concentrically laminated hyaline bodies, called corpora arenacea. These latter increase with age and may actually be derived from the cell clusters. They are not known to have clinical significance but they are similar to hyaline bodies on the disc, called drusen, which do have clinical significance (see p. 150).

2. Nerve Substance

The optic nerve consists of myelinated nerve fibers similar to those forming tracts of white matter elsewhere in the brain (Figure 89). They differ from peripheral nerve fibers in their absence of neurilemmal sheaths (the sheaths of Schwann) which are thought necessary for effective regeneration of nerves. At the same time the optic nerves differ from tracts of the brain in having relatively abundant connective tissue septa which give to these nerves pathologic reactions not shared by the intracranial portions of the central nervous system. These connective tissue septa are most conspicuous in the anterior portions of the optic nerve where they form dense cores containing the central vessels of the retina.

The nerve fibers are the axones of the retinal ganglion cells and comprise: (1) visual fibers destined for the lateral geniculate body;

(2) pupillary fibers destined for the pretectal nuclei of the midbrain; and probably (3) centrifugal fibers to the retinal blood vessels[1579]. The morphologic and topologic distinction of the visual and pupillary fibers in the optic nerve is debatable. Evidence from traumatic cases suggests that the pupillary fibers predominate in the nasal portions of the nerve as it passes through the optic foramen.

The myelin envelope of the individual nerve fibers is not known to differ from that of the rest of the central nervous system and it is similarly susceptible to demyelinating diseases and toxins that affect white matter.

The myelin stains lightly with eosin, moderately with Sudan Black, and heavily with Baker's stain (for phospholipid). With cresyl violet it stains metachromatically and shows a strikingly fine-grained birefringence so long as the sections have not been exposed to organic solvents.

A common artifact in histologic sections of the eye is the presence of myelin anterior to the lamina cribrosa and in the adjacent subretinal region[271]. This results from squeezing by enucleation scissors when the optic nerve is cut close to the globe. It is not found in eyes with atrophic nerves.

The glia of the optic nerve are similar to those in the white matter of the brain but tend to have larger nuclei. Predominant are the pleomorphic astrocytes which may be of the protoplasmic type with oval nuclei, considerable cytoplasm, and short processes, or the fibrillary type with sparse cytoplasm and long fibrous processes[984]. Best stained with Cajal's gold sublimate or Hortega's silver carbonate[291, 1580], these are the cells which form the scar tissue, known as gliosis, of various lesions of the optic nerve. Oligodendrocytes are also present in the optic nerve and are recognizable with ordinary stains by the characteristic arrangement of nuclei in rows. These oligodendrocytes are believed to be responsible for formation and regeneration of myelin.

3. Contiguous Structures

The relationship of the optic nerve to adjacent structures has practical importance.

In the posterior part of the orbit the optic nerve is separated from the sphenoid and ethmoid sinuses by only a thin lamina of bone; even this is occasionally absent so that the optic nerve is separated from the sinuses by mucous membrane only. On theoretical grounds one might expect infections of the sphenoid sinus to be a cause of optic neuritis. Such is often assumed but rarely proved to be the case. There can be no doubt, however, that this proximity accounts for the early involvement of the optic nerve and blindness with carcinoma of the sinuses.

The optic nerve sheath participates in the formation of the Annulus of Zinn to which the ocular muscles attach. This would seem to account for the characteristic pain which patients with optic neuritis experience on movement of the eye.

The intracranial portions of the optic nerve have an especially vulnerable relationship to the major arteries. The carotid arteries and ophthalmic arteries lie immediately beneath the optic nerves and when sclerosed are believed to be capable of damage either by direct trauma to the nerves or by pressure of the nerves against the unyielding edge of the optic foramen. The anterior communicating artery, which traverses the dorsal aspect of the optic nerve, is not known to affect it through sclerosis but may injure it, or even transect it when an expanding lesion pushes the nerve upward against the pulsating vessel. This constitutes one of the mechanisms of blindness with pituitary tumors. Dilatation of the 3rd ventricle is also thought to damage the nerves by pressing them against the anterior cerebral arteries[474]. Finally it should be noted that this intimate relationship between the optic nerves and the anterior portions of the circle of Willis exposes the visual system to damage by the saccular aneurysms which are so common in this region.

4. Lamina Cribrosa

The lamina cribrosa is a sieve-like portion of the sclera, modified to permit passage of the nerve fibers out of the eye (Figure 4). The diameter of the nerve as it passes through the lamina cribrosa is 1.5 mm. but it abruptly becomes 3 mm. or more immediately behind the lamina as it acquires myelin (Figure 91).

Myelination of the optic nerve develops embryologically in a

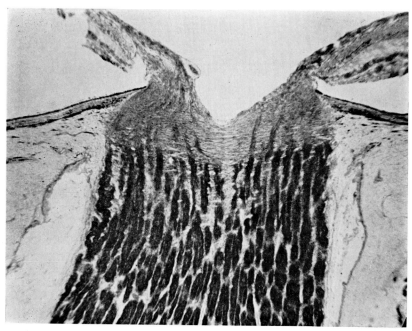

FIGURE 91. Horizontal section of the optic nerve to show the abrupt termination of myelination at the lamina cribrosa. Baker's phospholipid stain.

posterior to anterior direction. The fibers are grossly myelinated in the intracranial and intracanalicular portions of the optic nerve at 7 months of gestation but the myelin does not reach the lamina cribrosa until about term. The macular fibers are the first to be myelinated[92]. In some conditions, notably in oxycephaly and neurofibromatosis, but most often unassociated with other abnormality, myelination continues through the optic canal onto the retina (Figure 8). These radiating white patches are situated superficially on the disc and adjacent retina covering some of the vessels and terminating with characteristically fibrillated edges. These intraocular patches of myelinated fibres have been seen to undergo demyelination in life with the optic neuropathy of multiple sclerosis[522], and with retinal vascular disease[52, 510].

Reduction in size of the optic nerve as it traverses the sclera serves a mechanical purpose by minimizing this potentially weak spot in the outer covering of the eye. The sclera is normally a compact envelope that opposes distention of the eye by the intraocular pressure. The lamina cribrosa is the weakest point in this resistant envelope and is the first to give way with abnormal elevation of the intraocular pressure. In glaucomatous cupping the lamina may be bowed backward several millimeters (Figures 92 and 93). Clinical evidence suggests considerable variation in its rigidity; at times typical "glaucomatous" cupping may occur with normal intraocular pressures.

Isolated pits of the nerve heads may occasionally occur in otherwise normal eyes. Usually of no significance, they may on occasion be associated with sector field defects. Ophthalmoscopically they form small grey "holes" that may be several diopters deep. Although usually congenital, we and others[524] have had occasion to see typical pits develop spontaneously in both eyes of adults with normal intraocular pressure. Even when they occur later in life they are not necessarily progressive.

5. Blood Supply to Optic Nerve

The blood supply to the optic nerve has been the subject of many reviews. Discrepancies in the conclusions are probably attributable to variations in species studied and to variations among human

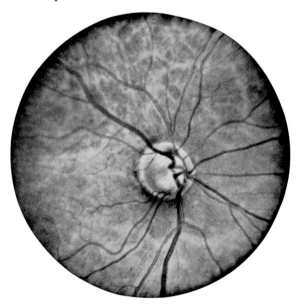

FIGURE 92. Glaucoma cup. The central cup of the nerve head has extended to the edge of the disc and displaced the vessels to the periphery.

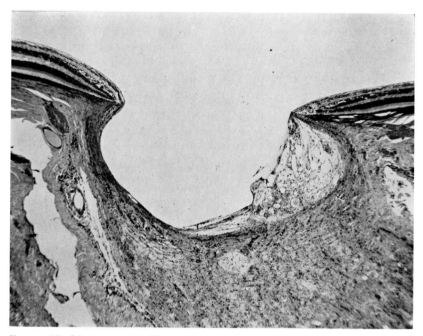

FIGURE 93. Glaucoma cup. The lamina cribrosa has been pushed backward and the nerve fibers impaled against the unyielding edge of the disc.

beings[703]. Blood vessel architecture is relatively constant only for the larger vessel systems.

In man the chief blood supply to the intracranial and intracanalicular portions of the nerve is from branches of the anterior cerebral and ophthalmic arteries; that to the orbital portion, from branches of the ophthalmic artery with probably a retrograde branch of the central retinal artery[1377, 1590, 481] (although this has been denied[478]); and that to the disc portion by branches from the Zinn-Haller anastomotic ring formed by both short ciliary and central retinal vessels. The questions are whether or not the arteries are end-arteries as is the rule for the rest of the nervous system, and how much each system contributes to the whole supply. But regardless of whether the arteries are end-arteries or not, the optic nerve is dependent on several systems and one might expect varied types of lesions with vascular disease.

One further consideration is the potentially abundant anastomosis between the ophthalmic artery and the external carotid artery about the rim of the orbit (Figure 24). While this may be of little significance normally, it may so develop with slow occlusions of the internal carotid artery as to form a major source of blood supply to the eye and even to the brain (see p. 187). In this latter case the direction of blood flow in the ophthalmic artery is reversed.

SUMMARY

The optic nerves comprise the axones of the retinal ganglion cells that extend from the lamina cribrosa anteriorly to the general region of the chiasm and optic tracts posteriorly. They are surrounded by sheaths similar to and continuous with the meninges of the cranium. Except for its considerable amount of connective tissue, the substance of the optic nerves is similar to tracts of white matter in the central nervous system. The fibers of the optic nerve differ from those of peripheral nerves in not having sheaths of Schwann.

The course of the optic nerves exposes them intimately to the sphenoid sinuses, from which they are separated by thin laminæ of bone, and to major vessels within the cranium. The optic nerves are also subjected to unusual confinement as they lose their myelin and pass through the lamina cribrosa.

The blood supply to the human optic nerve is derived from many and variable sources: directly from the large intracranial arteries; from the ophthalmic artery; from the ciliary arteries; and probably from the central retinal artery. At the same time the arteries of the orbit are the chief connections between the external carotid system (through the temporal arteries) and the internal carotid system (through the ophthalmic artery).

CHAPTER VIII

OPTIC NERVE: Atrophy and Papilledema

A. OPTIC ATROPHY

PALLOR of the disc (Figure 94) which is the clinician's criterion for optic atrophy is attributable to loss of the smaller blood vessels and to a variable amount of reactive gliosis and fibrosis. But since these are secondary changes they may not be evident for several weeks after the loss of vision. Although pallor is a useful index of atrophy, its value as a criterion is lessened by the wide variation in pinkness of normal discs and by the paradoxic finding of normal visual functions in some cases of extreme pallor. An alternative criterion,

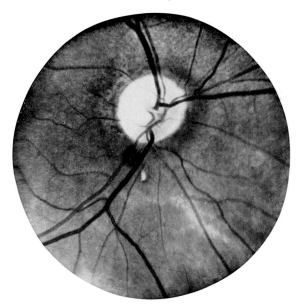

FIGURE 94. White disc with Leber's optic atrophy. The patient was a forty-nine year old man whose vision deteriorated rapidly over a period of several weeks two years previously. Examination revealed bilateral central scotomas and the discs eventually became pale. Two maternal male cousins and two maternal uncles have similar conditions.

which some believe to be more reliable is the diminution in number of arterioles traversing the disc margin (Kestenbaum's sign). Normally there are about ten such arterioles but in optic atrophy there are only six or seven.

Optic atrophy is said to be *primary* when the atrophic disc is white and has sharply defined edges. It is called *secondary* when the edges are blurred by proliferated, often grayish tissue. This terminology is confusing and sometimes meaningless but it has been irreversibly established by usage. More appropriate terms would be simple atrophy for the one and postpapilledema or postpapillitic atrophy for the other.

Changes in the vessels may also be of significance. Optic atrophy from arterial occlusion is often associated with extreme narrowing of the arteries; the vessels may even be replaced by white thread-like lines. On the other hand, optic atrophy may result from such a transient occlusion that the arteries retain a normal appearance. Or narrowing of the arteries may result from secondary optic atrophy where there is no vascular disease. Thus the presence or absence of arterial narrowing gives us little information on the type or etiology of the optic atrophy.

An important correlative of optic atrophy is the pupillary response to light. To be sure, traumatic lesions of the optic nerve, and possibly other acute lesions, produce a curious dissociation of pupillary and visual functions whereby the one may be abolished without the other, but by the time optic atrophy supervenes the loss in pupillomotor function parallels the loss of visual function. When it does not, the appearance of optic atrophy may be suspect because the pupillary reactions are a more objective and therefore more reliable sign.

The question as to whether an optic atrophy began in the retina or in the nerve must often go unanswered; primary optic atrophy will result either from loss of the ganglion cells or from transection of the nerve. The optic nerve fibers are the axones of the ganglion cells and lesions of the one will result in degeneration of the other with a common manifestation in primary optic atrophy.

Pathologically, optic atrophy consists of a selective loss of the nerve fibers and eventually of their myelin. When this occurs acutely the macrophages become distended over a period of several weeks with sudanophilic fat in the same manner as with acute lesions of white matter in the brain. With chronic lesions the neural elements may disappear without causing reactive changes. The end result is a fibroglial scaffolding which differs from atrophic lesions in the central nervous system by the abundance of connective tissue. With glaucomatous atrophy the spaces of this scaffold become distended with a mucoid substance to form holes in the nerve behind the lamina cribrosa (Schnabel's cavernous atrophy).

Causes of optic atrophy are legion. Analysis of any one case requires a knowledge of the age of the patient, the acuteness or chronicity of visual loss, the associated symptoms and laboratory findings, and especially the field changes.

In children optic atrophy is often a developmental defect and is then frequently accompanied by mental deficiency, cerebellar ataxia[580], cerebral palsy[171], or other neurologic defects[969]. Specific congenital syndromes are anencephaly, hydranencephaly, craniostenoses[1129] (such as oxycephaly and turricephaly[588]) and especially hydrocephalus[297]. Primary stationary optic atrophy may occur in families with typically dominant types of transmission[797]. Vision in such cases is usually no worse than 20/200. Certain heredo-degenerative diseases of children may involve the central nervous system and optic nerves together. Bielschowsky's disease characterized by epilepsy and visual loss is perhaps the best documented. The disease usually results in idiocy and blindness within a period of a year or two. Other cerebral degenerations of children which are accompanied by optic atrophy are Tay-Sach's disease (see p. 91), metachromatic leucoencepalopathy (see p. 163), spongy degeneration of the brain (Canavan's disease) and infantile neuronal axial dystrophy[303]. Optic atrophy is sometimes associated with the progressive neuropathy of the Charcot-Marie-Tooth disease[692]. Congenital syphilis was a common cause of optic atrophy but is now infrequent in this country. The acute exanthemata and various meningitides sometimes cause a retrobulbar neuritis which leads to optic atrophy. Of the metabolic diseases in childhood, idiopathic hyperparathyroidism may cause optic atrophy through excessive calcification of the optic foramina and consequent compression of the nerves. A similar overgrowth of bone and early optic atrophy occurs with osteopetrosis (marble-bone disease or the Albers-Schönberg disease) [1148, 1221, 409]. Lead poisoning was a not uncommon cause of optic atrophy at one time and should still be suspected when a child has unexplained papilledema, acute gastro-intestinal symptoms, muscular weakness, irritability and a dark line in the gums. Basophilic stippling of the red blood cells and serum-lead determinations will confirm the diagnosis.

But the most common cause of optic atrophy in children, as in adults, is expanding lesions within the orbit of cranium. Of the lesions in the orbit, gliomata of the optic nerve are foremost and should be the suspected diagnosis when a child presents with a combination of unilateral optic atrophy (especially when there is overgrowth of glia on the disc), exophthalmos, and x-ray evidence of an enlarged optic foramen. The common intracranial tumors of childhood that cause primary optic atrophy are craniopharyngiomas, gliomas, meningiomas, and ectopic pinealomas. On the other hand, the intracranial tumors of childhood that cause papilledema and secondary optic atrophy are more apt to be the cerebellar tumors in the posterior fossa or pinealomas and craniopharyngiomas in the region of the aqueduct.

The causes of optic atrophy in the adult will be described in some detail subsequently. For the present purposes optic atrophy in the adult may be said to result from any of the following: inflammation (optic neuritis); non-inflammatory swelling (papilledema); glaucoma; cicatrization (arachnoidal adhesions); compressive lesions (meningiomas, pituitary adenomas, craniopharyngiomas, nasopharyngeal carcinomas and metastases); poisons; trauma; aneurysms or other types of vascular disease.

Field defects may at times indicate the cause of an optic atrophy; at other times they may be deceptive. Bitemporal defects are of course the signature of a chiasmatic lesion (see p. 210). Blindness in one eye with optic atrophy and temporal hemianopia in the other eye with partial atrophy points to a lateralized lesion in the parachiasmic region, obliterating the function of one optic nerve and of the homolateral optic tract. This type of field defect is about as common and as characteristic of chiasmic involvement as is bitemporal hemianopia.

Tumors may cause atrophy of the optic nerve by strangulation or by competition for its blood supply. On the other hand, tumors may press the nerve upward against a pounding artery which thus ultimately transects it. The arteries most commonly responsible for transection of the optic nerves are the anterior cerebral[1041] and the anterior communicating[1444] arteries. It is apparent that the likelihood of optic atrophy occurring by this mechanism will depend on the local configuration of the circle of Willis and occasionally on the presence of abnormal arteries.

Central scotomas occur predominantly in inflammatory lesions of the optic nerve but they certainly are not limited to the neuritides. They are found occasionally with tumors and with vascular accidents. It is these compressive and vascular lesions producing sudden central scotomas which are often mistakenly diagnosed as optic neuritis. Central scotomas rarely occur with simple papilledema[765].

Altitudinal hemianopic defects due to optic nerve lesions including papilledema are almost always in the lower field. The reason for this predilection for the lower fields is not clear. It has been suggested that lesions in the intracranial area cause pressure against the upper rim of the optic foramen[1518] but this could not explain the inferior altitudinal hemianopia with lesions in the anterior portion of the optic nerve. In contrast to the preferential involvement of the upper fibers with lesions in the optic nerve, damage to the fibers with glaucomatous cupping is almost always greater in the lower portion of the nerve with consequent superior altitudinal hemianopia.

B. PAPILLEDEMA

1. Characteristics of Papilledema

To the clinician, papilledema is an abnormal elevation of the nerve head and obliteration of the disc margins without obvious signs of inflammation. It thus differs from papillitis in which, to be sure, there may be edema but in which there are inflammatory opacities in the vitreous, correlative visual disturbances, and often ocular pain and tenderness[690]. The elevation of the disc with papilledema is cylindric, unlike the sloping elevation with papillitis, and may mushroom forward into the vitreous 4-5 diopters; the physiologic cup is apt to be retained even when the papilledema is marked so that the disc comes to have the form of a truncated cone (Figure 95).

Measurement of the amount of papilledema is easy and reliable if one observes the following rules: start with a high plus

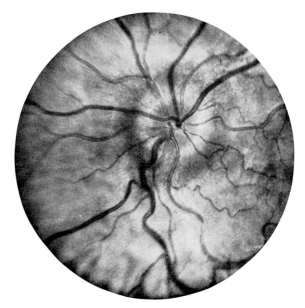

FIGURE 95. Chronic papilledema. The disc margins are obliterated and elevated in cylindric fashion with preservation of the central cup. The vessels show minimal engorgement.

lens in the ophthalmoscope and reduce the lens power until one just focuses on the top of the disc; then switch to the retina a short distance from the disc and again decrease the plus lens (or increase the minus lens) until the retinal vessels just come into focus. The difference in lens power indicates in dioptric units the amount of papilledema.

The common error in measurement of papilledema results from either failure to start with a high enough plus lens or failure to stop just when the disc or retina come into focus. One's own accommodative power then continues to maintain the focus and prevents accurate measurement of the disc's protruberance. This may be avoided by remembering to use the highest lens in all focusing.

Vascular changes, which are often a conspicuous feature, depend on the rate with which the papilledema develops rather than on the degree of the papilledema. With acute onset, the veins are greatly distended while hemorrhages and exudates form a radiating corona on and about the disc (Figure 96). At times the hemorrhages extend

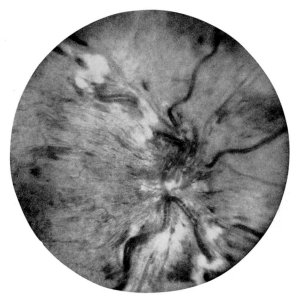

FIGURE 96. Acute papilledema with severe congestion of vessels, hemorrhage, and exudate centering about the disc.

into the vitreous overlying the disc. The predilection of hemorrhages for the peripapillary regions distinguishes the retinopathy of simple papilledema from that of hypertension and other conditions in which the hemorrhages and exudates are distributed widely over the retina. In contrast to the venous and hemorrhagic changes with acute papilledema, little or no stasis occurs with chronic papilledema of gradual onset even though the elevation of the disc may be much greater than that in the acute cases (Figure 95).

Minimal amounts of papilledema are often indistinguishable from normal variants (pseudopapilledema) or from certain pathologic variants (notably drusen) which produce elevation of the disc. One distinguishing feature is spontaneous pulsation of the central vein. When this is present, as it is in the majority of normal persons, the chances are that papilledema is not present[888]. The absence of pulsation, however, has no differential significance[690] and rarely venous pulsation may be present in spite of elevated intracranial pressure[1048].

A pathognomonic feature of papilledema is the presence of concentric ripples of the retina adjacent to the disc (Figure 97). Most evident on the temporal side they may occasionally surround the entire disc. They are best seen by transillumination with the ophthalmoscope beam directed to one side and can then be found in most cases of two or more diopters of papilledema. They may be the last sign to disappear with recession of papilledema. Occasionally subretinal hemorrhages with papilledema take on the same concentric arrangement.

To the pathologist papilledema is a swelling of the nerve fibers in front of the lamina cribrosa and of that portion of the retina immediately adjacent to the nerve head (Figure 98). The lateral swelling causes the inner surface of the retina to assume a convex shape and forces the outer surface into a series of undulating folds (Figure 99). These folds give rise to the ophthalmoscopic picture of concentric rings.

Another cardinal sign of papilledema, notable from a pathologist's point of view, is distention of the subarachnoid space about the optic nerve (Figure 100). This may be so marked that the optic nerve appears to have doubled its normal diameter.

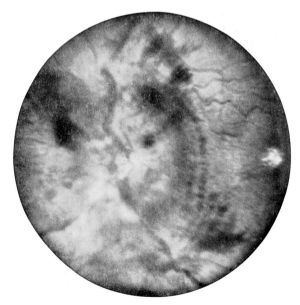

FIGURE 97. Papilledema of several diopters with concentric folds about the disc.

2. Pathogenesis

Our knowledge of the pathogenesis of papilledema is limited by the lack of an adequate model for its experimental production. Papilledema is most difficult to induce in the dog[1294] and is inconstantly induced in the monkey[545]. The concepts of the pathogenesis have therefore been based on observations in man wherein the factors necessarily lack the degree of control and variation desirable for definitive conclusions.

There is, of course, no doubt that the predominant cause for papilledema is increased intracranial pressure. The spaces about the optic nerves are known to be continuous with those about the brain and some of us find no difficulty in assuming the increased pressure forces fluid into the nerve head through the lamina cribrosa. We know, for instance, that myelin can be squeezed forward through the lamina with comparative ease[271] (see p. 127). However, others have felt constrained to postulate venous and lymphatic stasis as the cause of papilledema[49]. Perhaps venous stasis is a factor, especially

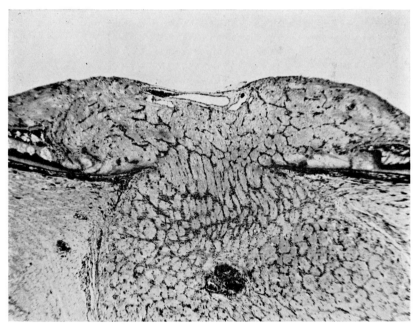

FIGURE 98. Papilledema. The interstitial tissue of the disc is much distended and the adjacent retina is pushed aside.

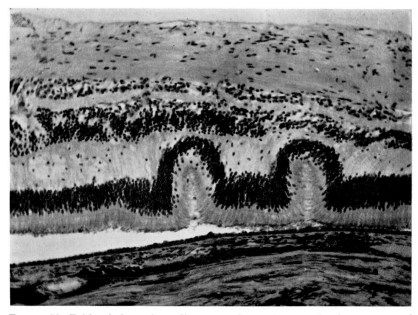

FIGURE 99. Folds of the retina adjacent to the optic nerve in the presence of papilledema. These are what give rise to the ophthalmoscopic appearance of concentric folds.

in cases of papilledema without increased intracranial pressure, but it can scarcely be the sole factor since instances of proved venous occlusion do not result in marked papilledema.

We have little information on the rate with which papilledema may develop and recede. While the degree of vascular congestion reflects the rapidity of onset we have little firm evidence to establish the minimum period for papilledema to develop or disappear[1010]. The question has obvious practical, and sometimes legal, significance, but the answer must depend on indeterminate variables such as rate of rise of the intracranial pressure, its absolute level, its constancy or inconstancy, and the condition of the eye. The one clinical condition which most nearly fulfills the experimental criteria is subarachnoid hemorrhage for here there is an acute rise in pressure in which the time and degree of rise of pressure may be established with some certainty. Since observations have been infrequently recorded we will cite three such cases: one patient had no papilledema at two hours after the onset but had a low degree of papilledema in one eye twelve hours after the onset at which

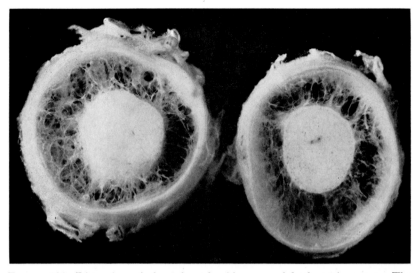

FIGURE 100. Distension of the subarachnoid space of both optic nerves. The patient was a ten year old boy with severe hydrocephalus resulting from a tumor in the pineal region.

time the spinal pressure measured 500 mm.; the patient died a few hours later. A second patient had one diopter of papilledema in both eyes twenty-four hours after the onset and the pressure was recorded as 460 mm. The third patient had 2 diopters of papilledema two days after the onset with a recorded pressure at that time of 500-600 mm. What one can say from this is that papilledema takes at least several hours and sometimes much longer[224] to develop even with excessively high pressures.

Although elevated intracranial pressure properly dominates any discussion of papilledema, it should be noted that typical papilledema may occur with normal levels of intracranial pressure; such cases should help us arrive at a reasonable understanding of its pathogenesis. Mild papilledema may result from hypotony of the eye[1397] as after intraocular surgery[1549]. The lowered intraocular pressure in the presence of normal intracranial pressure appears to have the same effect on the disc as a normal intraocular pressure does in the presence of increased intracranial pressure[1173]. There are, moreover, cases on record in which the fortuitous presence of an elevated intraocular pressure (glaucomatous) has prevented papilledema from occurring despite increased intracranial pressure. What appears to be important is the ratio of intraocular pressure to intracranial pressure rather than the absolute level of either. Then, too, there are conditions, to be discussed subsequently, in which papilledema results from neither lowered intraocular pressure nor elevated intracranial pressure but, apparently, from some local, edemogenic condition of the disc. Conspicuous among these are vascular abnormalities, contiguous infarcts (see p. 185), retrobulbar tumors, and orbital congestion.

3. Determining Factors in Development of Papilledema

Whether or not papilledema will occur in any one patient must depend on several factors other than the obvious ones of height and duration of intracranial pressure and the height of the intraocular pressure.

First, for papilledema to occur the spaces surrounding the optic nerve must be in free communication with those in the cranium[782, 325]. If there is a blockage at the optic foramen either by tumor or by arachnoid adhesions papilledema will not occur. The Foster-Kennedy syndrome in which partial blindness occurs in one eye and papilledema in the other is an illustration of this[782, 744] (see p. 197).

Secondly, the condition at the nerve head is important. Atrophic discs may show little papilledema and no measurable elevation of tissue despite high intracranial pressure. To use papilledema for detection of elevated intracranial pressure is, therefore, unreliable in the presence of optic atrophy. Myopic discs show a similar, although less rigid, resistance to development of papilledema whereas hyperopic eyes with normally protruberant nerve fibers show papilledema more easily.

Thirdly, the constancy of the elevated intracranial pressure appears to be of importance. If the intracranial pressure intermittently returns to normal at sufficiently frequent intervals, papilledema will not develop. Thus it is not only the height of intracranial pressure which is important, but also the maintenance of that pressure.

4. Effects on Vision

Papilledema is, of course, a serious sign insofar as it reflects underlying disease of the central nervous system or of the optic nerves. But it is also serious in itself as it may cause visual loss and secondary optic atrophy.

Minor visual disturbances may result from wrinkles of the retina extending to the macula or damage to the nerve fibers at the disc. This latter may manifest itself in a sector defect, a Bjerrum's scotoma, altitudinal hemianopia, or complete blindness. With chronic papilledema the blindness frequently comes on after a series of blackouts and is at first accompanied by only minimal optic atrophy.

The blackouts that occur with papilledema result from transient ischemia of the nerve head (although no changes in the retinal arteries can be seen with the ophthalmoscope during the attack). The blackouts, which are described variously as a "shade being drawn over the eye" or "like going into a darkened room," rarely last more than a few seconds (in constrast to the blackouts of carotid ischemia which last 5-10 minutes). Some persons deny the blackout but say it is a "patchy blur" and some liken it to the sensation which is produced when pressure is exerted on the eye. Posture sometimes affects the blackouts. Sudden standing up will at times precipitate them and, conversely, lying down will relieve them. Excitement or nervous tension will occasionally increase them. Rarely they are associated with flashes of light or colored sensations. One or both eyes may develop the blackouts but the pattern tends to be repetitively similar for any one person.

While blackouts are portentous of permanent blindness and warrant prompt attention, it must be admitted that they may be frequent, occurring many times a day, for long periods of time without resulting in permanent damage. However, when a lasting blackout does occur, it is too late to do anything about it; indeed craniotomy then may seem to establish a permanent defect.

Venous congestion does not appear to be a factor in the optic atrophy resulting from papilledema. In fact, the acute congestive papilledemas seem to be relatively immune to optic atrophy. Nor have we been able to enhance or otherwise affect the blackouts by inducing venous congestion with a blood pressure cuff applied about the neck so as to induce a pressure of 40 mm. Hg.

The optic atrophy due to papilledema is of the secondary variety in which the disc margins are rendered hazy by the overgrowth of glial tissue. The disc may be white or grayish-white and the arteries may be either normal or narrow. The veins often show an ensheathing that extends several millimeters from the disc.

5. Causes of Papilledema

Papilledema may result from any one of the many causes of increased intracranial pressure or from some local abnormality at the disc. The former is suggested when the papilledema is bilateral and associated with such symptoms of increased intracranial pressure as headaches, nausea and vomiting, stiffness of neck, abducens palsies, drowsiness, confusion, and stupor. The following list includes those causes which have been reported frequently in the literature or have occurred repeatedly among the author's patients.

(a) *Tumors.* Papilledema is especially apt to occur in children with tumors of the 4th ventricle and cerebellum[139] and in adults with meningiomas of the middle or anterior cranial fossa. Cerebellar tumors and acoustic neuromas are always to be suspected when papilledema is accompanied by vertical nystagmus, ataxia, and auditory symptoms. Meningiomas that cause papilledema, on the other hand, may produce little in the way of neurologic symptoms. Pinealomas and craniopharyngiomas may also cause few neurologic symptoms other than those due to increased intracranial pressure but are apt to be associated with papilledema and mid-brain signs (Parinaud's syndrome with pinealomas) and diencephalic signs (diabetes insipidus and disturbances of growth with craniopharyngiomas). Metastatic tumors also cause papilledema frequently[868]. In all cases the papilledema results from obstruction to flow of the cerebrospinal fluid and consequent hydrocephalus. The papilledema may be asymmetric and is then usually greater on the side of the lesion.

Of some practical importance is the fact that tumors in the region of the sella turcica (pituitary adenomas and meningiomas of the tuberculum sellæ) do not ordinarily produce papilledema. It is an ominous sign when papilledema does occur with lesions in this area and ordinarily signifies huge tumors projecting precariously into the third ventricle.

Less common tumors causing papilledema are the diffuse carcinomatoses of the meninges, leukemia[698], Hodgkin's disease and, curiously, tumors of the spinal cord[521, 934, 874].

(b) *Subarachnoid hemorrhage, subdural hematoma, and other vascular accidents.* Subarachnoid hemorrhage, usually resulting from rupture of a saccular aneurysm, causes an acute and congestive type of papilledema. More than any other type this is apt to have hemorrhage extending into the vitreous. It will be described further subsequently (see p. 181). Subdural hematoma produces a chronic type of papilledema which, except for the history of antecedent trauma, suggests a tumor. Vascular accidents occurring in the nerve (as with temporal arteritis) also cause papilledema but rarely affect the two eyes simultaneously and do not have the other stigmata of increased intracranial pressure.

(c) *Systemic disease and papilledema.* This group includes a large number of inflammatory, metabolic, and toxic diseases that have in common the occasional occurrence of increased intracranial pressure.

Conspicuous among the inflammatory diseases are infectious polyneuritis (Guillain-Barré Syndrome)[464, 387, 435, 509, 757, 1164], poliomyelitis[1541, 1418], and less commonly, infectious mononucleosis. This does not mean that an infectious agent is present in the cerebrospinal space. Indeed, in the case of poliomyelitis, the rise in intracranial pressure comes on usually only when the rest of the symptoms are subsiding[855]. It has been suggested that the rise in protein of the spinal fluid causes an obstructive hydrocephalus by blocking the outflow channels.

Of the metabolic diseases, hypertension is perhaps the most significant cause of papilledema. As will be described subsequently, the noteworthy concomitants of hypertensive papilledema are the morphologic changes in the retinal arteries[699] and the lack of correlation with the level of the cerebrospinal pressure[350, 1235]. Other metabolic and toxic causes of papilledema are hypoparathyroidism in children[710, 1109, 181], anemia[937, 1296], massive blood loss[1125], congestive dysthyroid exophthalmos[180, 632], vitamin A intoxication[1454, 1049], pulmonary emphysema (carbon dioxide poisoning)[45, 1021, 248, 974, 1382, 1365, 495], cystic fibrosis of pancreas[495] (with associated pulmonary disease[1365]) and lead poisoning[562].

(d) *Arachnoidal adhesions.* Adhesions blocking the flow of cerebrospinal fluid may result from meningitis, from trauma, from lumbar anesthesia, or may represent congenital heterotopic gliosis[223]. Whatever the cause, they will result in an internal hydrocephalus and papilledema when they are in a position to obstruct the flow of spinal fluid. Exceptions are those cases in which optic atrophy is present or in which the arachnoid spaces about the optic nerves are also obliterated by arachnoidal adhesions[898]. Papilledema does not then occur.

(e) *Meningeal hydrops.* This condition called by a variety of names (otitic hydrocephalus, pseudotumor cerebri, benign intracranial hypertension)[537, 504] merits a separate listing since papilledema is often the sole objective manifestation. Meningeal hydrops occurs idiopathically in young[1023] to middle aged adults (especially fat females) and produces headaches, sixth nerve palsy, papilledema, occasionally field defects and rarely blindness[537]. Characteristic is the negative neurologic examination, the alertness of the patient, and the finding on ventriculography of normal sized ventricles[520]. It thus differs from almost all other instances of obstructive hydrocephalus. Except for elevated pressure, the cerebrospinal fluid is normal.

The pathogenesis of meningeal hydrops is either an obstruction of outflow or a hypersecretion[1537] of cerebrospinal fluid. Thrombosis of the saggital and lateral sinuses has been found in most cases which have come to autopsy[537, 1402], but meningeal hydrops has also resulted from extensive venous occlusion in the neck[993]. Otitis media may be an antecedent cause of this thrombosis in children[162, 1023] but is infrequent. The prognosis for eventual recovery is good so long as damage does not result from the papilledema per se[504].

Blockage of the drainage channels by excessive protein in the cerebrospinal fluid (in the Guillain-Barré syndrome) is said to cause a similar elevation of spinal fluid pressure and papilledema[435] (see p. 147).

SUMMARY

Optic atrophy is characterized clinically by pallor of the disc. It is said to be primary when the disc edges are distinct and secondary when the edges are indistinct. Primary atrophy results from lesions behind the eye whereas secondary atrophy results from lesions on the nerve head (papillitis and papilledema). Diminution or loss of the pupillary reflex is an important objective correlate of optic atrophy. Pathologically, atrophy of the optic nerve shows the same loss of myelin, lipid phagocytosis, gliosis, and lacunar formation that accompanies disappearance of white matter in the brain.

In infants and children optic atrophy may result from congenital and hereditary anomalies (anencephaly, hydranencephaly, hydrocephalus and craniostenosis), from specific metabolic and degenerative disease (hyperparathyroidism, Bielschowsky's type of amaurotic family idiocy, and the marble bones of the Albers-Schönberg syndrome), from inflammatory lesions in the orbit and cranium, or from tumors (gliomata of the optic nerve, craniopharyngiomata, or ectopic pinealomas). Secondary atrophy results especially from tumors of the posterior fossa (cerebellar gliomas or medulloblastomas) and tumors obstructing the aqueduct (craniopharyngiomas).

In the adult, optic atrophy results more commonly from optic neuritis (multiple sclerosis), intracranial tumors (pituitary adenomas, suprasellar meningiomas, and sphenoidal ridge meningiomas), aneurysms, vascular accidents, and trauma. Only by an evaluation of the fields, ophthalmoscopic appearances, and other cognate signs can one approach a reasonable etiologic diagnosis.

Papilledema is a swelling of the nerve head that differs from papillitis in the absence of inflammatory signs (cells in the vitreous, loss of central vision, pain on movement of the eye or tenderness to pressure against the globe). It presents as a protrusion of the disc into the vitreous with an amount of congestion of veins (and hemorrhage) that increases with the rapidity of onset. The prime cause of papilledema is increased intracranial pressure but the amount depends on the ratio of intracranial to intraocular pressure. Other determining factors are the amount of glial tissue on the disc, and the communication at the optic foramen between the spaces about the optic nerve and subarachnoid space within the cranium.

The conditions which cause papilledema are chiefly those which produce an elevation in intracranial pressure: obstruction to the flow of cerebrospinal fluid by tumors (craniopharyngiomas, acoustic neuromas, cerebellar tumors, though not ordinarily the tumors in the region of the chiasm) and a miscellany of conditions in which the pathogenesis is only partially understood (infectious polyneuritis, hypertension, arachnoidal adhesions, pulmonary emphysema, and meningeal hydrops).

CHAPTER IX

OPTIC NERVE: Lesions

A. PATHOLOGIC VARIANTS

1. Drusen

THE NAME drusen, literally clusters of crystals, refers in the case of the optic nerve to conglomerate bodies seen on the disc (Figure 101). When visualized by the ophthalmoscope they appear as white or yellow white spheres having a characteristic translucence when the light is directed to the side of the disc. The entire nerve head is often elevated and the disc margins obliterated. When deep in the nerve substance, the drusen may not be apparent and the

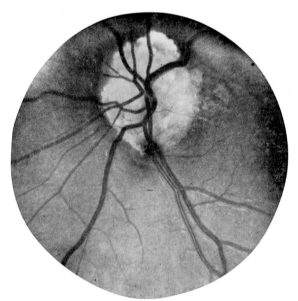

FIGURE 101. Drusen of the nerve head. The patient was a twenty-four year old woman who had been known to have the drusen for nine years. They were associated with some defect in visual acuity (20/70) and irregular field defects. The patient had no other ocular or neurologic abnormality.

[150]

elevated disc then simulates papilledema[1283, 237, 233]. Drusen are usually present in both eyes but are frequently more conspicuous in one eye than in the other. They are only slowly progressive.

Pathologically, drusen of the nerve head consist of concentrically laminated hyaline bodies of varying sizes and shapes, situated in front of the lamina cribrosa, preferentially on the nasal side[238] (Figure 102). At first they are eosinophilic but become basophilic with the development of calcification and siderosis[1601].

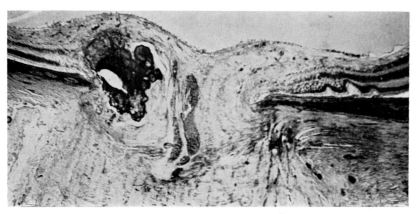

FIGURE 102. Section showing calcified drusen on the nasal half of the nerve head. The drusen were an incidental finding in an eye removed on account of injury. Mild papilledema was also present.

The pathogenesis of drusen is not clear[1495]. They have obvious similarity to corpora arenacea of the meninges but are much larger than these and differ in that they are situated within the nerve substance. Moreover, meningeal corpora arenacea are not unusually prominent in cases with drusen of the optic nerve[512]. These drusen of the nerve head are somewhat similar to hyaline excrescences of Bruch's membrane which are also called drusen and believed to derive from aberrant secretion by the pigment epithelium. One theory to account for drusen of the nerve head is that they result from pigment epithelial cells which have been misplaced in the disc.

The clinical significance of drusen revolves in part about their frequent confusion with papilledema[961] (sometimes resulting in needless neurosurgery[695]), in part about the field defects which are occasionally associated with them[1246], and in part about the diseases of the eye and central nervous system with which they are sometimes associated.

The field defects follow no one pattern[658, 1246]. Usually there is merely enlargement of the blind spots[1495] but there may be sector scotomas, arcuate scotomas, binasal hemianopic defects, or generalized constrictions[1525c] (Figure 103). Occasionally they involve central vision but this is fortunately infrequent[1384]. Their rate of progression is very slow[862].

Drusen usually occur without other evident ocular or nervous system disease; that is, they are idopathic and they may be hereditary[931]. They also occur occasionally with retinitis pigmentosa and are said to occur with tuberous sclerosis[658, 1185] (sometimes with little other evidence of this disease[1268]) and in association with angioid streaks[1525b]. We and others[1249, 1098] have also seen drusen with several cases of meningioma; they have been reported once with a pituitary tumor[1384]. They may be found with non-specific optic atrophy but it is a question whether the optic atrophy caused the drusen[1304] or the drusen caused the optic atrophy. Although similar bodies do not occur in the orbital part of the optic nerve (except in the vicinity of the papilla), they are said to be frequent in the intracranial portions of the optic nerves, chiasm and tracts of elderly persons; they may then be associated with loss of vision[512].

2. Pits, Colobomas, and Staphylomas

Anomalies of the disc include a wide assortment of aberrations ranging from merely an unusually large physiologic cup to gross excavation of the entire disc and peripapillary region. Eyes with these congenital anomalies are particularly vulnerable to the further excavations of glaucoma cupping[1571].

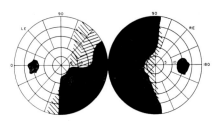

FIGURE 103. Predominantly binasal field defects in a patient with drusen of the nerve head.

Pits have already been described in connection with the lamina cribrosa (see p. 130) (Figure 104). They are isolated holes which are generally thought to be congenital and stationary but may be acquired. They usually have little or no clinical significance but may produce arcuate scotomas[26, 1470, 1572, 406] and on rare occasion they may be associated with central serous retinopathy[830].

A severe form of excavation of the disc occurs occasionally in association with what appears to be an inherently weak lamina cribrosa[517]. We have under observation several cases of this in one family in which the cupping is so extensive as to have pulled the retina into the disc and produced traction folds in the retina. The cupping is like that of glaucoma but the intraocular pressure is not elevated (Figure 105).

Colobomas of the nerve head, always situated in the lower pole of the disc, vary from simple, inferior crescents to gross defects that extend into the retina and choroid[55] (Figures 106 and 19). Abortive

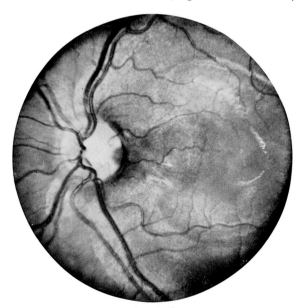

Figure 104. Pit of nerve head. This appears in the photograph as a dark semi-circle on the temporal edge of the disc. In the present case the patient also had central serous retinopathy evidenced by the sharply demarcated circular area surrounding the macula.

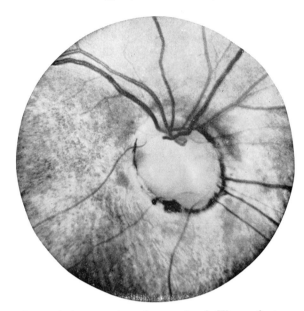

FIGURE 105. Congenital excavation of nerve head. The patient was a fifty-two year old woman who had had poor vision in the right eye all her life. The nerve head was severely excavated and the major vessels were anomalously situated in the upper portion of the disc. The intraocular pressure was normal.

forms of this produce no symptoms and have no clinical significance, but severe forms are usually associated with microphthalmos, extrabulbar evaginations (so-called cysts), and blindness.

Staphylomas are circumscribed outpouchings of the papillary and peripapillary regions. The disc, which may be surprisingly normal in appearance, is situated several diopters deep in the excavation. The edges of this excavation are sharp, like those of a buckle following a retinopexy operation, and cause a sharp angulation of the retinal vessels as they dip into the staphyloma. Vision is usually poor in such eyes. A variant of this is the frank meningocele of the optic disc[1587].

3. Aplasia of the Optic Nerve

The optic nerve may fail to develop altogether (aplasia)[1357] or may show various deficiencies in growth (hypoplasia)[1343]. This may result from an hereditary defect[854] or it may be a sporadic developmental anomaly in one[1065] or both eyes. In the latter case other anomalies such as ectopic brain tissue in the orbit and bony defects in the skull are often present.

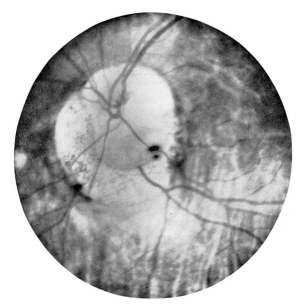

FIGURE 106. Coloboma and staphyloma. The sclera below and nasal to the nerve head shows an absence of pigment epithelium and choroid with a bulging backward of the crescent shaped area. (The different level is indicated by the blurred fundus outside the crescent.)

B. DEMYELINATIVE AND INFLAMMATORY DISEASES

Several syndromes characterized by loss of myelin are included under the collective term demyelinative disease. Little is known of their etiology; only fragments of their pathogenesis are understood; and they are neither clearly differentiated among themselves nor from some of the inflammatory neuritides. Because of this overlap these demyelinative diseases and certain of the inflammatory diseases of the optic nerve will be considered together in this section.

The comprehensive term demyelinative disease is sometimes used in a restricted sense to refer to that recurrent disease or group of diseases having focal lesions throughout the nervous system and known as *multiple (disseminated) sclerosis*. Demyelination, however, is equally characteristic of other diseases which are typically progressive and widespread. These, by contrast with multiple sclerosis, are collectively called *diffuse scleroses* and include the special types known as Schilder's disease and various leukodystrophies. Both multiple sclerosis and the diffuse scleroses may involve the optic nerves. Also noteworthy are opticomyelitis and hereditary optic atrophy which in turn include several overlapping subtypes. Indeed, the best one can expect of our present classification is that it will serve a useful purpose until our knowledge of the pathogenesis provides us with a more rational basis for differentiation.

Some of the terms used for demyelinative and inflammatory processes of the optic nerve warrant clarification. *Retrobulbar neuritis* refers to inflammatory or demyelinative lesions of the nerve that show no abnormality in the fundus. *Papillitis,* on the other hand, refers to lesions in which the disc is swollen and shows other signs of an exudative process (Figure 107). These other signs comprise hyperemia of the disc, fine opacities in the vitreous, and central scotomas. *Neuroretinitis* has the same connotation as papillitis but suggests a process extending farther into the adjacent retina (and uvea).

These clinical terms should not necessarily imply an inflammatory process. Some of the underlying diseases are certainly inflammatory but some are primarily demyelinative, and some are vascular. All these processes are included under the general heading of *optic neuritis.* On the other hand, the term *papilledema* is restricted to purely passive swelling of the disc, most especially to that associated with increased intracranial pressure (see Papilledema, p. 137).

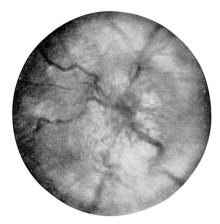

FIGURE 107. Papillitis. The disc is partially blurred by the exudate in the vitreous but sufficient details can be seen to illustrate the swelling of the entire disc region, the obliteration of the physiologic cup, and the congestion of the vessels. The patient was a thirty-four year old woman whose vision in the affected eye was 20/150.

The one symptom common to all optic neuritides is loss of vision. With retrobulbar neuritis this usually takes the form of a central scotoma. With papillitis there may be a central scotoma but frequently there is complete amaurosis. For reasons unknown the papillomacular bundle is especially vulnerable to demyelinative, inflammatory and compressive lesions. Another conspicuous, although variable symptom of optic neuritis is pain on movement of the eye and tenderness on pressure against the globe. The pain on movement presumably reflects involvement of the meninges at the apex of the orbit. It is less frequent with papillitis than with retrobulbar neuritis but may be absent, or severe, with either. Occasionally it precedes the visual symptoms by several days and may sometimes occur without the development of visual loss.

Analysis of optic neuritis requires evaluation not only of such ocular factors as visual acuity, field changes, ophthalmoscopic appearances, laterality, manner of onset and course, but also of such non-ocular factors as age of patient, evidence of other neurologic or systemic disease, composition of the cerebrospinal fluid, and, of course, the pertinent history. Probably no branch of neuro-ophthalmology has to its discredit the abundance of erroneous diagnoses as has optic neuritis (see Pseudo-optic neuritis, p. 177).

All the demyelinative diseases have certain pathologic features in common[1602]. As myelin breaks down, sudanophilic globules, presumably consisting of triglycerides and cholesterol esters, accumulate in the microglia. These microglial cells, often grotesquely distended with fat, tend to accumulate about blood vessels and are believed to transport their lipid cargo to the blood stream. With acute demyelination the cells accumulate in vast numbers. With subacute demyelination or in the late stage of all demyelination, astrocytic glia replace the macrophages. With multiple sclerosis this gliosis forms discrete plaques; with diffuse sclerosis the gliosis is widespread and less well demarcated; not infrequently the glial reaction is slight and the holes left in the tissue indicate a process known as cavitation. The extent to which the phagocytic, glial, or cavitation reactions predominate depend on the duration and severity of the lesions. The degree of phagocytosis increases with acuteness of onset and severity of the disease.

Some of the demyelinative diseases are said to show a significant paucity of oligodendrocytes. Since these cells are believed to be responsible for the normal formation and regeneration of myelin, their alleged absence in these diseases is currently the subject of much histopathologic investigation.

1. Primarily Demyelinative and Degenerative Diseases

(a) *Multiple sclerosis.* The name multiple sclerosis derives from the characteristic formation of multiple plaques of demyelination. Although scattered widely throughout the white matter of the central nervous system, certain sites are more frequently affected than others; two of these sites are of particular concern to neuro-ophthalomology. These are: the medial longitudinal fasciculus, lesions of which produce internuclear ophthalmoplegia; and the papillomacular bundle, lesions of which produce optic neuritis.

Typically the optic neuritis of multiple sclerosis comes on without apparent cause, affects one eye, reduces visual acuity to 20/100 or less, and is accompanied by pain on movement of the eye. Most characteristic, although not invariably present, is a central scotoma; less common are sector scotomas, altitudinal hemianopias, and complete amaurosis. Photophobia and headache are occasional symptoms.

The first attack usually clears up completely within a few weeks, although the duration is widely variable. Recurrences may affect the same or other eye and repeated attacks often culminate in optic atrophy and some degree of blindness.

A severe and unremitting form of demyelinative disease is the acute disseminated encephalomyelitis. Like multiple sclerosis or opticomyelitis, of which it may be merely a severe form, it affects predominantly the optic nerves, brain stem, and spinal cord, but in comparison with these diseases it is more necrotizing and less limited to the white matter. Most of the patients die within a few weeks after the onset. Of those who survive, many develop typical symptoms of multiple sclerosis later[1434, 144].

The objective findings in the retrobulbar neuritis of multiple sclerosis may be few. The pupillary reaction to light is depressed to the same degree as the visual acuity. Abnormal ensheathing of the veins has been reported to occur commonly[1247, 480, 925, 1540,596] but most of us have seen it infrequently[438]. With papillitis the disc margins are blurred and the process extends into the peripapillary retina; occasionally uveitis is present with inflammatory deposits on the back of the cornea[161, 1326, 1053, 597, 1589].

Multiple sclerosis is perhaps the most frequent cause of classifiable optic neuritis. Approximately one half of all patients with optic neuritis have or will have other manifestations of multiple sclerosis[1438, 1416, 842]. In a chronic disease hospital the incidence is much higher[1284]. On the other hand, about 15 per cent of patients with multiple sclerosis begin their disease with optic neuritis and as many as 40 per cent will have optic neuritis as one of their symptoms during the course of the disease[103].

Optic neuritis that affects both eyes at the start is less likely to be due to multiple sclerosis[645] and less likely to have remissions than is unilateral optic neuritis. This is not because multiple sclerosis spares the two eyes but because it rarely affects them both simultaneously. On the other hand, various systemic diseases and poisons do involve the two eyes at the same time.

Only fragmentary data is available on predisposing causes for the optic neuritis of multiple sclerosis. Antecedent infections are common[1525e], and the disease is particularly prevalent in cold climates. Overheating of the body or strenuous exercise will often precipitate an attack or worsen the symptoms which are already present[173, 560] (Uhthoff's symptom[1204]). A significant number of attacks have come on post-partum[1263, 1084, 1045] and are therefore called lactation optic neuritis (but in one of our post-partum cases it came on even though lactation had been suppressed by diethylstilbesterol).

In three of our patients with optic neuritis due to multiple sclerosis the transient worsening of vision with physical exercise was the presenting complaint. One patient who subsequently developed a full blown bilateral optic neuritis showed a transient deterioration of vision from 20/40 in one eye to 20/200 on climbing a flight of stairs. This reduction in vision persisted for five to ten minutes. Another patient who had had several attacks of optic neuritis in both eyes showed a regular drop in vision from 20/100 to 20/200 in one eye and from 20/30 to 20/50 in the other eye on running up and down the corridor (40 feet) several times. These effects lasted five to ten minutes. A similar drop occurred on taking a hot drink or hot bath. A third patient initially developed blurring of vision for two to three hours while playing a vigorous game of football. Although subjective, these observations seemed genuine and valid.

The age of the patient at the onset of optic neuritis is important. Most neuritides beginning in the twenty to forty age group are due to multiple sclerosis[1416]. Those occurring in persons younger than age twenty are more apt to be idiopathic[780] or attributable to one of a miscellany of systemic diseases or poisons, frequently in association with encephalitis[921], while those in persons over forty-four years of age are usually vascular in origin. Nevertheless, the optic neuritis of multiple sclerosis may occur at a young age[935]. The disease then tends to run a particularly malignant course and is apt to be bilateral[781].

The general symptoms associated with retrobulbar neuritis are those classically associated with multiple sclerosis. Frequently occurring are the paresthesias of arms and legs, spasticity of gait, internuclear ophthalmoplegia, and scanning speech. But more characteristic than any one of these individual symptoms is the history of intermittency in their occurrence.

The pathology of optic neuritis is similar to that of the rest of the nervous system in patients who have died with multiple sclerosis (Figure 108). Spotty loss of myelin occurs in the white matter with remarkable preservation of many of the axis fibers[1236, 1603]. This preservation accounts for the typical recovery of function (although not of myelin) after an attack. It also has a bearing on the fact that many patients with multiple sclerosis who are found at autopsy to have involvement of the optic nerves, had no subjective disturbance of vision during life[522]. There appears to be little or no tendency for the myelin to regenerate and eventually the demyelinated areas are replaced by glial plaques.

Since central scotomas are such regular occurrences with optic neuritis one might expect preferential demyelination in the papillomacular bundle. Yet by the time these patients come to autopsy this is not usually the case; the plaques are found scattered widely in the optic nerves without predilection for the central fibres. From the pathologic point of view, therefore, it would appear that the especial vulnerability of the papillomacular fibres was not due to their demyelination but was functional, possibly associated with swelling of the nerve. There is ample evidence not only that simple pressure on the optic nerve will cause a central scotoma but that

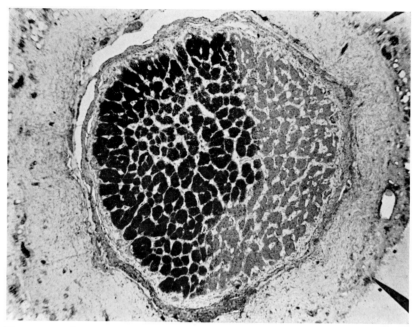

FIGURE 108. Cross section showing demyelination of temporal half of nerve. The patient was a forty-two year old woman who had had various neurologic symptoms since the age of eighteen, thought to be due to multiple sclerosis. Cresyl violet stain of gelatine embedded tissue.

retrobulbar neuritis produces sufficient swelling of the nerve in the optic canal to cause compression[339, 1196].

The pathogenesis of the optic neuritis with multiple sclerosis is no more clear than the pathogenesis of multiple sclerosis itself. The theories (of which there is no lack) might be categorized into the viral, allergic, vascular, thrombotic and metabolic hypotheses. None can be said to have been established and the eye findings add little to our total knowledge of the underlying process.

The optic neuritis of multiple sclerosis must be differentiated from that occurring with other demyelinative and inflammatory disease. In general, unilaterality of optic neuritis favors the diagnosis of multiple sclerosis[645]. The disease is all the more likely to be multiple sclerosis if the symptoms resolve spontaneously and it is almost certainly multiple sclerosis if a history is obtained of prior attacks of this or other typical syndromes. On the other hand, central scotomas may be the presenting symptom in various compressive lesions in the anterior cranial fossa, notably with tumors[870], aneurysms and sclerotic internal carotid arteries[1217]. Thus before making a diagnosis of retrobulbar neuritis it is of the utmost importance to rule out an intracranial lesion when an isolated central scotoma presents without pain or tenderness and especially when the cerebrospinal fluid shows increased protein or pressure.

There is no effective treatment for the acute optic neuritis of multiple sclerosis. Controlled studies have shown no benefit from steroids[535].

(b) *Diffuse sclerosis.* In contrast to multiple sclerosis, those diseases categorized under the heading of diffuse sclerosis tend to show large areas of demyelination and have a greater tendency to involve the cerebral hemispheres. They include most especially a demyelinative syndrome known as Schilder's disease[1280] and various leucodystrophies. All may involve the optic nerve at times.

Schilder's disease (encephalitis periaxialis diffusa) has diverse clinical manifestations. Coming on in the first few decades of life[156], it may mimic multiple sclerosis[903, 1167] but differs insofar as signs point conspicuously to the cerebral hemispheres; it also runs a more rapid, and often fatal, course. Some have postulated that Schilder's disease is the infantile or childhood counterpart of multiple sclerosis but it would appear to have a closer similarity to acute disseminated encephalomyelitis and opticomyelitis[143].

Optic neuritis may be the initial manifestation of Schilder's disease[290] and optic atrophy eventually occurs in many cases. The optic nerves are, however, less frequently involved than are the visual pathways within the brain. An optic neuritis due to Schilder's disease is, therefore, to be suspected only in patients with mental changes or with those visual field defects that point to cerebral involvement as well as to optic nerve involvement.

Even with typical symptoms the diagnosis is not always clear-cut and the findings at autopsy may be inconclusive. An illustrative case, which we had occasion to study, was analyzed by Walsh[222]. The patient was a thirty-year-old woman who developed typical, but severe, optic neuritis as her initial symptom. As vision returned in the previously blind eye, the patient developed homonymous hemianopia, progressive dementia, and convulsions; she died four years after the onset. On post-mortem examination the widespread demyelination was compatible with any of the demyelinative diseases.

Leucodystrophies, so-called because of preferential involvement of white matter, generally belong to the category of inborn errors of metabolism. They are usually familial and frequently begin in childhood. The age of onset is variable, however, and has been the basis for classification into infantile types of Krabbe and of Canavan, juvenile type of Scholz, adult type of Ferraro, late adult type of van Bogært and Nyssen, and the chronic type of Pelizæus and Merzbacher. Obviously such a classification has little pathogenic meaning; current studies are directed toward histochemical and biochemical differentiations of the subtypes (see Poser and van Bogært)[1167].

The general symptoms of the leucodystrophies are disturbances of gait progressing to quadriplegia, apathy progressing to dementia, and visual deterioration culminating in blindness. Psychiatric disturbances are prominent in the older age group.

Although optic atrophy is frequent in all types, and papilledema occurs occasionally, a history of typical optic neuritis is rarely obtained. Possibly the demented state of the patients and the coexistence of lesions in the visual pathways in the brain mask the presence of optic neuritis.

Differentiation of the leucodystrophies from Schilder's disease is often difficult and accounts for much confusion in the literature. Indeed, one of Schilder's original three cases may have been one of leucodystrophy. Foremost distinguishing features are the familial occurrence of the dystrophies and their tendency for bilateral and symmetric involvement of the nervous system.

One of the types which has been distinguished with a measure of clarity is that which is called metachromatic leucoencephalopathy because of the brownish metachromasia of its myelin breakdown products[1127, 367]. Formerly a strictly pathologic diagnosis, it can now be established clinically by the finding of metachromatic substances in the urine of affected patients[47].

Optic atrophy may occur in metachromatic leucoencephalopathy[47] but is usually a late manifestation. Even when atrophy is not evident clinically the optic nerve may show abnormal clumping of its myelin and characteristic metachromasia of the retinal ganglion cells[278]. Optic atrophy may also occur with other clinical syndromes that have only a quasi-relationship to the leucodystrophies (e.g., Charcot-Marie-Tooth muscular atrophy[176, 692]).

(c) *Opticomyelitis (Devic's disease)*. For historical reasons, if for no other, opticomyelitis is considered separately. Individual cases may well be manifestations of multiple sclerosis, diffuse sclerosis[726], or one of the inflammatory encephalitides. It is a clinical syndrome that may belong to any one of these several categories. It may even occur secondary to meningeal neoplasia[1101].

The optic neuritis of opticomyelitis is typically bilateral[168] and accompanied by paraplegia, segmental loss of sensation, and incontinence[1370, 774]. Abortive forms are said to occur in which spinal cord signs are absent[1525f]. The initial manifestation may be either optic neuritis or myelitis although an upper respiratory infection may precede either[338]. In comparison with typical multiple and diffuse sclerosis, opticomyelitis runs a more rapid and severe (often fatal) course[1405] but the prognosis is less dire than would be inferred from the literature[1298, 1339]. Short of death, the end result is either complete recovery or optic atrophy and paraplegia. Recurrences are relatively infrequent[1298].

Autopsied cases of opticomyelitis have shown acute demyelination and perivascular cuffing by round cells[1371]. The gray matter and nerve axes are involved to a greater extent than in multiple or diffuse sclerosis and many specimens seem to be those of a necrotizing encephalomyelitis[498]. It must be conceded, however, that cases which come to autopsy represent only the most severe types. The milder cases show no clearcut separation of the pathology from that of multiple sclerosis[1405].

(d) *Hereditary optic atrophy*. Hereditary forms of optic atrophy occur with various modes of transmission. The sex-linked type known as Leber's optic atrophy is the best known but the dominant type is the most frequent. Less is known of recessive and congenital types but it seems altogether probable that some cases diagnosed as chiasmatic arachnoiditis belong in these categories.

Characteristic of some of the hereditary optic atrophies is the spontaneous and often sudden occurrence of blurred vision in the two eyes. An upper respiratory infection may precede the optic neuritis[663]. The acuity is usually reduced to 20/200 or less and the fields show bilateral central scotomas. After this abrupt onset the vision deteriorates only slightly and is rarely lost completely. Although the early course and central scotomas are compatible with optic neuritis, pain, tenderness and other evidence of inflammation are generally lacking. The ophthalmoscopic appearance is simply that of primary optic atrophy with normal retinal vessels (Figure 94).

In contrast to the foregoing, one form of hereditary optic atrophy occurs so early in life as to suggest congenital optic atrophy[591, 586,1431, 923, 728]. Yet the frequent absence of nystagmus may suggest a postnatal onset[1300]. This early type shows pale discs bilaterally, reduction of acuity to 20/200 or worse, and central scotomas[733, 797]. It is often transmitted as a dominant trait[1300, 820] affecting one half the progeny and is usually non-progressive although progressive types do occur[796]. Other dominant types may occur in older age groups, even in midlife, but the time of onset is approximately constant for any one family.

The best known hereditary example is Leber's optic atrophy[881] having a typically sex-linked transmission in which half the male progeny show the defect[1431]. It may develop at any age but is most frequent in the late teens or early twenties and may be associated with hereditary ataxia[1584].

The diagnosis of hereditary optic atrophy is not obvious unless other members of the family are known to be affected. Thus the first members recognized are thought to have atypical retrobulbar neuritis, toxic amblyopia or opticomyelitis. Several cases which had surgical exploration or roentgenographic studies were said to have typical chiasmatic arachnoiditis[1130, 718].

The confusion in diagnosis is illustrated by the case of three brothers whom we had occasion to study with the benefit of hindsight. All three suddenly developed central scotomas in their late thirties or early forties and suffered over the ensuing several years some further loss of vision to the level of seeing hand movements only. The first patient was operated upon by Harvey Cushing for a supposed suprasellar meningioma but was reported to show only chiasmatic arachnoiditis. The second brother "forgot" to mention to his doctor that his brother had had a loss of vision similar to his own; he was diagnosed as having toxic amblyopia. Only when the third brother developed the same condition at about the same age was the diagnosis made of Leber's optic atrophy.

Pathologically, hereditary optic atrophy shows, as one would predict, disappearance of retinal ganglion cells, loss of fibers in the optic nerve, and, what one might not expect, gliosis of the geniculate bodies[852]. It thus represents a primarily neuronal degeneration of the retina and optic nerve.

2. Vasculitis

Vasculitis may be a manifestation of a strictly local inflammation in the vessels of the optic nerve or it may be part of a wider process affecting cranial (most particularly temporal) and other vessels.

Local vasculitis is not always easy to differentiate during life from optic neuritis. Perhaps the two are at times one and the same disease. Suggestive of a local vasculitis is the clinical appearance of a papillitis with extensive ensheathing of retinal vessels and neovasculogenesis at the nerve head. This latter may be so conspicuous as to warrant the designation rete mirabile (Figure 109). The reduction in visual acuity, the pain and the photophobia which may be severe, are of the type seen with optic neuritis. The visual field, however, is apt to show an altitudinal hemianopia or a complete amaurosis rather than a central scotoma and the defect is less apt to remit than is the case with optic neuritis.

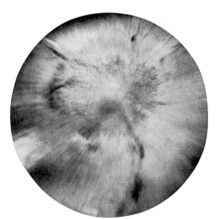

FIGURE 109. Vasculitis of nerve head with marked neovasculogenesis. The patient was a twenty-five year old man who first developed blurring of vision in the right eye four months previously. Subsequently he lost all vision in this eye and developed severe pain. Three months after the photograph was taken the eye was removed on account of secondary glaucoma. The sections showed persistent inflammation and destruction of the optic nerve.

The etiology of local arteritis or vasculitis in the optic nerve is generally obscure. Except for the occasional increase in sedimentation rate of the blood or elevation of the protein in the spinal fluid, little or nothing is generally revealed on systemic examination. At times there is a suggestive relationship to Raynaud's disease and occasionally to multiple sclerosis. Rare causes are trypanosomiasis[1441] and rheumatic fever[1275].

Few pathologic studies of vasculitis of the optic nerve are available (Figure 110). One patient whom we had an opportunity to study clinically and pathologically showed occlusion of the artery by an eosinophilic material (possibly fibrinoid) and an intense round cell infiltration about the veins. When the specimen became available, three months after the onset, the optic nerve fibres were being replaced by microglial phagocytes and fibroglial overgrowth.

In contrast to purely local disease, the vasculitis of *temporal* or giant cell arteritis is a well defined clinical entity. Occurring exclusively

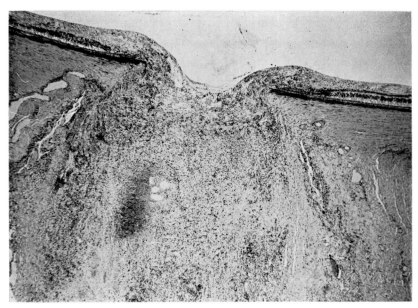

FIGURE 110. Section of nerve head showing vasculitis. The patient had had loss of vision and pain in eye beginning three months previously. The nerve and meninges showed extensive lymphocytic infiltration, especially about the blood vessels, and one area of focal necrosis (AFIP 184267).

in the older age group, this disease is characterized by headache, pain and tenderness in the temporal region (often most evident on chewing), elevation of sedimentation rate, and fever (see p.   ). Generally bilateral, involvement of one side may precede that of the other by several weeks.

About half the cases of temporal arteritis develop blindness in one or both eyes[317, 1503] and the visual symptoms may be the presenting complaint[1116] (see p. 40). At times this is associated with papilledema and obstruction to blood flow but often it shows only the residuum of a former obstruction, that is opacification of the perimacular retina and eventual optic atrophy. Rarely, if ever, does one see clinically the evidence of inflammation or the typical fundus picture of arterial vasculitis[1503]. The disease lasts a few weeks or months and then spontaneously remits, but vision does not return even when paracentesis is done promptly. Ocular motor palsies occur frequently with it[449, 669].

The pathologic changes in the temporal arteries have been abundantly studied since biopsies are regularly obtained (Figure 111). Granulomatous reactions with giant cells ("giant cell arteritis") seem to center about fragments of the internal elastic lamina. The few pathologic studies on the orbital arteries have shown similar granulomatous arteritis of the ophthalmic and ciliary arteries[294, 639, 315, 1367, 1395]. The retinal arteries show thrombotic occlusion without inflammation[294, 210].

The etiology and pathogenesis of temporal arteritis are debatable. Pathologic evidence suggests an antigen-antibody reaction involving elastic tissue of the arteries. This would account for the sparing of the retinal arteries, which have no internal elastic lamina, and for the absence of intraocular inflammation. It leaves out of account, however, the predilection for the temporal and ophthalmic arteries and the remarkable sparing of other cranial arteries[1050].

The differential diagnosis of the optic neuropathy of temporal arteritis revolves about the causes of sudden blindness in older persons. The age rules out typical optic neuritis due to multiple sclerosis. The interval of days or weeks separating involvement of the two eyes makes poisoning unlikely. The absence of hemiplegic or hemianesthetic symptoms militates against carotid artery occlusion but does not exclude it. The suspicion of an operable lesion about the chiasm has occasionally led to craniotomy[1395]. Headaches are sometimes absent

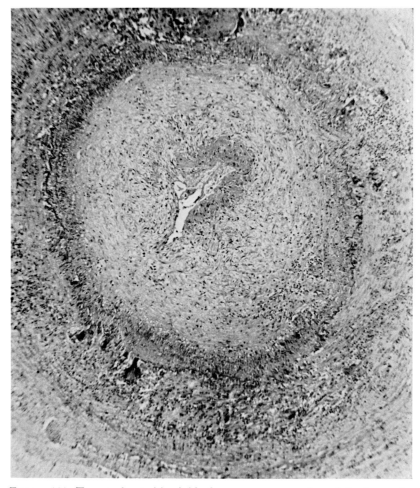

FIGURE 111. Temporal arteritis. Aside from severe narrowing of the lumen by intimal proliferation, the media shows considerable infiltration by inflammatory cells and a number of giant cells just outside the elastic lamina. Verhoeff's elastic stain.

and the clinical symptoms alone often do not permit differentiation from the ischemic optic neuropathy of local arteriosclerosis[449]. Suggestive of temporal arteritis is the combination of tenderness along the temporal arteries, pain on chewing, increased sedimentation rate, and headache. Definitive diagnosis can usually be made by biopsy of the temporal arteries; at times this is positive even when no tenderness or pain has been present to suggest the diagnosis[1329].

Finally vasculitis probably underlies the occasional lesions of the optic nerve with periarteritis nodosa[559], some cases of syphilis, drug reactions and other systemic diseases of blood vessels. The lack of reliable pathologic studies, however, makes conclusions little more than tentative speculations.

3. Secondary Inflammatory Processes

Optic neuritis may result from inflammatory processes in contiguous structures or from systemic disease. In the former category is spread of inflammation from sinuses, meninges, brain or orbit[216] while in the latter category is a variety of systemic processes that affect the optic nerves by way of the blood stream or by sensitization. Those which have been reported or discussed sufficiently often will be presented in the following few paragraphs.

Proximity of the optic nerves to the sphenoidal sinuses and to the posterior ethmoidal sinuses makes it highly probable[1596, 130] that inflammation from a sinusitis could extend into the nerve in the region of the optic foramen. At one time this was thought to be a common cause for retrobulbar neuritis of otherwise obscure origin[206, 659] but the evidence was rarely secure; now that many of these patients have developed multiple sclerosis[711], the general thesis of sinusitis as a cause of optic neuritis has lost favor. Perhaps the pendulum has swung too far in the counter balance but the fact remains that optic neuritis is rarely found in persons with severe sinusitis.

Optic neuritis is relatively common with meningitis and encephalitis. Within the cranium the optic nerves are not protected by dura or arachnoid sheaths; lying in the base of the middle fossa, they are exposed to all inflammatory processes in this region. Optic neuritis thus occurs with purulent meningitis of bacterial or fungal origin and may occur with tuberculous or viral meningitis and encephalitis. This meningitic optic neuritis is most common in children and probably accounts for the majority of bilateral optic neuritides in the first decade of life. The prognosis is variable but recovery of vision may occur months after the onset even though the nerves remain partially atrophic.

Allied to this contiguous spread of viral disease is the optic neuritis (and occasional ophthalmoplegia) that occasionally follows herpes zoster infections of the gasserian ganglion[142, 1468, 1281, 837, 1490, 1128].

The term opticoarachnoiditis suggests an inflammatory process that affects the optic nerve by contiguity with the meninges. Actually this is a term which has limited meaning. It refers to a proliferation of meninges at the base of the skull which may result from trauma or from any of a number of inflammatory processes (see Chiasmic Arachnoiditis, p. 217). The question is whether the optic atrophy results from the original trauma and inflammation or from the meningeal adhesions. The answer is not clear-cut.

Syphilitic optic neuritis is a special case probably compounding several types. One type is that resulting from direct involvement of the outermost portions of the nerve[190] in its intracranial course[715]. This is probably the most common and is thought to be attributable to a toxic cerebrospinal fluid. Another type of syphilitic optic atrophy is that due to spirochetal invasion of the pia and arachnoid (although not of the parenchyma[715]). This is the type seen with tabes and general paresis. Other types result from gummas of the orbit, from syphilitic arterial disease, and still further types from the treatment (tryparsamide) used for the syphilis. Occasionally optic neuritis results from an adjacent gumma in the orbit or within the cranium.

Except in association with meningitis[1040, 1607] tuberculosis would appear to be an infrequent cause for optic neuritis. A tuberculous granuloma has, however, been demonstrated on the nerve head[220] and, as previously noted, a tubercle, interpreted as tuberculous, has been demonstrated within the retinal vein[1485]. Sarcoid has also presented with blindness in one eye due to local granuloma in the optic nerve[1376].

Involvement of the optic nerves from orbital abscesses (including abscesses within the nerve itself), from cellulitis, and from midline granulomas[326, 915, 393] is so obvious that further discussion is unwarranted. Worth mentioning, however, is the orbital syndrome, *opticociliary neuritis*. This rare entity of undetermined etiology is characterized by the symptoms of retrobulbar neuritis (central scotoma, pain on movement of the eye, etc.) with iridoplegia and cycloplegia[360, 116, 1207, 972].

Although isolated optic neuritis cannot be shown by antigen tests[361] to be of specific viral etiology, it does occur in the wake of such childhood diseases as measles[621, 1319, 1013, 1560, 208, 85, 1387], chicken pox[617, 1108], mumps[1583, 1424, 420, 149, 1211], pertusis[878], equine encephalitis, poliomyelitis, and occasionally following diseases not necessarily in the childhood category such as infectious mononucleosis[151, 1310, 150, 419], torula meningitis, Asiatic influenza[253], small pox[1000], and small pox vaccination[963]. The optic neuritis may occur early in the disease but the characteristic time is one to two weeks after onset of the clinical symptoms. It may resolve completely but occasionally leads to profound loss of vision with optic atrophy and ophthalmoscopic evidence of retinal degeneration. These severe cases are usually associated with evidence of encephalitis or meningitis and sometimes with ophthalmoplegia. The pathogenesis of the optic neuritis, like that of the encephalitis, may involve a direct invasion by the virus—such as has been shown to occur frequently in animals[758, 1270] and occasionally in man[1424]—but the delayed type probably represents a sensitization phenomenon[465]. This latter has its experimental counterpart in allergic encephalomyelitis[1506].

The possibility of optic nerve substance being specifically sensitizing and capable of inducing a selective optic neuritis has been investigated[194, 1492] and found to be unconvincing. While sensitization by optic nerve substance (both homologous and heterologous) did lead occasionally to involvement of the optic nerves, it also led to involvement of the spinal cord such as occurs with inoculation of any white matter of the central nervous system. Conversely, injection of brain substance may induce optic neuritis on occasion[465]. Thus the optic nerve substance was antigenically non-selective.

Peripheral polyneuritis (often called infectious) of the Guillian-Barré variety is occasionally accompanied by optic neuritis. The diagnosis is made by the characteristic paralyses, anesthesias, and especially by the high protein content of the spinal fluid. Optic neuritis has also been reported with epidemic myositis (Bornholm's disease)[1450], erythema multiforme[368], botulism[896], and other systemic diseases, but it is not always possible to decide whether the disease or its treatment caused the optic neuritis.

One systemic condition in which optic neuritis is a frequent and prominent feature is that curious combination of symptoms known as Behcet's disease[599]. This consists of relapsing ulcers of the mouth, eye, and genitalia with chronic uveitis and recurrent hypopyon. Because of its relapsing nature and association with optic neuritis[741, 1307] and other neurologic disease[597], Behcet's syndrome is occasionally diagnosed as multiple sclerosis[817, 1146]. Currently thought to be a virus disease[1562, 1307] as originally assumed by Behcet[86], little is known of its pathogenesis or curious tropisms. Blindness is the usual outcome, either by complications of the uveitis or because of bilateral optic atrophy.

4. Metabolic Diseases and Poisons

Several of the so-called metabolic diseases are associated with optic neuropathy sufficiently often to warrant the suggestion of a causal relationship. These diseases include diabetes, dysthyroidism, possibly hyperparathyroidism, Paget's disease, fibrous dysplasia[1258, 654], certain nutritional disorders, and probably others. They will be described separately since the symptomatology and pathogenesis differ for each disease.

The optic neuropathy of diabetes is generally that of an optic neuritis associated with a peripheral neuritis[1400]. It may be uni-lateral[1440] or bilateral[1334] and some evidence suggests a familial predisposition to optic nerve involvement[1372, 1309]. Occasionally it is the initial manifestation of diabetes[1334].

The optic neuropathy of dysthyroidism ("optic neuropathy of Graves' disease")[632] occurs with that form of thyroid-pituitary disease in which the orbit and periorbital structures show excessive con-gestion[331]. This form usually follows thyroidectomy or other anti-thyroid treatment and at the time of the eye involvement may be associated with hyperthyroidism, hypothyroidism, or euthyroidism[627, 346]. It is most common in women[632]. Aside from exophthalmos and congestion, the ocular symptoms are reduction in vision and scotomas. The latter may be central but tend to be spotty and lack the symmetry associated with central scotomas of the usual optic neuritis. Although no pathologic study has been done on the optic nerves of these patients, one would expect by analogy with the proved changes in the extra-ocular muscles and other orbital structures that the abnormality in the optic nerves would also consist of edema and lymphocytic infiltra-tion. Such a finding, if confirmed, would provide a sufficient explana-tion for the field changes. Nevertheless, one cannot deny at present that pressure[716] or ischemia[1064, 632] may play a role in their patho-genesis. Most of these scotomas clear up without surgery[331, 632]. The exceptions are those which are accompanied by considerable papilledema; some of these patients develop optic atrophy with permanent loss of vision. Once vision has been lost, surgical decompression is ineffective in restoring it[627]; nor will decompression necessarily prevent the optic neuropathy from developing.

Hyperparathyroidism is a rare and little documented cause of optic neuropathy. Two patients called to our attention developed optic atrophy as the result, apparently, of excessive calcification of the optic foramina. Both were children who had been on high calcium diets for a long time. Paget's disease may also lead to optic atrophy through overgrowth of bone.

An optic neuritis of nutritional origin was frequently reported after the Second World War in prisoners[1006, 78, 136, 1054, 506, 1226]. It is a manifestation of beriberi in which other symptoms (paresthesias, burning of feet) point to a generalized peripheral neuritis. A similar optic neuropathy has been observed in half-starved children of the West Indies[1555, 215]

The visual symptoms in this ocular manifestation of beriberi come on a few months after the individuals have been placed on the deficient diet. The vision drops within a day or two to 20/200 in both eyes and the visual fields show central scotomas. As optic atrophy supervenes the vision may deteriorate further and is then unaffected by restoration of an adequate diet[1226].

In some of the camps where the diet consisted largely of polished rice, optic neuritis was so common that the entity became known as "camp eye"[1055, 1322, 1044, 354]. Aside from the lack of thiamine which specifically underlies beriberi the food intake of these camp inmates provided only about 1,000 calories and most of this was in the form of carbohydrates which enhance the need for thiamine.

Megaloblastic (pernicious) anemia is sometimes associated with optic neuritis[1099]; smokers with this anemia are particularly vulnerable[889, 81, 496].

The cyanides of tobacco are normally converted to harmless thiocyanates by hydroxycobalamin of the liver[622]. The source of hydroxycobalamin is vitamin B_{12} and when this is deficient, as in megaloblastic anemia, the patient is liable to chronic cyanide poisoning. This is said to be the basis for optic neuritis in smokers with megaloblastic anemia and to constitute the rationale for treatment with vitamin B_{12}[895].

Optic neuritis and optic atrophy have been reported to result from various poisons. Some of these reports should be accepted cautiously as it is natural and sometimes profitable for a patient to claim an exogenous cause for his otherwise enigmatic optic neuritis. Conclusions should be particularly cautious in unilateral cases of optic neuritis, for exogenous poisons characteristically affect both eyes about the same time.

Of the optic neuropathies due to poisons the most frequent is that occurring in alcoholics. One type, known as toxic amblyopia, occurs most commonly in persons who both drink and smoke excessively. The question whether the alcohol or the tobacco is responsible is debatable but apparently excess of either can alone cause the neuropathy[217]. The typical history is that of a long-time social drinker and habitual smoker who, over the period of a few days, develops painless blurring of vision in both eyes. Sometimes this is noted first for reading; sometimes it is first evidenced by difficulty in distinguishing traffic lights. The fundi are for a long time normal but the visual fields show an egg-shaped scotoma with most dense involvement of the cecocentral area and a disproportionately greater scotoma for red and green test objects. Pathologically the optic nerves show loss of myelin in those portions of the nerve corresponding to the central fibers (Figure 112).

That toxic amblyopia is due to alcohol and tobacco is established by the facts that continuation of these agents leads to irreversible optic atrophy whereas early discontinuation results in restoration of vision to normal. It does not necessarily follow, however, that the toxic effect is the direct result of the drugs. Much evidence suggests that the toxic amblyopia is attributable to the associated dietary deficiency[213, 889, 1488] or hepatic disease[179]. There is further evidence that it is attributable to vitamin B_{12} deficiency[622, 496].

What constitutes excessive alcohol and tobacco consumption probably varies with the individual person. Certainly we all know excessive drinkers and smokers who never develop optic neuritis. The claim has been made that at least one quart of whiskey must be consumed daily. On the other hand, one patient of ours developed typical toxic amblyopia on a regime which was reliably found to be only four to five highballs and one to two packages of cigarettes daily.

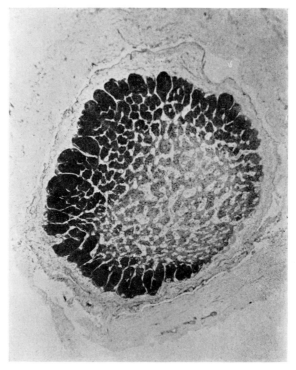

FIGURE 112. Demyelination of papillo-macular fibers from long-standing toxic amblyopia. The patient was a sixty-seven year old man who had been a chronic alcoholic with inadequate diet for many years. He also smoked one package of cigarettes daily. He had had symptoms of polyneuropathy (pain and tremor) and central scotomas for ten years with an acuity of 20/200 in both eyes. The eyes and optic nerves were obtained after he died of hepatic cirrhosis and cardiac decompensation.

A second form of visual difficulty in alcoholics is the acute amaurosis following an episodic debauch[218]. This clears up in twenty-four hours. Its pathogenesis is obscure but since the pupillary reactions are said to be retained despite temporary loss of all vision, the site of involvement may well be in the cerebrum rather than in the optic nerves.

A third type of visual impairment in alcoholics is that which is due to methyl alcohol. After a sufficient intake of methyl alcohol (approximately 10 grams is cited as the minimum[1171]) the patient lapses into a stupor or coma that may be confused with ordinary drunkenness. On recovery in a day or so the patient is found to be partially or completely blind. For a few days vision may improve but is then apt to worsen and optic atrophy becomes apparent. Although this is the typical course of events, there is a great deal of variability and poor correlation of the intake and subsequent symptoms[107].

One of the peculiarities of optic neuropathy from methyl alcohol poisoning is the exclusive susceptibility of primates. Extensive studies in rabbits and other lower animals have failed to produce an experimental counterpart of the human disease[1227]. This species variability is presumably attributable to differences in acid-base balance of the blood and on the different capacity to detoxify the methyl alcohol rather than to any inherent differences in the optic nerves[578].

It is difficult to present a useful classification of the other poisons which are believed to affect the optic nerves. Those which have been reported to cause central scotomas include thallium salts[138, 861], carbon disulphide[1067], chloramphenicol[288, 756], and sulfonamides[1415]. Those which produce predominantly peripheral constriction of the visual fields or generalized visual loss are pentavalent arsenicals (tryparsamide[499], acetylarsan[518]) quinine[115, 385, 913, 1453], plasmocid[827, 550], felix mas[154, 581], hair dyes (p. phenylenediamine)[789] and various chlorinated hydrocarbons[1340, 519, 473]. Other substances produce transient functional disturbances. Thus digitalis and digitoxin produce subjective color disturbances and a blur that is variously described as simple whiteness or hoar-frost appearance. Rarely do they cause optic neuritis[1399, 492]. Isoniazid and streptomycin have been stated to cause optic neuritis[766, 1033] and optic atrophy[1491, 1392, 140], but whether it is those agents or the underlying disease that is causing the neuropathy is not always apparent[730, 104].

5. Pseudo-optic Neuritis

This term encompasses all those conditions which mimic optic neuritis. Such a category serves the useful and important purpose of emphasizing alternative diagnoses in cases of atypical optic neuritis.

Producing central scotomas and therefore foremost among pseudo-optic neuritides are expanding lesions in the anterior and middle cranial fossæ (sometimes as remote as the interparietal falx[811]). These expanding lesions include meningiomas[1249], pituitary adenomas[1523], nasopharyngeal carcinomas, lymphomas, Hodgkin's disease[831], craniopharyngiomas, metastatic carcinomas[335,871] and occasionally ectopic pinealomas[1523]. Each has its characteristic symptomatology (see Chapter XII). Inasmuch as a central scotoma, often of sudden onset, may be the presenting symptom, an erroneous diagnosis of retrobulbar neuritis is easy to make[782, 1526, 845]. Signs suggestive of a diagnosis other than optic neuritis are a gradual onset, progressive course, and absence of pain. More decisive evidence of an underlying expansive lesion is elevation of protein level in the spinal fluid, abnormal roentgenographic or arteriographic changes in the skull, and, of course, associated neurologic symptoms.

The compressive lesions that produce purely central scotomas are usually those within the cranium or optic canal. Lesions of the orbit are apt to produce visual field defects that extend to the periphery as well.

Blurring of the disc from contained drusen[555, 945] or from papilledema[54] may lead to the erroneous impression of optic neuritis. This is especially the case when vision is reduced for any reason. This form of pseudo-optic neuritis differs from the true form, however, in being bilateral, unassociated with central scotomas, and, in the case of true papilledema, of having an elevation of the cerebrospinal pressure.

The reverse situation may also exist wherein an optic neuritis (papillitis) is mistaken for papilledema. This has been called pseudo-choked discs ("pseudostauungs papille"[992]).

Perhaps the most common cause of pseudo-optic neuritis is *ischemic optic neuropathy* (see p. 185). Mimicking optic neuritis in almost every detail, ischemic lesions may produce central scotomas and pain on movements of the eye. One or both eyes may be affected. A diagnosis of ischemic optic neuritis is to be suspected in all patients who have their initial attack in middle life or later. Actually the differentiation from true optic neuritis is not of great importance since treatment of either is simply palliative.

Occasionally, retinal lesions are mistaken for optic neuritis. The chief distinguishing symptom is metamorphopsia; distortion of images is common with retinal lesions but rare with optic nerve lesions. The most frequent retinal lesion to be confused with optic neuritis is that type which is called serous or angiospastic retinopathy. The confusion exists when the retinal lesions are not looked for.

SUMMARY

Drusen of the nerve head are conglomerate bodies that have a characteristic translucence by ophthalmoscopy and blur the disc margins to simulate papilledema. Their pathogenesis is not understood and except for a superficial resemblance to the corpora arenacea of the meninges, they have no counterpart in the nervous system. They usually produce no symptoms and are discovered accidentally but they may produce enlargement of the blind spot, irregular field defects, and occasionally loss of visual acuity. The majority are idiopathic but they do occur with significant frequency in retinitis pigmentosa and tuberous sclerosis.

Pits are discrete "holes" in the nerve head; colobomas are defects in the nerve substance resulting from failure of the fetal cleft to close; staphylomas are frank outpouchings of the disc and adjacent ocular structures. All are congenital anomalies with considerable variation in ophthalmoscopic appearance and visual impairment. A most severe variant often associated with anomalies of the brain and skull is aplasia of the optic nerves.

Demyelinative and inflammatory diseases of the optic nerve include an ill-defined group of entities that are clinically termed papillitis when the lesion is apparent on the nerve head, retrobulbar neuritis when it involves the nerve behind the globe and optic neuritis in reference to either. The chief symptom is loss of vision that usually takes the form of a central scotoma but may be a complete amaurosis. The other frequent symptom is pain on movement of the eye.

Of the primarily demyelinative diseases, multiple sclerosis accounts for about one half of all cases of optic neuritis. It characteristically affects one eye at a time, is recurrent, and frequently leaves permanent optic atrophy. It is most common in the twenty to forty-four year age group and is frequently associated with recurrent paresthesias, spasticity, and other signs of multiple sclerosis. Multiple sclerosis is characterized by relatively discrete plaques of demyelination in which the axis cylinders are preserved. The more diffuse forms of sclerosis, known as Schilder's disease, and various leucodystrophies may also involve the optic nerves. The symptoms in these diseases, however, focus on the cerebral hemispheres (apathy, dementia, convulsions) and much of the visual defect results from involvement of the geniculocalcarine radiation. The course of the disease in diffuse sclerosis is also usually more continuous and rapid than is the case with multiple sclerosis.

Opticomyelitis (Devic's disease) is a clinically separate entity in which an optic neuritis, usually involving both eyes, is associated with symptoms of a transverse myelitis. Hereditary optic atrophy is another form of optic neuritis, sometimes transmitted as a sex-linked trait (Leber's optic atrophy) but appearing under several guises.

Vasculitis produces one form of optic neuritis. This may be a local manifestation in the eye, though alterations in the sedimentation rate suggest a general disease, or it may be part of a widespread giant cell arteritis. The ciliary, ophthalmic, and temporal arteries are particularly prone to show the giant cell arteritis and induce a syndrome in elderly persons known as temporal arteritis.

Optic neuritis may result from direct extension of an inflammatory process from adjacent sinuses or orbital and intracranial structures. It may also be part of a systemic disease. In the past, syphilis has been a particularly prolific cause of optic nerve inflammation. Optic neuritis may occur in the wake of the childhood exanthemata, meningitis, viral encephalitis, and other infectious diseases. Metabolic disturbances may also produce the clinical and pathologic syndrome of optic neuritis. Most notable are: diabetes; that form of dysthyroidism associated with exophthalmos and orbital congestion; the alcohol-tobacco syndrome; thiamine deficiency; and poisons such as methyl alcohol.

Pseudo-optic neuritis simulates optic neuritis clinically but is distinct etiologically. It includes the syndrome produced by intracranial tumors pressing on the optic nerve, non-specific swelling of the disc, some cases of ischemic optic neuropathy, and sometimes retinal lesions. The importance of pseudo-optic neuritis lies in the confusion which it occasions with true optic neuritis.

CHAPTER X

OPTIC NERVE: Lesions (Continued)

A. VASCULAR OPTIC NEUROPATHY

VASCULAR disease may affect the optic nerves in various ways depending on the type, site, and mode of onset of the lesion. Aside from inflammatory lesions of the vessels which have already been discussed, the chief types of vascular disease are: (1) aneurysms and subarachnoid hemorrhage; (2) ischemia and infarction of the optic nerve; and (3) sclerotic plaques of the major arteries.

Characteristic, but by no means pathognomonic of vascular optic neuropathy, are sudden onset of symptoms and reasonable basis for the assumption of underlying vascular disease. Neither the fundus nor field changes are characteristic of all vascular lesions and frequently the diagnosis must be made by exclusion.

1. Aneurysms and Subarachnoid Hemorrhage

Saccular aneurysms which involve the optic nerves are those arising from the internal carotid, from the anterior cerebral, and from the anterior communicating, and occasionally from the ophthalmic artery. When they exert their effect by slow expansion, aneurysms give rise to the same symptoms as do tumors; when they bleed they cause the symptoms of subarachnoid hemorrhage (Figure 113). Definitive diagnosis is made by arteriography[1139] although this may have to be done on both sides to discover the aneurysm[302].

Unruptured aneurysms may exert pressure on the optic nerves, chiasm or tracts[742]. The symptoms of these compressive lesions are simply blurred vision and primary optic atrophy[996, 1529, 1559]. Since the presenting symptom is sometimes a central scotoma, the initial impression may be that of a retrobulbar neuritis or meningioma[1526]. Typical Foster-Kennedy syndromes with central scotoma in one eye and papilledema in the other eye have been reported[783]. Suggestive of an aneurysm is a sudden onset and variation of symptoms from day to day[1008], but the etiologic diagnosis can be established

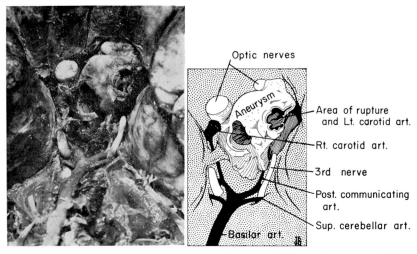

Optic nerves

Aneurysm

Area of rupture and Lt. carotid art.

Rt. carotid art.

3rd nerve

Post. communicating art.

Sup. cerebellar art.

Basilar art.

FIGURE 113. Aneurysm pressing on left optic nerve. The patient was a thirty-five year old man whose initial complaint was loss of vision with optic atrophy in the left eye. Five months after the loss of vision he developed a severe frontal headache, convulsion and coma. The left common carotid artery was ligated but the patient died.

only by arteriography. Most of the aneurysms compressing the optic nerve arise from either the internal carotid or anterior cerebral artery but some have appeared to arise from the ophthalmic artery[1094, 1142].

The sites of aneurysms which impinge on the visual pathways have been illustrated by Jefferson[742]. They are usually supraclinoid aneurysms situated in the parachiasmic region above the cavernous sinus. Aneurysms arising within the cavernous sinus, the infraclinoid aneurysms, rarely produce visual symptoms[1009].

Less well characterized but none the less important are fusiform or cirsoid aneurysms of the internal carotid artery resulting from arteriosclerosis and occasionally from congenital anomalies[1556]. These fusiform aneurysms also cause visual loss by pressure against the optic nerves[816, 7, 1414, 902, 1378, 1177] but, in contrast to the saccular aneurysms, they are usually bilateral and are found chiefly in older patients (see subsequent section on Sclerosis of Internal Carotid Arteries p. 188).

Rupture of an aneurysm is typically characterized by sudden and severe headache, stiff neck, and frequently by loss of consciousness. Convulsions, nausea, and vomiting occur occasionally. The focal signs vary with the site of the rupture but it should be observed that this site may be some distance from the origin of the aneurysm—at times on the opposite side. The chief ophthalmic feature of ruptured aneurysms, aside from visual loss, is the occasional presence of blood about the disc and in front of the retina. Papilledema develops in some cases and is said to indicate a poor prognosis[76]; sometimes the papilledema develops several weeks after the hemorrhage[247].

The route by which blood enters the eye with subarachnoid hemorrhage is a subject of controversy. The two major hypotheses are: first, that the venous drainage from the retina is suddenly obstructed in the vaginal space by the acute rise in intracranial

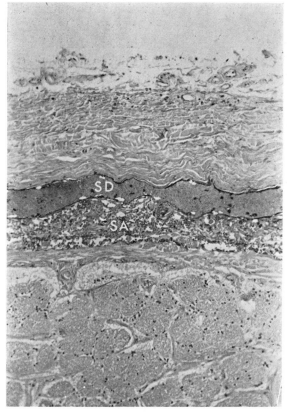

FIGURE 114. Blood in the subdural (SD) and subarachnoid (SA) spaces with intracranial hemorrhage. The patient was a young man who died as the result of a subdural hemorrhage following an automobile accident.

pressure[63, 1528, 1342, 1536]; and secondly, that blood extends directly into the vaginal spaces and thence into the eye from the subarachnoid space [983, 980] (Figure 114).

Without wishing to enter the controversy too vigorously, it would seem that the evidence favors the latter hypothesis. Blood may reach the interior of the eye by traversing the spaces about the central retinal vessels (as we have observed in a post-mortem specimen) or possibly by direct intrusion through the nerve substance as occurs when myelin is forced forward[271].

In establishing the diagnosis of subarachnoid hemorrhage in a patient who suddenly becomes unconscious, the finding of peripapillary and preretinal hemorrhages is a valuable diagnostic sign. Lumbar puncture will usually reveal an elevation of pressure and blood in the spinal fluid. The puncture, however, may be hazardous because of the danger of herniation of the brain stem. Arteriography yields the greatest information and can now be done with relative safety. Treatment consists either simply of observation or of ligation of the internal carotid artery in the neck or within the cranium. In either case the mortality with ruptured aneurysms is still about 50 per cent.

Aside from rupture of an areurysm, subarachnoid hemorrhage may result from trauma, from tumors, from the break-through of an intracerebral hemorrhage or spontaneously (syndrome of Terson[494]). In either case the blood can extend about the optic nerve and present in the interior of the eye[950, 1449, 979, 1436, 298, 980]. Occasionally one may find hemorrhage in the optic nerve sheath and in the eye without appreciable blood in the subarachnoid space about the brain[628].

A special case of subarachnoid hemorrhage is that which occurs in infants either spontaneously or following trauma. Unlike adults, infants develop subarachnoid hemorrhage as a complication of subdural hemorrhage[1316, 721, 569, 1375, 594, 671]. Massive retinal and subhyaloid hemorrhage is common in these cases and may result in permanent ocular damage. Then, too, spontaneous subarachnoid hemorrhages in children are more likely to result from arteriovenous anomalies than from berry aneurysms. It seems probable that the optic atrophy of many infants diagnosed as opticochiasmatic arachnoiditis or otherwise unexplained is due to organization of subarachnoid blood about the chiasm and optic nerves.

2. Ischemia and Infarction

Occlusive disease of the arterioles in the optic nerve is undoubtedly a frequent cause of optic neuritis in older patients[714, 501, 483, 1141, 74, 1217]. It has been called variously arteriosclerotic papillitis, opticomalacia, vascular pseudopapillitis, papillary apoplexy, and ischemic optic neuropathy. The symptoms are those of blurred vision (with or without pain), swelling of the disc (often segmental), and peripapillary hemorrhages[846] (Figure 115). The varied field changes include central scotomas, inferior altitudinal hemianopias[1153], sector defects, and peripheral constrictions[1111, 703, 1141] (especially peripheral constrictions that are not as sharply demarcated by the horizontal line as are field defects with retinal infarcts). Scintillations or transient blurs may precede the final scotoma. In the course of a few days vision may improve but, unlike the primarily inflammatory type, ischemic optic neuropathy does not usually show complete recovery;

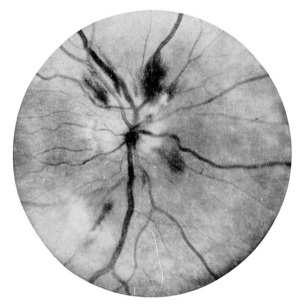

FIGURE 115. Ischemic optic neuropathy. The patient was a fifty year old woman with cirrhosis of the liver and severe hypochromic anemia from blood loss. The optic disc showed papilledema with peripapillary hemorrhages and exudate. The fundus became normal as the anemia resolved.

vision may, in fact, worsen progressively. Arteriosclerosis is by far the most common cause of ischemic optic neuropathy at present but syphilis has been a major cause in the past. Less frequent causes are sickle cell trait, embolism[836], pernicious anemia[1069, 408, 604], temporal arteritis (see p. 167), and circulatory disturbances following intraocular surgery[1188, 877].

Pathologically, ischemic optic neuropathy may show a well-defined opticomalacia (Figure 116) but the identifiable vessel changes are minimal. The vascular changes in the optic nerve show little or no correlation with those in the retina[713, 1141].

Opticomalacia is one of the causes of cavernous atrophy behind the lamina cribrosa[926, 1216] and probably accounts for some, but not all[959, 1155, 869] of the cases of cupping in low tension glaucoma[111, 942].

On quite another basis, ischemic optic neuropathy may follow massive loss of blood[987]. This is seen following excessive hemorrhage from a gastrointestinal ulcer[897, 153, 1578, 1125], from metrorrhagia[929,

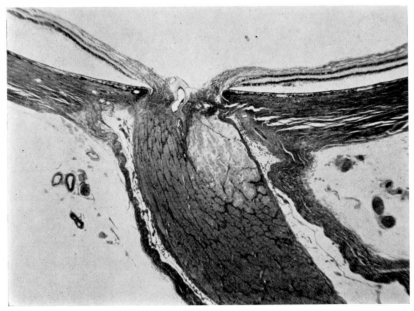

Figure 116. Infarct of optic nerve. Noteworthy is the loss of nerve structure from entire temporal half of nerve.

[471], or following injury. The visual loss is bilateral and generally irreversible but not necessarily complete[1153].

Sclerotic or thrombotic occlusion of the carotid arteries also produces a characteristic syndrome leading to optic atrophy and blindness (see p. 37). The full syndrome consists of blindness in one eye with hemiplegia, hemianesthesia, and hemianopia[1525g, 566] on the opposite side of the body. Preceding the final "stroke," the patient has transient blackouts with paresthesias in the opposite arm and leg. The diagnosis can frequently be established even without symptoms by finding a significantly lower retinal arterial pressure on the affected side than on the opposite side[1501]. The site of occlusion is determined by angiography[1308].

Although arteriosclerosis is the most frequent cause of carotid occlusion, young persons may have the disease. In fact, one substantial series[514] showed the average age to be only forty-seven; at least seventeen cases have been recorded less than fifteen years of age[456]. It may even occur in infants[1381]. It is more common in males than females and is said to involve the left side more often than the right side[1390].

> Since the occlusion affects the internal carotid artery and is slow in development, effective by-passes to the eye and brain[444, 886, 539] may be established by way of the external carotid and ophthalmic arteries[1260, 1529] (Figure 24). The chief blood supply to the anterior portion of the brain then traverses the ophthalmic artery in a direction the reverse of the normal flow. Collateral circulation through the orbit is, however, less effective in maintaining brain function than is collateral circulation through the vertebral system[1157].

Bilateral occlusion of the carotid arteries occurs with a systemic condition appropriately called "pulseless disease" (see p. 38). This results usually from a widespread sclerosis of all the major arteries. Also called pulseless disease and having most of the same symptoms is a generalized arteritis of young (especially Japanese) women (see p. 42).

Blackouts may occur, of course, independent of carotid occlusion. Those occurring in both eyes simultaneously are symptomatic of fainting or of any condition in which the drop in systemic blood pressure causes local ischemia in the eyes. The term "blackouts" is also liberally used by patients when they mean dizziness, blurred vision, or confusion. True unilateral blackouts not due to carotid occlusion may also occur: with impending vascular occlusion as in temporal arteritis; with intracranial tumors that intermittently interfere with the blood supply to the optic nerve; with papilledema that obstructs the blood supply at the nerve head; with arteriosclerosis and hypertension; and with a miscellany of conditions including psychogenic disturbances and so-called migraine equivalents. The most important sign in differentiating these cases not due to carotid occlusion from those due to carotid occlusion is the bilaterally equal retinal blood pressure in the former.

3. Sclerotic Plaques of the Major Arteries

In addition to the foregoing ischemic optic neuropathy, some sclerosed vessels cause visual impairment by direct pressure on the optic nerves[1199]. Best documented is sclerosis of the internal carotid arteries but sclerotic plaques of the anterior cerebral arteries may also damage the optic nerves[1593]. The pulsatile thrust of the arteries pressing the nerves against an unyielding ligament of the optic foramen results in damage to the upper and temporal portions of the nerve[512, 959, 1599, 902]. The visual fields show accordingly inferior altitudinal hemianopias[1111], Foster-Kennedy syndrome[21], binasal scotomas[1111, 474, 1199], central scotomas (suggesting retrobulbar neuritis[1217]) or irregular defects in the lower fields. The visual loss may occur episodically or progressively but rarely does it result in complete blindness; at times it may be transient and non-recurrent[21]. There is nothing in the fields[378] or course of the symptoms which can be said to be absolutely diagnostic. Even roentgenographic demonstration of calcification of the carotid arteries intracranially is not pathognomonic since this is a common finding in the elderly who have no symptoms of optic neuropathy. The diagnosis can be established with reasonable certainty only by neurosurgical exploration[1286].

B. TRAUMA

The optic nerves are implicated in somewhat less than 1 per cent of all head injuries[163, 286, 226]. In most of these cases the injury is thought to occur at the optic foramen[858, 943, 1530]. Yet x-rays reveal a fracture of the foramen only occasionally and a displacement of bone rarely[967] (Figure 117). The injury is nevertheless thought to result in either a transection of the nerve or interruption of its blood supply[704]. Vision is often lost completely and permanently but some patients recover a degree of function within the first few weeks after the injury. A few patients have been reported to benefit from surgical decompression of the optic foramen[879, 891] but most have not[995].

Orbital wounds may injure the optic nerve directly. Bullet wounds, as from attempted suicide, may transect the optic nerves and spare the intracranium. Sticks, cows' horns and other foreign bodies may enter the orbit between the globe and wall and tear the optic nerves; or the optic nerve may be torn apart by injuries which proptose the eye

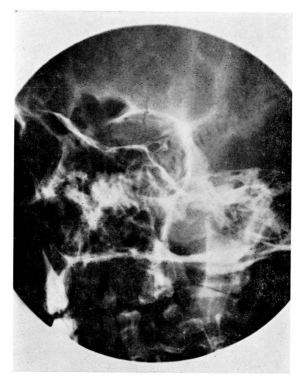

FIGURE 117. Fracture of the sphenoid bone passing through the optic foramen. The patient was injured in an automobile accident and found to be blind in the left eye on regaining consciousness.

excessively[821]. It seems unlikely that orbital hemorrhage by itself or by pressure could cause an optic nerve lesion.

Injuries to the retro-orbital part of the nerve may induce no ophthalmoscopic abnormality but lesions in the orbit frequently show papilledema, peripapillary hemorrhage, and vitreous hemorrhage. The most chaotic abnormalities of the fundus are found with avulsion of the nerve from the globe[589].

Pupillary reactions after injuries to the optic nerve are sometimes paradoxic. Despite loss of vision the pupillary response to light may be retained for several days. On the other hand, the pupil may remain areflexic to light when partial vision returns[476]. This curious dissociation of vision and pupillary reactivity following injury has not been satsfactorily explained.

C. TUMORS

Tumors affecting the optic nerves arise intrinsically within the nerve substance or extrinsically to it. In the latter case they exert an effect on the nerves by pressure. Of the *intrinsic tumors,* gliomas and meningiomas of the optic nerve comprise the majority; also included occasionally in this category are benign congenital tumors of the nerve head, hemangiomas, and a special type of melanoma at the nerve head. Of the *extrinsic tumors,* meningiomas of the sphenoidal ridge and of the olfactory groove are the most frequent; less common extrinsic tumors are anteriorly situated pituitary adenomas, craniopharyngiomas, nasopharyngeal tumors, metastatic tumors, ectopic pinealomas and frontal lobe gliomas.

The prime symptoms of tumors involving the optic nerves are progressive, painless loss of vision and optic atrophy but there are exceptions where, due to hemorrhage or swelling, the onset is so sudden as to suggest a vascular lesion or retrobulbar neuritis[1007]. Exophthalmos is present when the tumor is situated in the orbit and may be the presenting symptom in children who are too young to have observed the visual loss. The exophthalmic globe shows a lack of resilience when an attempt is made to press it backward into the orbit. Paralyses of the extraocular muscles occur variably; they are more frequent with extrinsic than with intrinsic tumors of the optic nerve[1091]. The optic foramen is enlarged with tumors of the optic nerve.

1. Gliomas

These tumors, generally classified with the astrocytomas, occur predominantly in girls[372] during the first decade of life[1366]. The patients present with unilateral loss of vision, optic atrophy, and exophthalmos (Figures 118 and 119). In exceptional cases vision may be remarkably preserved. The blurring of the disc, suggestive of papilledema, is usually due to gliosis or to tumor on the nerve head with, at times, considerable extension into the retina[147]. Strabismus and sometimes unilateral vertical nystagmus may result from the amblyopia but ocular motility is usually normal since the tumor is situated within the muscle cone. When tumor extends into the cranium the x-rays show characteristically an enlargement of the optic foramen[676] and at times a "gourd-like" deformation of the sella turcica[997] (Figure 148).

Gliomas of the optic nerve contain fine or coarse fibrillary cells (Figure 120), similar to those seen with astrocytomas of the central nervous system, but the optic nerve tumors differ from astrocytomas

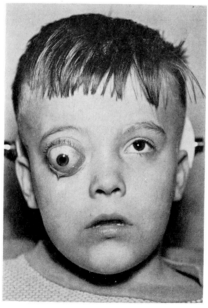

FIGURE 118. Exophthalmos due to glioma of the optic nerve. The patient was a six year old boy who developed proptosis and blindness of the right eye over a six month period.

elsewhere in having conspicuous septa of connective tissue[791] and in showing proliferation of the overlying meningeal sheaths[585]. This

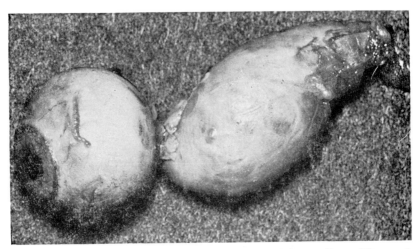

FIGURE 119. Eye ball and attached optic nerve containing a glioma. The specimen was from a three year old girl who had noted blindness and progressive proptosis over a four months period.

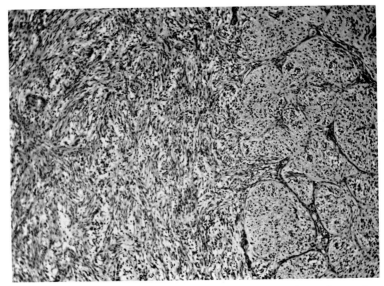

FIGURE 120. Cross section of portion of optic nerve and meninges showing gliomatous proliferation. The tumor cells were thought to be astrocytes.

latter may constitute such a dominant feature immediately behind the eye as to suggest a meningioma when only the retrobulbar portion of the nerve is examined. Occasionally the neoplastic cells appear to be oligodendrocytes and sometimes, when less well differentiated, suggest a spongioblastoma[1610] or glioblastoma multiforme. This dedifferentiation is more commonly seen in patients of the older age group.

The classification of these gliomas of the optic nerve is open to question. Some pathologists have called them all spongioblastomas[1610, 585]; some prefer to think most are oligodendrocytomas[941, 1220, 917]; the majority feel they are most like astrocytomas[193, 372, 1366, 1500]. The fact is that most of these tumors are not easily categorized[1478, 193]. Indeed, some observers doubt that they are truly neoplastic, suggesting they represent aberrant rests[1478, 1219], reactive glioses[1478], or fibrogliomatoses[700, 193]. They have a less dense and less anaplastic cell population than other supratentorial gliomas, a greater fibrous tissue component, and are associated with a unique proliferation of the meninges.

Gliomas of the optic nerve may arise in either the orbital portion or the intracranial portion of the nerve. Whatever their origin, the tumors are slow growing and do not metastasize. With involvement of the chiasm a temporal field defect appears in the other eye while involvement of the diencephalon results in diabetes insipidus and other hypothalamic signs. The prognosis for such advanced cases is obviously poor.

Special cases of optic nerve gliomas are those occurring with neurofibromatosis (von Recklinghausen's disease)[343, 994, 1500] and tuberous sclerosis (Bourneville's disease)[1156]. These familial abnormalities are classified as hamartomas[1038] or phakomatoses.

About 10 per cent of all optic nerve gliomas occur in the entity having neurofibromatosis and café-au-lait pigmentation of the skin (von Recklinghausen's disease)[343, 1497, 994]. Other ocular manifestations of this disease are: multiple tumors of the lids, optic atrophy[1311, 1022], papilledema, orbital deformity with pulsating exophthalmos[1145, 682, 191], myelinated nerve fibers[267], buphthalmos, choroidal melanomas[994], iris nodules[1149] and limbal neurofibromatosis. Common systemic manifestations of the disease, to be thought of in cases of gliomas of the optic nerve, are multiple neurofibromas of the skin, more than the usual number of café-au-lait spots, skeletal deformities (scoliosis) and acoustic neuromas[558]. These associated abnormalities may develop some time after the tumor of the optic nerve[91].

The optic nerve gliomas with tuberous sclerosis (Bourneville's disease)[1012, 1185, 1413] usually present on the nerve head as conglomerate drusen (likened to mulberry clusters) often associated with gliomas of the retina[1215, 1295, 747]. They do not ordinarily cause blindness. Tuberous sclerosis derives its name from the multiple gliomas of the brain and is characterized clinically by epilepsy, increased density of the bones of the skull[363], mental deficiency and adenoma sebaceum of the face.

Treatment of optic nerve gliomas is surgical excision through either a transfrontal approach[329], orbital approach[997, 994], or, as is usually necessary, through a combination of intracranial and orbital procedures[924, 1225] in which the eye may[933, 372], or may not be spared. Each of these procedures has its enthusiastic advocates. Once the tumor has involved the chiasm, however, it is a question of one's outlook on life whether any surgical procedure is warranted[997].

The differential diagnosis of a glioma of the optic nerve revolves about the causes of unilateral blindness, exophthalmos, and optic atrophy in a child. Occasionally granulomas present the typical signs of optic nerve gliomas. Sparing of the extraocular muscles suggests a distinction from other orbital tumors, while the combination of anomalous tissue on the nerve head and enlargement of the optic foramen makes the diagnosis of glioma practically certain.

2. Meningiomas

These are the second most common tumors of the optic nerve. The incidence is said to be about half that of the gliomas but this estimate would vary with the arbitrary limits of classification. Meningiomas arising from the sheaths of the optic nerve within the orbit[486] or optic foramen[36, 1439] are rare. Those arising within the cranium and involving the nerve secondarily are common. In any case they are slow growing and, in contrast to the gliomas, occur predominantly in the twenty to forty age group. They are more common in women than in men.

The chief symptoms of meningiomas affecting the optic nerve

are loss of vision and optic atrophy[772]. Usually the visual fields reveal a peripheral or sector defect initially. Central scotomas are, however, relatively frequent[234] and may give rise to the erroneous impression of retrobulbar neuritis[864, 1249] (Figure 121).

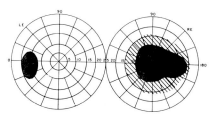

FIGURE 121. Central scotoma due to meningioma. The patient was a thirty-four year old man who presented with anosmia, right-sided headaches, and poor vision in the right eye. Examination showed optic atrophy in the right eye and papilledema in the left (Foster-Kennedy syndrome). Craniotomy revealed a meningioma of the olfactory groove compressing the right optic nerve.

Meningiomas arising within the orbit produce exophthalmos and various ocular motor palsies early (Figure 122). Meningiomas arising within the cranium produce different syndromes depending on whether they are the diffuse meningiome-en-plaque arising from the

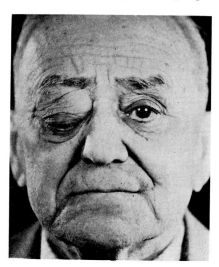

FIGURE 122. Meningioma of the orbit. The patient was an eighty-three year old man with exophthalmos, total ophthalmoplegia, and blindness of the right eye. Surgery disclosed extensive meningioma.

outer wing of the sphenoid or the localized variety, simulating an osteoma, that arises from the inner aspect of the sphenoid. Meningiome-en-plaque (or pterional meningioma) grows by diffuse invasion and thickening of bone. It is the secondary bony changes, rather than the tumor, which cause the optic nerve lesion. In addition to visual loss and optic atrophy, these tumors induce a slowly progressive exophthalmos, downward displacement of the eye, unilateral palsy of upward gaze, and a bulge on the temporal side of the face (Figure 123).

The other, relatively localized, type of intracranial meningioma affecting the optic nerve produces blindness and optic atrophy by direct compression of the nerve. It also produces extraocular muscle palsies but not usually the exophthalmos or temporal bulge of the meningiome-en-plaque.

Other meningiomas potentially affecting the optic nerve by contiguity are those derived from the olfactory groove[228] and from the tuberculum sellæ (see section on chiasm, p.   ).

Aside from these visual symptoms, meningiomas of this region commonly produce anosmia, headache, and frontal lobe signs (especially with tumors on the left side). An especially frequent

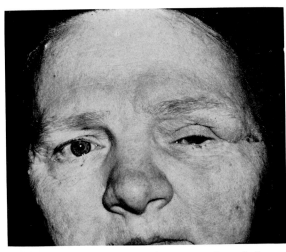

FIGURE 123. Meningioma arising from the outer wing of the sphenoid bone (pterional meningioma). The patient was a forty year old woman whose symptoms were blurring of vision, congestion about the left eye and increasing bulge of the left temple. Surgery disclosed meningiome-en-plaque.

symptom complex, although not necessarily a diagnostic one, is the Foster-Kennedy syndrome consisting of primary optic atrophy in one eye and papilledema from increased intracranial pressure in the other eye[1122, 782, 1014, 744] (Figures 124 and 125).

The association of optic atrophy with cerebral symptoms from remote (parasagittal) meningiomas is an occasional source of confusion. Such cases are usually found at autopsy to have multiple or widespread meningiomatosis[83, 1553].

Pathologically, meningiomas consist of compact masses of benign cells simulating endothelial cells (whence the name endothelioma) having characteristic whorls or psammoma bodies. Sometimes the overgrowth of bone with meningiome-en-plaque is so conspicuous that the histologic appearance simulates fibrous dysplasia of bone[221].

The prognosis with meningiomas affecting the optic nerve is, of course, variable depending on the site and extent of the tumor. Rarely is it possible to remove a meningioma entirely but growth is so slow that significant symptoms may not recur for many years after partial removal.

The differential diagnosis for these meningiomas is that of the causes of any optic atrophy. Suggestive of a meningioma is gradual blindness and exophthalmos in one eye of a patient in the third to

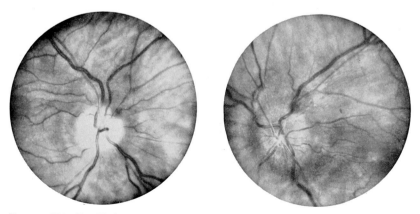

FIGURE 124. Papilledema in one eye and optic atrophy with blindness in the other eye (Foster-Kennedy syndrome).

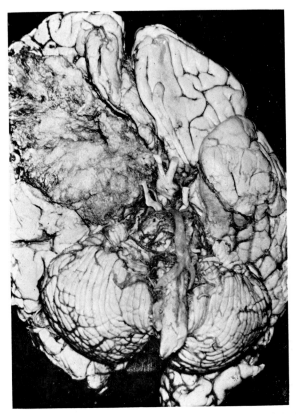

FIGURE 125. Large meningioma arising from the right sphenoidal ridge region and causing a Foster-Kennedy syndrome.

fifth decade of life. The rare case occuring in a child may be clinically indistinguishable from a glioma[1255]. The meningiomas arising within the cranium and not having typical x-ray evidence may be confused with retrobulbar neuritis[864], frontal lobe gliomas, aneurysms, craniopharyngiomas, or other slow growing tumors.

3. Extrinsic Tumors

Various *extrinsic tumors* involve the optic nerve secondarily. These include the congenital heterotopias and a miscellany of infrequent but often malignant tumors.

Of the congenital heterotopias, most common are the glial metaplasias and other aberrations of growth. In such cases ectopic or evaginated brain tissue may be inextricably bound in with the optic nerve. The eyes are of course blind and often microphthalmic. Another congenital "tumor" results from the insinuation of pigment epithelium into the nerve head causing a pigmented mass which may be mistaken for a melanoma (Figure 126). Other cases consist simply of gliosis.

Of the miscellany of *extrinsic tumors,* the following are the most common. A type of melanoma of the nerve head occurs in Negroes and dark complectioned persons[299, 1604]. This presents as a globular black mass extending several diopters into the vitreous. It is benign and, despite its formidable appearance, is compatible with normal vision[835]. Histologically it consists of large, highly pigmented cells which, in bleached preparations, are foam-like; they are quite dissimilar to cells in the usual choroidal melanomas although the latter may invade the optic nerve secondarily. Retinoblastomas commonly extend into the optic nerves. *Metastatic carcinomas* and *nasopharyngeal tumors* are occasional causes of blindness and of pseudo-optic neuritis[870, 242, 1075, 767, 1421]. These are usually associated with other cranial nerve lesions. Occasionally tumors metastasize to the optic nerve directly[1421, 1547].

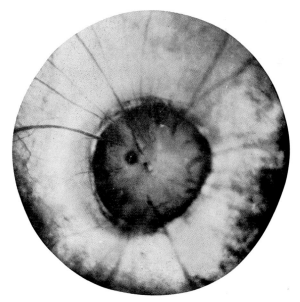

FIGURE 126. Congenital pigmented mass of optic disc. The patient was a three year old boy with esotropia and poor vision in this eye. The mass did not change over a subsequent follow-up period of four years. It is believed to be due to aberrant pigment epithelial tissue in the nerve head.

An infrequent cause of optic nerve disease is the *neoplastic lepto-meningitis* that occurs with metastatic malignancy of the meninges (carcinomatosis; lymphomatosis)[335, 1523].

Of the benign extrinsic tumors, gliomas of the frontal lobe or adjacent structures frequently produce optic nerve compression early[744]; craniopharyngiomas and ectopic pinealomas may also present with optic nerve involvement as an initial sign. Craniopharyngiomas are to be suspected when there is typical intracranial calcification. Ectopic pinealomas produce a characteristic syndrome[760] of optic atrophy, diabetes insipidus, and round cells in the cerebrospinal fluid[787]. Finally there are a few other extrinsic tumors of such infrequency as to warrant mention by name only: myxochondroma[336], hemangioma[824, 1519], medullo epithelioma[1137, 1187], and extension of a melanoma from the intracranial meninges[429, 1289].

SUMMARY

Saccular or fusiform aneurysms of the intracranial vessels may involve the optic nerves by compression, as tumors do, or by rupture with consequent hemorrhage. Arteriography is usually necessary for definitive diagnosis but the presence of retinal and preretinal hemorrhage, together with symptoms of sudden headache and stiff neck, is always suggestive of a subarachnoid hemorrhage from an aneurysm. Non-aneurysmal causes of subarachnoid hemorrhage with bleeding into the eye are trauma, tumors, extensions of a cerebral hemorrhage and occasionally subdural hemorrhage.

Ischemia with occlusive disease of the small vessels is a common cause of optic neuropathy, producing the symptoms of optic neuritis in elderly people. Ischemia may result from massive blood loss or from occlusion of the carotid arteries. The latter produces the typical syndrome of blackouts in one eye and hemiplegic or paresthetic symptoms in the opposite hand. It is frequently diagnosed by finding pathologically low retinal arterial pressures on the affected side. Occlusion of both carotid arteries, together with sclerosis of the aorta and of other arteries produces the syndrome of pulseless disease.

Sclerotic plaques of the intracranial arteries, most especially of the carotid arteries, may involve the optic nerves by pressure. Such lesions cause bizarre and varied field defects.

Injuries involve the optic nerve either by transection, by interference with blood supply or by avulsion of the nerve from the globe.

The most common tumors affecting the optic nerve are the gliomas in children and meningiomas in adults. The gliomas of the optic nerve are usually most similar to astrocytomas and give rise to painless loss of vision with optic atrophy and slowly developing exophthalmos. Enlargement of the optic foramen, visualized roentgenographically, is an important correlative sign. Occasionally gliomas of the optic nerve occur in patients with café-au-lait spots and neurofibromatosis (von Recklinghausen's disease) and sometimes with tuberous sclerosis.

Meningiomas may arise in the sheaths about the optic nerve but more commonly arise from either the sphenoidal ridge or olfactory groove within the cranium. They produce painless loss of vision, optic atrophy, and slowly developing exophthalmos. Those arising from the outer portion of the ridge are particularly apt to induce bony overgrowth and marked exophthalmos.

Less common tumors affecting the optic nerve are the congenital heterotopias, the benign melanomas of the nerve head, nasopharyngeal tumors, metastatic carcinomas, craniopharyngiomas, ectopic pinealomas and a miscellany of less frequent types.

CHAPTER XI

CHIASM (Continued)

A. ANATOMY

THE CHIASM and parachiasmic portions of the visual pathways occupy the plateau region between the temporal fossæ extending from the optic foramina anteriorly to the attachments of the tentorium porteriorly. Included in this area (a region known as the cisterna basalis) are the intracranial portions of the optic nerves, the chiasm proper, and most of the optic tracts (Figures 127 and 128).

In the chiasm decussating fibers from the two retinas approach one another in alternate laminæ[184, 1163, 694]. The nerve fibers from the nasal portions of each retina, constituting in human beings about 60 per cent of all fibers, cross over to intermingle with uncrossed fibers from the temporal portion of the opposite eye. Some of the more ventral of these decussating fibers form a short loop extending into the optic nerve of the opposite side before passing backward into the optic tract while the more dorsal fibers form a similarly short loop extending into the homolateral optic tract before decussating to the opposite side. Thus, field defects from lesions of this area are often asymmetric and bizarre[703]. Clean-cut bitemporal hemianopia results only from lesions that transect the chiasm sagittally.

The macular fibers decussate in the same manner as do those from the more peripheral portions of the retinas. The decussation of the macular fibers occurs, however, in the postero-superior portion of the chiasm[694] so that lesions limited to this region may produce a bitemporal field defect limited to the central area.

Aside from the visual fibers the chiasm and optic tract contain commissural fibers (the tracts of Meynert and Gudden) connecting diencephalic and midbrain centers on one side with those on the other side. These tracts are probably connected with the auditory system and have no known neuro-ophthalmic significance.

The clinical importance of chiasmic lesions requires a knowledge

[202]

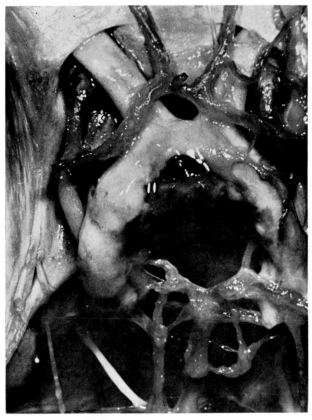

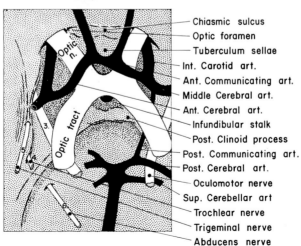

Chiasmic sulcus
Optic foramen
Tuberculum sellae
Int. Carotid art.
Ant. Communicating art.
Middle Cerebral art.
Ant. Cerebral art.
Infundibular stalk
Post. Clinoid process
Post. Communicating art.
Post. Cerebral art.
Oculomotor nerve
Sup. Cerebellar art
Trochlear nerve
Trigeminal nerve
Abducens nerve

Optic n.

Optic tract

3.

FIGURE 127. Normal chiasm and adjacent structures

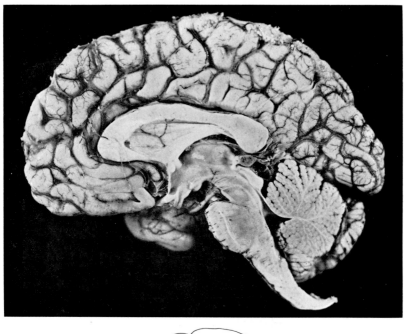

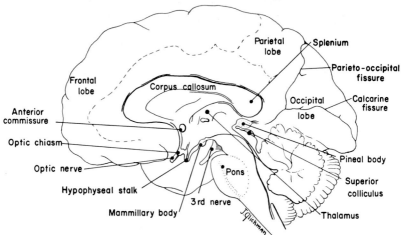

FIGURE 128. Medial surface of brain.

of the structures in the immediate vicinity of the chiasm (Figure 129). Most important is the relation of the chiasm to the sella turcica. This bony structure which derives its name from an alleged similarity to a Turkish saddle is a fossa containing the pituitary gland. It is bounded inferiorly by the sphenoid sinus, laterally and inferiorly by the carotid

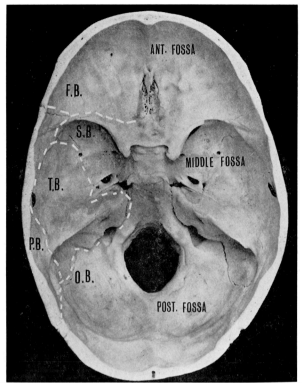

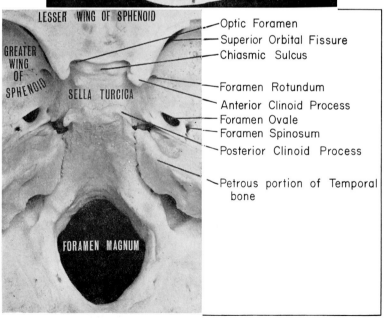

FIGURE 129. Sella turcica and adjacent bony structures. FB, frontal bone; SB, sphenoid bone; TB, temporal bone; PB, parietal bone; and OB, occipital bone.

sulcus, posteriorly by the dorsum sellæ and anteriorly by the tuberculum sellæ or olivary eminence. The sella abuts laterally and inferiorly the cavernous sinus and superiorly a portion of the dura called the diaphragma sellæ. The chiasm lies above this diaphragma occupying usually a region just behind the tuberculum sellæ. Anterior to the chiasm is a potential space, erroneously called the chiasmic sulcus, while posterior to the chiasm is the infundibular stalk connecting the diencephalon with the pituitary gland. Superiorly and posteriorly the chiasm is in contact with the thin plate of hypothalamus comprising the floor of the third ventricle.

> The anatomic relationship of the chiasm to the sella turcica, important as it is for interpretation of signs and symptoms of pituitary tumors, varies considerably. In the majority (79%) the posterior border of the chiasm lies directly over the dorsum sellæ but in some (12%) the chiasm lies on the diaphragm, in others (5%) partially on the tubercle, and in still others (1-2%) behind the dorsum sellæ[1271]. Moreover the distance between the chiasm and dorsum sellæ may vary as widely as 0-10 mm while the angle made by the chiasm with the optic nerves and optic tracts varies with the length of the skull. These anatomic variations will influence the nature of the field defect resulting from expansive lesions in the chiasmic region.

The relationship of the chiasm to the internal carotid artery and to the circle of Willis is also significant. The internal carotid artery, entering the skull through the foramen just lateral to the posterior clinoid process, traverses that intradural structure called the cavernous sinus. This sinus contains a large venous plexus, all of the ocular motor nerves, and the ophthalmic branch of the trigeminal nerve. Taking a sinuous course through the cavernous sinus, the internal carotid enters into the subarachnoid space just lateral, and in close proximity, to the optic nerves and chiasm. It gives off the ophthalmic artery which joins the inferior portion of the optic nerve to enter the orbit through the optic foramen. Continuing its sinuous course, the internal carotid artery passes posteriorly and laterally giving off the posterior communicating and choroidal arteries, then dividing into the middle and anterior cerebral arteries. The carotid artery thus forms the lateral boundary of the chiasm and parachiasmic portions of the visual pathways.

The circle of Willis, which plays a major role in chiasmic lesions, is formed anteriorly by the anterior cerebral arteries connected through the anterior communicating artery and posteriorly by the posterior communicating and the posterior cerebral arteries connected through the basilar artery. The anterior portion of the circle of Willis (that is the anterior cerebral arteries), lies dorsal to the optic nerves, the middle portion lies lateral to the chiasm, while the posterior portion lies beneath and behind the optic tracts.

The sella turcica lying immediately below the chiasm is well seen in routine roentgenograms of the skull (Figure 130). Visualization of soft tissue masses or abnormalities which do not involve bone require filling the ventricular spaces with air, a process known as ventriculography when done through the skull and pneumoencephalography when performed by introducing air into the spinal subarachnoid space (Figure 131). Normally the third ventricle including the prechiasmic sulcus and a space between the chiasm and the diaphragma sellæ may be visualized. Portions of the infundibulum can often be seen bridging this latter space. The chiasm itself is frequently seen

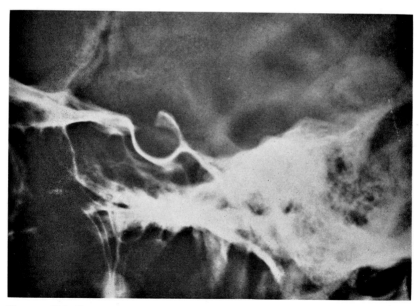

FIGURE 130. Roentgenogram of normal skull. The sella turcica is positioned directly over and behind the sphenoid sinus and is bounded by the anterior and posterior clinoid processes.

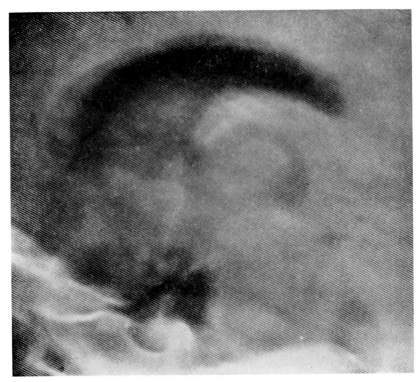

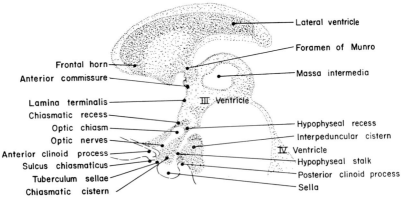

Frontal horn
Anterior commissure

Lamina terminalis
Chiasmatic recess
Optic chiasm
Optic nerves
Anterior clinoid process
Sulcus chiasmaticus
Tuberculum sellae
Chiasmatic cistern

III Ventricle

Lateral ventricle
Foramen of Munro
Massa intermedia

Hypophyseal recess
Interpeduncular cistern
IV Ventricle
Hypophyseal stalk
Posterior clinoid process
Sella

FIGURE 131. Pneumoencephalogram showing normal structures about the chiasm.

directed backward and upward at an angle of 45°. Tumor masses such as suprasellar pituitary adenomas, meningiomas, and craniopharyngiomas will prevent complete filling of the third ventricle and the mass itself may be effectively outlined. On the other hand, some abnormalities such as chiasmic arachnoiditis will be evident only through the obliteration of the potential spaces in the suprasellar regions. Experienced radiologic opinion is necessary to interpret the x-ray films, since they are fraught with abundant artefacts.

Knowledge of the anatomy and functions of the chiasm has an illustrious history. The earliest illustration of the chiasm was drawn by Leonardo da Vinci about 1505 followed fifty years later by that of Vesalius in the famous *Fabrica* and somewhat more than a century later by that of the architect, Christopher Wren, in Dr. Thomas Willis' *Anatomy of the Brain*. But the original intimation of a decussation of fibers was in the form of a query by Sir Isaac Newton appended to his first edition of *Opticks* in 1704[1248]. Nevertheless, the first illustration of the semidecussation did not appear until publication of the book on ocular anatomy by that famous, or infamous, itinerant Chevalier Taylor (1738).

That the visual fibers should decussate and represent the two "halves" of each retina on opposite sides of the brain is of great practical significance. The representation is such that a vertical line drawn through the macula will cleanly and completely divide the elements projecting onto the homolateral and contralateral portions of the brain. This is, of course, part of the general law which states that functions referable to localization in space are represented contralaterally in the brain. In accordance with this, visual sensations are represented on the same side of the brain as are the tactile and motor sensations for the corresponding halves of the body. The amount of decussation is predictable phylogenetically by the amount of overlap in the visual fields of the two eyes. In fishes and birds, where there is little overlap, the decussation is essentially complete, while in mammals the decussation becomes less complete as the eyes assume a more forward position in the head. In man the amount of decussation is about 60 per cent. The fact that the ratio of decussated to undecussated fibers is not 50-50 is because much of the temporal field of each eye does not overlap with the nasal field of the other eye.

The chiasmic blood supply is provided not by any one artery but by an arterial plexus derived from multiple branches of the anterior cerebral and anterior communicating arteries anteriorly and from branches of the internal carotid, the hypophyseal, and the posterior communicating arteries posteriorly[345, 1377, 479, 703].

B. SYMPTOMS OF CHIASMIC LESIONS

The chiasmic area is of neuro-ophthalmic importance not only because visual symptoms are conspicuous with lesions in this region but because they are frequently the sole symptoms[6]. Only when lesions involve the third ventricle, the cavernous sinus, or the pituitary gland do they produce symptoms other than visual. It behooves the neuro-ophthalmologist to be aware, therefore, of the protean ways by which chiasmic lesions become manifest. With chiasmic disease errors in diagnosis—and they are frequent—result from failure to suspect a lesion in this region. Diagnostic procedures are fortunately available to rule in or out most lesions that are suspected.

Ocular symptoms of chiasmic and parachiasmic disease are *chiefly visual field defects* and *loss of acuity* (Figure 132). Bitemporal hemianopia is the signature (as Harvey Cushing called it) of chiasmic lesions but only when the chiasm is completely transected will the hemianopia be total. Incomplete transections will result in partial bitemporal hemianopias; these are paracentral when the lesion involves the posterior angle of the chiasm and peripheral when it involves the more anterior part of the chiasm. Just as characteristic of chiasmic disease as the bitemporal hemianopias is the combination of temporal hemianopia in one eye with complete blindness in the other eye. This indicates a lateralized lesion that affects not only the chiasm but one optic nerve as well. Less common are the irregular altitudinal and totally asymmetric scotomas that cannot be readily allocated to any one anatomic part of the chiasm[99, 703]. The rare binasal hemianopias—more properly, binasal defects since they are never precise hemianopias—are attributable to selective involvement of the lateral portions of the chiasm.

Loss of acuity is an important sign with chiasmic lesions and often serves to differentiate a chiasmic from a retrochiasmic lesion. Usually associated with peripheral field loss, a chiasmic lesion may present with central scotomas in one or both eyes. The loss of acuity is of importance not only because this is what often calls the patient's attention to his disease but because when present it serves to distinguish a hemianopia due to a chiasmic lesion from one that is due to a tract or geniculocalcarine lesion. These latter do not impair visual acuity unless the lesion is bilateral.

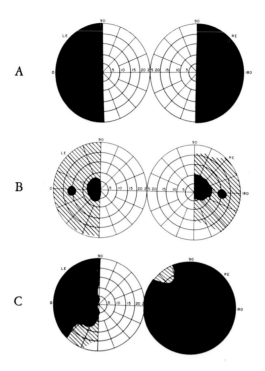

FIGURE 132. Visual field defects with lesions in the region of the chiasm:

A. Complete bitemporal hemianopia in a patient with a suprasellar cyst. This results from interruption of all the decussating fibers.

B. Predominantly paracentral bitemporal hemianopia in a patient with a pituitary tumor. The field defect results from interruption of fibers in the posterior crotch of the chiasm.

C. Blindness in one eye and temporal hemianopia in the other eye in a patient with a pituitary adenoma. Such a combination of field defect results from involvement of the chiasm and of the optic nerve on the side of the blind eye.

It is a common error to believe that splitting of the point of fixation will by itself cause a reduction of visual acuity. This is not so. Visual acuity as recorded with the usual test objects may be normal when the macula is halved by the hemianopia.

Optic atrophy, revealed by pallor of the discs, is a notoriously variable sign of chiasmic lesions. Destruction of the nerve fibers will eventually produce pallor of the discs but inasmuch as this may be delayed the vision will, for some time, be much worse than the ophthalmoscopic appearances would suggest. Conversely, one also encounters at times patients in whom visual acuity is remarkably well preserved despite gross optic atrophy.

The optic atrophy may be bitemporal whereas one would expect it to be binasal. The reason for this paradoxic and often confusing finding is that the temporal halves of the discs are normally paler than the nasal halves and a general decrease in vascularity results in the accentuation of the normal bitemporal pallor.

Hallucinations are unusual with chiasmic lesions but they do occur in the form of either vague phenomena ("whiteness," "visual glow," "film of water") or as formed images. These latter, occurring predominantly in blind persons and sometimes associated with vivid colors, are probably a manifestation of what has been called peduncular hallucinosis (occurring with lesions in the region of the cerebral peduncles[995]) and may be due to coincidental involvement of the temporal lobes.

Headaches are common with some lesions (especially tumors) in

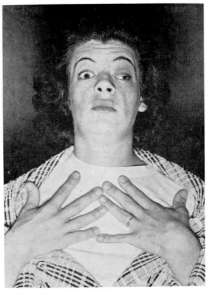

FIGURE 133. Acromegaly and ophthalmoplegia. The patient was a twenty-seven year old woman whose chief complaints were diplopia and ptosis of the left eye for four to five months, increasing size of hands and head, and amenorrhea. Examination showed left third nerve paralysis, bitemporal hemianopia, and ballooning of the sella turcica.

the chiasmic region. They are usually mild, intermittent, and referred to the area of the orbits. When they become severe or associated with nausea and vomiting, one should suspect elevation of the intracranial pressure. The most common lesions about the chiasm that produce this elevation of intracranial pressure are craniopharyngiomas.

Ocular motor palsies occur frequently with those parachiasmic lesions that involve the cavernous sinus (Figure 133). Especially noteworthy are the retro-orbital lesions producing total ophthalmoplegia with blindness in one eye and temporal hemianopia in the other eye. Bilateral total ophthalmoplegia with blindness is a variation of this syndrome resulting from bilateral involvement of the cavernous sinuses, optic nerves, and optic chiasm.

The *non-visual symptoms* of chiasmic lesions depend, of course, on the type of lesion and on its local extent. Lesions invading the

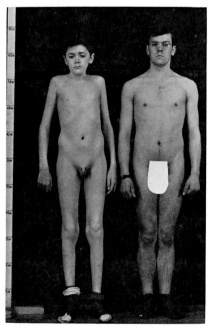

FIGURE 134. Maldevelopment in a patient *(on the left)* with a suprasellar cyst as compared with normal development in a person of the same age *(on the right)*. The patient was a nineteen year old boy whose chief symptom was failing vision of six to seven months duration. Campimetry revealed bitemporal hemianopia. The photograph shows poor physical development, a child-like face, and absence of hirsute.

hypothalamus are particularly apt to manifest diabetes insipidus (polydipsia and polyuria), drowsiness, stupor, and sometimes coma. Those destructive lesions which involve the pituitary gland (at least the anterior lobe) manifest growth disturbances (infantilism) (Figure 134), physical inability to withstand stress (hypoadrenalism), hypoglycemic unresponsiveness, and such endocrine abnormalities as amenorrhea, impotence, and loss of libido. Mental changes, convulsions, and uncinate fits are less common and probably indicate

A   B

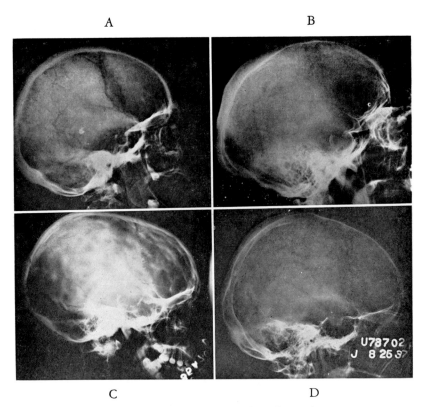

C   D

FIGURE 135. Several types of abnormalities of the sella turcica.
A. Normal sella turcica. Of incidental interest is the calcified pineal gland.
B. Balloon-like enlargement of the sella due to a pituitary tumor.
C. Enlargement of the sella turcica with erosion of the clinoid processes due to a suprasellar cyst.
D. Destruction of the clinoid processes in a patient with a suprasellar meningioma.

correlative involvement of contiguous brain structures. The prominence of these non-visual symptoms is, in some measure, a function of the rate of development of the lesion: slow growing tumors, for instance, may attain tremendous proportions with considerable compression of neighboring structures without necessarily giving rise to symptoms other than visual loss.

Differentiation of chiasmic disease from involvement of the intra-cranial portion of the optic nerves is not always easy, nor important. But differentiation of either from involvement of the orbital portions of the optic nerves is important. Orbital lesions that may be confused with chiasmic defects are bilateral vascular disease (opticomalacia) and occult drusen of the nerve head. Both may produce the bizarre types of field defects sometimes seen with chiasmic disease. Conversely the central or cecocentral scotomas that occasionally occur with chiasmic disease are often misinterpreted as optic neuritis or toxic amblyopia[1505, 6, 1041, 755, 652]. Here the differentiation depends on evaluation of other signs and symptoms.

Roentgenographic visualization of the chiasmic region is frequently crucial (Figure 135). This is especially true for tumors which may otherwise masquerade as inflammatory or vascular lesions. Pituitary adenomas cause a ballooning of the sella; craniopharyngiomas show a rim of calcification; and suprasellar meningiomas show erosion of the clinoids. Failure to get a skull film in atypical cases diagnosed as optic neuritis or vascular neuropathy is one of the greatest mistakes in neuro-ophthalmology; many expanding lesions are thereby over-looked.

To be looked for in x-rays of the sellar region are: (1) evidence of enlargement, such as might occur with intrasellar tumors and cysts; (2) erosion of the clinoid processes as occurs with tumors or aneurysms dorsal to the sella turcica; (3) calcification within or above the sella as occurs with craniopharyngiomatous cysts and aneurysms, and (4) either thinning or thickening of the tuberculum sellæ as occurs with suprasellar meningiomas. The sphenoidal ridge region and the orbital fissures are also important areas for disclosing lesions that involve the optic nerves and chiasm. While thinning or thickening of the sphenoidal bone may result from meningiomas, frank erosion occurs more frequently with nasopharyngeal tumors and metastatic carcinomas.

C. DEMYELINATIVE AND INFLAMMATORY LESIONS

1. Multiple Sclerosis (Disseminated Sclerosis)

Chiasmic lesions are frequently present with multiple sclerosis and its variants, opticomyelitis (Devic's disease) and acute disseminated encephalomyelitis. The symptoms of early chiasmic involvement are asymmetric field defects in the two eyes with a bitemporal distribution[1445, 1231, 1232, 199]. The pathology of the plaques is the same as that of the optic nerves: loss of myelin sheaths with relative sparing of nerve fibers, formation of sudanophilic droplets and lipid phagocytosis.

2. Diffuse Sclerosis

The few cases of Schilder's disease and other diffuse scleroses in which the chiasm has been studied, have shown the same pathologic changes as are found in the optic nerve and similar to what one sees in multiple sclerosis[222]; but the clinical manifestations of chiasmic involvement with these diffuse scleroses have never been clearly described.

3. Inflammation

Meningitis and meningoencephalitis are not uncommon causes of chiasmic and optic nerve disease that, prior to the antibiotic era, culminated in blindness. Occasional cases show extraordinary recovery after a few weeks. With the acute exanthemata of childhood and even more with the less acute meningitis of tuberculosis and syphilis, inflammation is prone to be especially severe about the base of the brain, literally bathing the chiasm in exudate.

Meningitis may be a solitary process in the cranium or may be part of a general infection. Those specific diseases which have been reported to have an associated meningitis involving the chiasm and optic nerve are influenza[567], scarlet fever, rheumatic fever[188] and poliomyelitis[866]. Considerable evidence also supports the possibility of a parachiasmic meningitis resulting from sphenoidal sinusitis[322, 1585, 148, 1464, 614].

Tuberculous meningitis is a special case as it may involve the chiasm (and often the ocular motor nerves) without displaying other clinical evidence of its presence[204]. Treatment of tuberculosis with the chemotherapeutic agents, (streptomycin, para amino salicylic acid and isoniazid), has possibly resulted in an increase of those cases which show chiasmic disease since many of these patients would have otherwise succumbed to the meningitis[1059]. The chiasmic involvement may result from contiguous granulomatous inflammation or the chiasm may be the site of caseous necrosis[1124, 795].

Sarcoidosis in the region of the chiasm has been reported to cause several cases of visual loss, hypopituitarism, and diabetes insipidus[205, 1222, 1158, 1306].

Syphilis may affect the chiasm, as it does the intracranial portions of the optic nerve, by a relatively quiescent meningitis (or leptomeningitis). Rarer is the direct involvement of the chiasm by a syphilitic gumma at the base of the brain[489].

4. Chiasmic Arachnoiditis

This is a name which includes chiasmic disease from chronic inflammation or arachnoidal adhesions of whatever source (inflammation or trauma), and a miscellany of clinical syndromes which do not fit into other classifications[341, 1427].

The usual clinical manifestation of what is called chiasmic arachnoiditis is loss of visual field (including central vision) with eventual optic atrophy but without other neurologic or ophthalmologic abnormalities. The visual field defects may be a bitemporal hemianopia[322, 305, 330, 1527] (pointing unequivocally to the optic chiasm), a binasal hemianopia[474], a central scotoma[148, 1464] (which is hard to explain on the basis of the chiasmic lesion), a generalized constriction of the field, or a bizarre combination of peripheral and central defects affecting both eyes but not otherwise following any one pattern (Figure 136). The visual loss is usually progressive but may be precipitous in

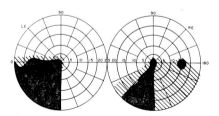

FIGURE 136. Bizarre field defects with chiasmic arachnoiditis. The patient was a fifty-nine year old man with gradual loss of vision and headache over a nine month period. A craniotomy revealed extensive arachnoidal adhesions about the optic nerve and chiasm.

onset and cease spontaneously at any one stage[407]. The only other symptom commonly encountered is headache. This may be in the frontal area, in the vertex, or, when the visual symptoms are on one side, it may be lateralized. Exophthalmos and ophthalmoplegia have also been noted on occasion[1076].

The symptoms of chiasmic arachnoiditis following injury may develop at the same time or within a few days after the trauma but more commonly develop months later. In any case the symptoms are apt to develop precipitously and be bewildering if the relationship to the original trauma is not recognized.

When, as is often the case, the arachnoidal adhesions obstruct the foramina of Munro or other portals of cerebrospinal drainage, the intracranial pressure rises, the headaches become severe, and a papilledema develops, sometimes presenting as a Foster-Kennedy syndrome[57, 1593, 1459]. But papilledema is not always present; it may be absent despite severe elevation of the intracranial pressure when the subarachnoid space about the optic nerves is occluded.

The heterogeneous causes of chiasmic arachnoiditis include trauma, spinal anesthesia[973], syphilis, and a miscellany of local meningitic processes not clearly distinguishable from the acute meningitides previously described. In all probability the entity is analogous to the localized arachnoiditis of the cerebrum associated with Jacksonian fits, or the circumscribed arachnoiditis of the cerebellum (which often simulates tumors[685]) or the arachnoiditis of the spinal cord.

Trauma is the most common cause of chiasmic arachnoiditis[148, 778, 557, 330]. This does not result from a direct tear since the visual symptoms do not necessarily come on until later. The suggested mechanisms are pressure of constrictive bands, organization of a hematoma[189] or cicatrical interference with the blood supply[124, 543].

Inflammatory or post-inflammatory chiasmic arachnoiditis may follow an overt meningitis but more frequently it results from a basilar meningitis in which the non-visual symptoms are minimal or absent. The pathogenesis of this chiasmic lesion is debatable but the suggested mechanisms are constrictive adhesions, vascular occlusion[364, 1040] or direct invasion by inflammation[305,614]. Tuberculous[1040, 1598] and syphilitic[619, 189] meningitis have played prominent roles in the etiology while spinal anesthesia[973] and myelography (with iodized oil[540]) have been responsible for some cases[973].

Routine roentgenograms show nothing abnormal[341]. Unlike tumors in this region, chiasmic arachnoiditis causes no enlargement of the sella, no erosion of the clinoids (except when the intracranial pressure is elevated) and no abnormal calcification. Carotid arteriography, however, may reveal a characteristically acute angulation or distortion of the ophthalmic artery[415] and pneumoencephalography (cisterno-graphy[1240, 225]) usually shows an obliteration of the chiasmic cistern[1130] along with absence of a space-taking lesion.

Despite frequent surgical lysis of the adhesions, few cases of chiasmic arachnoiditis have been studied pathologically. The few microscopic studies which have been reported merely indicated fibrous thickening of the meninges, round cell invasion, circumscribed collections of fluid (pseudocysts), and cellular necrosis[344, 973, 717].

The *differential diagnosis* of chiasmic archnoiditis is often subtle as the symptoms may simulate any lesion of the chiasmic region. Central scotomas lead to confusion with retrobulbar neuritis and some patients who have been reported to have chiasmic arachnoiditis later develop typical multiple sclerosis[189]. Unlike ordinary retrobulbar neuritis, however, chiasmic arachnoiditis is usually progressive. The visual field changes, which are predominantly bitemporal, may suggest tumor but the normal skull films and absence of endocrine or hypothalamic symptoms make either pituitary tumor or craniopharyngioma un-likely. Confusion with those cases of meningioma that show little abnormality of the tuberculum sellæ is a real problem and differentia-tion may have to depend on pneumoencephalography. The rare cases of glioma of the chiasm also offer difficulty in differentiation from arachnoiditis of that region since visual loss may be the only con-spicuous finding in either. The age of the patient may, however, be a helpful indication of one or the other since gliomas are found almost exclusively in childhood.

In another category is the confusion of chiasmic arachnoiditis with occult changes in the optic nerve or nerve head. Thus drusen of the nerve heads may produce bilateral field defects that simulate those of a chiasmic lesion. Conversely, some lesions generally thought to be in the optic nerves may in fact be part of a chiasmic arachnoiditis. Thus, patients originally presumed to have had Leber's optic atrophy have shown typical chiasmic arachnoiditis at surgery[344, 148, 30].

The *treatment* of chiasmic arachnoiditis is controversial. Some authorities have recommended surgical lysis of parachiasmic adhesions[642, 911, 1254, 833, 1076, 973]; others have been less than enthusiastic[614, 439]. Some cases have improved following the use of steroids but others have improved spontaneously[856]. Perhaps the most important consideration is the exclusion of other, treatable causes for visual loss and to this end surgery is indicated in all doubtful cases.

SUMMARY

The chiasm is a biconcave body formed by decussation of the nerve fibers from the nasal portions of both retinas. It is not a neuronal relay and the fibers which constitute it are almost entirely the axones of the ganglion cells of the retina. The postero-superior portions of the chiasm contain the macular fibers.

The neuro-ophthalmic importance of the chiasm depends largely on its proximity to structures that are clinically important. Lying over the sella turcica, the chiasm is close to the pituitary gland, to the cavernous sinuses and to the sphenoid sinus. These lie on its ventral and ventrolateral surfaces. It is also contiguous dorsally to the 3rd ventricle and laterally and dorsolaterally to the circle of Willis. Lesions in this area produce bitemporal field defects but are often otherwise neurologically silent and do not cause elevation of the intracranial pressure until far advanced. Roentgenography, which is of particular importance with lesions in this area, reveals informative enlargement of the sella turcica (pituitary tumors), erosion of the clinoids (from various causes), thinning or thickening of the tuberculum sellae (suprasellar meningiomas), or suprasellar calcification (craniopharyngiomas). These findings when supplemented by pneumoencephalography or arteriography are frequently pathognomonic.

Aside from bitemporal hemianopia, which is called the signature of chiasmic lesions, blindness in one eye with predominantly temporal field defects in the other eye is a common finding with lesions in the region of the chiasm. So are asymmetric bitemporal field defects with loss of acuity in one eye. (Bitemporal hemianopia does not reduce the acuity unless some of the nasal central field is also involved). Optic atrophy occurs with chiasmic lesions but is a late and unreliable sign in evaluating clinical cases. Inconstant signs are headache, ocular motor palsies, hallucinations and signs due to endocrinopathy (amenorrhea and loss of libido from pituitary deficiency) or due to involvement of the diencephalon (excessive thirst and drowsiness).

The optic chiasm is susceptible to multiple sclerosis and to the diffuse scleroses in the same way as are the optic nerves. Usually symptoms from involvement of the nerves mask those due to the chiasm, but it may well be that many cases diagnosed clinically as bilateral retrobulbar neuritis actually represent chiasmic disease. The chiasm also shares with the optic nerve a susceptibility to damage from basilar meningitis caused by tuberculosis, syphilis and sometimes by more acute diseases. An ill defined syndrome termed chiasmic arachnoiditis is thought to cause a slow attrition of the chiasm and optic nerves by formation of arachnoidal adhesions; this arachnoiditis frequently follows trauma. It is a diagnosis that is commonly, and often erroneously, made when no specific disease of the chiasm is found.

CHAPTER XII

CHIASM (Continued)

D. VASCULAR LESIONS OF THE CHIASM

1. Opticomalacia

A S IS THE CASE with the optic nerve, primary vascular occlusion in the chiasm would be expected to produce discrete foci of softening with corresponding scotomas in the visual field. A few such cases have been recorded[1445, 160, 703] but surprisingly few. Vascular occlusions are also thought to underlie much of the visual loss from tumors and arachnoiditis.

Although the anatomy of the arteriolar and capillary supply to the chiasm has been studied extensively with modern techniques of injection and microangiography little has yet been learned that is clinically useful. Nor have any substantial attempts been made to correlate the clinical and pathologic manifestations of vascular disease in the chiasm.

2. Aneurysms

Saccular aneurysms may give rise to typical chiasmic syndromes. Those situated within the sella (intrasellar aneurysms) and those presenting between the anterior cerebral arteries may cause bitemporal hemianopia, panhypopituitarism, and enlargement of the sella turcica —signs typical of pituitary tumor[1606, 516, 1354, 1047, 1557] (Figure 137). They are then distinguishable only by arteriography. Failure to obtain a carotid arteriogram preoperatively in such cases has resulted in more than one fatality. Signs and symptoms suggestive of aneurysm in distinction to adenoma are: supraorbital pain; episodes of intense headache; sudden blindness in one eye and temporal field defect in the other eye; anesthesia in region of one eye and forehead; unilateral ophthalmoplegia[1557]; and x-ray evidence of intracranial calcification. On rare occasions normal carotid arteries that are anomalously positioned in relation to the chiasm will produce typical bitemporal hemianopia by pressure[1199, 109].

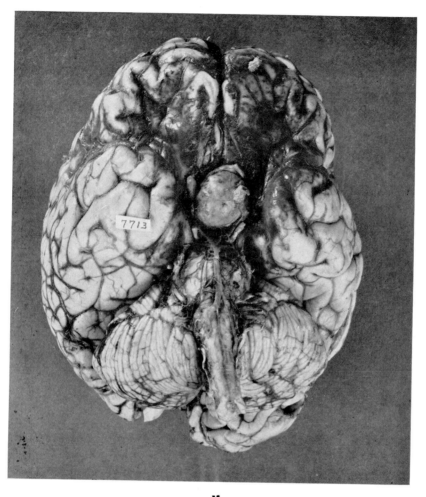

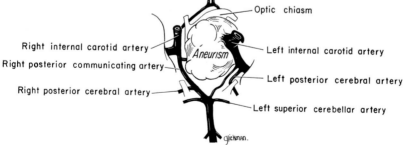

Optic chiasm

Right internal carotid artery

Right posterior communicating artery

Right posterior cerebral artery

Aneurism

Left internal carotid artery

Left posterior cerebral artery

Left superior cerebellar artery

glickman.

FIGURE 137. Aneurysm which had given rise to chiasmic symptoms suggestive of tumor. The patient was a forty-four year old man who had had progressive failure of vision for the previous year. He had been completely blind in the left eye for six months and had lost central vision of the right eye. While being studied he suddenly became comatose and died of subarachnoid hemorrhage. Autopsy disclosed an intrasellar aneurysm extending upward through the diaphragma sellae and impinging on the chiasm.

One of the earliest and best documented cases of intrasellar aneurysms was that recorded by S. Weir Mitchell in 1888. A forty-three-year-old man, who had had transitory hemiparesis four years previously, developed headache and bitemporal hemianopia. Following a severe exacerbation of the headache the patient became comatose and died. Autopsy revealed an aneurysm, one inch in diameter, arising from the internal carotid artery and lodged within the sella turcica. The chiasm had been elevated and "parted in the middle, leaving a nerve on either side."

Supraclinoid aneurysms, derived from the internal carotid artery or its major branches, are usually situated lateral to the chiasm and optic nerve. They may produce blindness in the homolateral eye and temporal hemianopia in the other eye (see p. 181). Rupture of these aneurysms (or of other vascular anomalies) at the base of the skull often precipitates blindness and collapse.

Fusiform aneurysms are usually atherosclerotic in origin, although occasionally congenital[1556], and tend to cause asymmetric binasal or inferior altitudinal defects by pressure against the lateral halves of the optic chiasm or optic nerves[959, 1199].

E. TRAUMA

Chiasmic syndromes with bitemporal hemianopia, or blindness in one eye and temporal hemianopia in the other eye, may result from head injuries[1588, 1530]. The injuries are usually blunt blows, such as are encountered in traffic accidents, and result in fracture of the frontal bone or bones of the sella turcica[330]. The visual loss is typically present immediately after the injury (or is discovered as soon as the patient is alert enough to permit testing), but it may be delayed with a subsequently variable course. Sometimes the visual defect is permanent, or may improve (Figure 138), or in some patients it may worsen over a period of months.

Frequent associated symptoms are seizures, anosmia due to involvement of the olfactory nerves, diabetes insipidus due to hypothalamic injury and, sometimes, panhypopituitarism due to involvement of the sella turcica[1386, 1605].

The pathogenesis of these chiasmic lesions undoubtedly varies from case to case. Actual tear of the chiasm[1180, 1106] is probably unusual[706] but can be produced experimentally[1104]. It has been

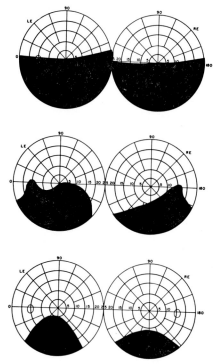

FIGURE 138. Series of field defects charted over a period of months in a patient who had sustained skull injury. The patient was a twenty-four year old man who was completely blinded, with loss of light perception, after being struck on the head with a clothes pole. X-rays revealed a parietal bone fracture through the groove of the middle meningeal artery.

The visual acuity spontaneously returned to normal but the optic nerves became pale. The uppermost pair of fields were charted three days after the injury, the middle pair seven weeks after the injury, and the lower pair six months after the injury.

suggested that most lesions result from hemorrhage[1386], ischemia, or thrombosis[1446, 705, 704]. Those in which the vision deteriorates late fall into the category of chiasmic arachnoiditis (see p. 217).

F. TUMORS

Tumors arising in the vicinity of the chiasm are frequent and important. One in four of all intracranial tumors is said to arise in this region[1551] and, in the majority, visual symptoms constitute the initial manifestation. While most of these tumors are cytologically benign, they are hazardous by reason of their proximity to vital diencephalic and brain stem centers. Their early recognition and treatment is therefore of paramount importance.

The three common tumors of this area are pituitary adenoma, craniopharyngioma, and suprasellar meningioma. On occasion all three may induce identical chiasmic syndromes, being clinically indistinguishable among themselves or indistinguishable from other compressive lesions (aneurysms and less common tumors); more frequently each produces its own distinguishing signs. Age is one of these suggestive features. Craniopharyngiomas predominate in childhood although they may occur at any age; pituitary tumors are most common in the twenty to forty age group[1609, 916]; suprasellar meningiomas occur preferentially in the middle aged or older group. Sex is a further distinctive feature: suprasellar meningiomas occur most commonly in women. Especially helpful, although sometimes deceptive, are the roentgenologic findings in these three types of tumors (Figure 135). Typically, pituitary adenomas produce a ballooning of the sella turcica while craniopharyngiomas produce an erosion of the clinoids. (The situation may be reversed, however, when the growth of the pituitary is directed outside the sella or when the craniopharyngioma is situated within the sella.) Meningiomas of the tuberculum sellae usually produce either a destruction or overgrowth of the tuberculum sellae. But these tumors may produce only slight or inconspicuous changes in routine skull films and therefore give the greatest difficulty in diagnosis and the highest score of misdiagnoses.

Further differentiation is suggested by the fact that craniopharyngiomas commonly induce diabetes insipidus and infantilism whereas pituitary adenomas induce either excessive growth (gigantism and acromegaly) or panhypopituitarism.

Because of their great importance for neuro-ophthalmology, each of these classes of tumors will be discussed separately. Reference to the less common tumors and pseudotumors will follow.

1. Pituitary Adenoma

Three types of pituitary tumors are classically distinguished by their histologic affinity for certain dyes: the chromophobic, the acidophilic, and the basophilic adenomas. This cellular differentiation is reputed to have functional significance in that chromophobic adenomas appear to be non-secretory and produce either no endocrine symptoms or only pituitary deficiency (panhypopituitarism); the acidophilic adenomas produce excessive growth hormone that causes gigantism in the first two decades of life or acromegaly thereafter; and the basophilic adenomas which induce hyperadrenalism (Cushing's disease[323]) characterized by moon facies, hypertension, acne and insulin-resistant diabetes mellitus. Of the three types of pituitary tumors the chromophobic adenomas are the most common and the ones which grow to a size that cause visual symptoms without necessarily manifesting endocrine disturbances (Figures 139 and 140). Acidophilic adenomas produce the chiasmal syndrome less commonly[241] and basophilic adenomas only rarely before they have made themselves apparent by the endocrinopathy. Except for occasional seeding within the cerebrospinal space[283, 463, 1312, 770], pituitary tumors are limited to the parachiasmic region; rarely are they malignant.

This classical division into three functional types of tumors must be accepted with reservations. It is true that the majority of

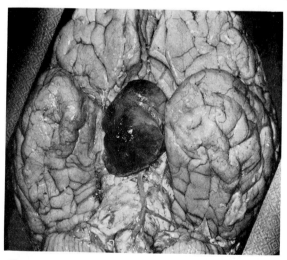

FIGURE 139. Chromophobe pituitary adenoma. The patient was a fifty-six year old woman who had had progressive loss of vision and occipital headaches for two years. On examination she was found to have complete blindness in one eye and hemianopia in the other eye. The sella turcica was enlarged and a large tumor mass was shown by pneumoencephalography projecting into the third ventricle. Following pneumoencephalography the patient became decerebrate, comatose and died with what was interpreted as acute brain stem compression.

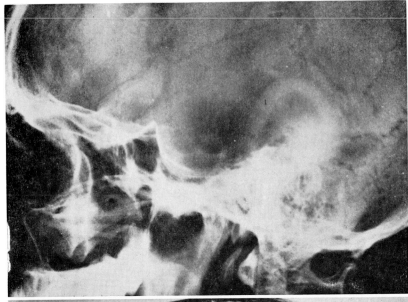

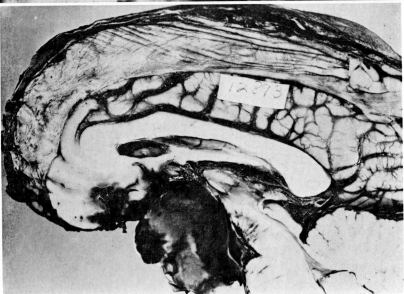

Figure 140. X-ray and sagittal view of brain illustrating a large chromophobe pituitary adenoma. The x-rays show massive "ballooning" of the sella turcica. The specimen shows a tumor growing upward to obliterate the third ventricle.

The patient was a fifty-two year old man who presented initially with "blind spots" in the lateral fields of both eyes. Examination showed complete bitemporal hemianopia and optic atrophy but no other neurologic abnormality. The patient was operated upon with removal of the lower portion of the tumor mass but he died shortly thereafter.

chromophobic adenomas manifest hypopituitarism but some are associated with acromegaly, some with Cushing's disease[770, 991, 1063], and some with a lactation syndrome[462]. Then there are mixed tumors having both chromophobic and chromophilic cells and sometimes one obtains clinical histories suggesting that a secretory type of tumor may metamorphose into a non-secretory type (the "fugitive acromegalic").

The relationship between basophilic adenomas of the pituitary and secretory tumors of the adrenal gland has been especially questioned[770]. Following Cushing's exposition of these tumors in patients with hyperadrenalism[323], it was thought the pituitary tumor caused the overactivity of the adenal gland. Well documented cases and experiments have now been reported, however, which suggest that hypoadrenalism may be the cause of the pituitary tumor[1068] or at least make the pituitary tumor take on accelerated growth[770, 1262, 991, 477]. Moreover, some pituitary tumors have been reported to diminish with appropriate steroid therapy[1333]. On the other hand, patients with Addison's disease do not have an unusually high incidence of pituitary adenomas[1237] as would be expected if the cause of the tumors were simply hypoadrenalism.

The initial symptoms of pituitary adenomas may be either visual or endocrine. Bitemporal hemianopia appears to be due to a stretching, and tearing apart, of the chiasm by the mass extending out of the chiasm. It typically begins in the upper temporal quadrant, progresses into the lower temporal quadrant, with or without involvement of central vision, then extends into the lower nasal quadrant and finally involves the upper nasal quadrant[1445, 702]. Tumors that involve preferentially the posterior crotch of the chiasm induce a bitemporal hemianopic defect limited to the central region of the visual field.

The reason for this relative sparing of the upper nasal quadrant is unknown. Some have suggested that it is related to a separate arterial supply of the inferolateral portion of the chiasm[703].

This clinical course of symptoms with pituitary tumors shows wide variations and a common variant is blindness in one eye with temporal hemianopia in the other (the "junction scotoma" of Traquair). Another variant comprises central scotomas[634, 743] simulating retrobulbar neuritis[426]. Papilledema is unusual with pituitary adenomas[650, 652,

[241]; and pallor of the discs, while variable, may be absent even with dense and prolonged field defects.

The degree of visual involvement depends not only on the direction and growth of the tumor but on the particular anatomic relationship of the chiasm to the sella turcica. It gives no indication of the size of the tumor[1408] nor of its operability.

There are undoubtedly a variety of mechanisms by which vision is lost with chiasmic lesions. Stretching and laceration of the chiasm over a protruding tumor is well established in some cases. This could give rise to clean-cut bitemporal hemianopias. Pressure of the chiasm upward against pulsating anterior cerebral arteries with consequent notching of the superolateral portions[1251], and even severance of the optic nerve from the chiasm, are also well authenticated in some cases. (Strangulation of the optic chiasm by the circle of Willis was described as early as 1852[1448].) Other mechanisms include interference with the vascular supply[1444, 1361, 6, 482], post radiation necrosis[316] and post-radiation scarring[287]. The variability of field changes would seem to be related to the differing mechanisms for damage to the chiasm with pituitary tumors.

The endocrine symptoms of pituitary adenomas follow the pattern associated with either excess growth hormone or insufficiency of hormones (panhypopituitarism). The former, typically associated with acidophilic adenomas, consists of gigantism when the onset coincides with the growth period of a child or acromegaly in the adult (Figure 141). The syndrome of acromegaly comprises prominence of jaw, thickness of tongue, enlargement of hands and feet, separation of teeth, coarseness of hair, deepening of voice, insulin-resistant diabetes mellitus and an elevation of the serum phosphorous. The first symptoms are often tightness of a wedding ring and increasing size of one's hat or shoes. The pattern of endocrine deficiency on the other hand classically associated with chromophobic adenomas includes amenorrhea, frigidity, impotence, loss of libido, fatigue, drowsiness and, less manifestly, hypoglycemia, low excretion of 17 ketosteroids, and collapse under stressful situations. Since these tumors occur frequently in middle life the endocrine symptoms are often passed off as menopausal and disregarded[946]. Rarely the presenting symptom may be a collapse due to adrenal insufficiency; this simulates

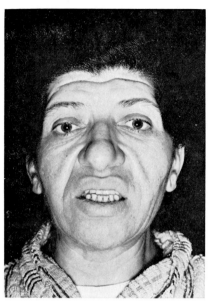

FIGURE 141. Acromegaly. The patient was a forty-two year old woman who had headache, dizziness and gradual change in her appearance over a six to seven year period. X-rays showed enlargement of the sella turcica. Noteworthy are the furrows of the forehead, prominent frontal ridges, coarseness of the skin, separation of the teeth and prominent nose and lower jaw.

coma from stroke but can be differentiated from it by the low blood pressure.

Large pituitary tumors may cause psychotic symptoms[1558], denial of blindness (Anton's symptom), hallucinations (peduncular hallucinosis) and uncinate fits. These are obviously attributable to involvement of the adjacent portions of the brain and are not particularly suggestive of a pituitary tumor. They are, however, unfavorable signs insofar as they occur only with large tumors.

The roentgenologic abnormalities of pituitary adenomas are usually diagnostic. The sella balloons out; the clinoids disappear; and the floor of the sella may erode into the sphenoid sinus. These changes occur with either malignant or benign adenomas[1073]. Yet this same picture may be found on occasion with intrasellar craniopharyngiomas and intrasellar aneurysms. At times pituitary adenomas will extend through the diaphragm at an early stage and grow suprasellarly without producing the characteristic roentgenologic pictures[341].

Pneumoencephalography is of great value in detecting a suprasellar extension of the pituitary adenoma. It is recommended for diagnostic purposes and essential prior to surgery for an estimation of the size of the lesion[341, 1166].

An infrequent but nevertheless well documented syndrome associated with pituitary adenomas is that resulting from hemorrhage and necrosis in the tumor[183, 468,919, 1313, 301, 1527, 922]. Called pituitary apoplexy, and said to occur most especially with acidophilic adenomas[183], it produces sudden severe headaches, visual loss, sometimes ophthalmoplegia, stiff neck, collapse and coma. At times it results from x-ray therapy to the tumor[379, 1360, 13, 267, 316] and may be precipitated by surgery[1456]. The rare cases in which pituitary apoplexy is the presenting symptom of tumor may be mistaken for aneurysm and subarachnoid hemorrhage. Prompt surgical release of the hematoma is said to result in a considerable return of vision[1313].

The differential diagnosis of pituitary adenomas varies with each individual case. Many instances have been diagnosed erroneously as retrobulbar neuritis or chiasmic arachnoiditis simply because no skull x-rays had been taken[240]. Those few cases in which the tumor grows extrasellarly and in which the skull x-rays are consequently normal, cannot be differentiated without surgery from craniopharyngioma, meningioma or other less common tumors.

The indication for treatment of pituitary adenomas is usually threat of visual loss, and the urgency for treatment is a function of the rate with which the symptoms come on. Acute lesions require prompt treatment and usually have a better prognosis[477]. Small tumors may be approached through either the frontal or transphenoidal route[651, 605]. Tumors that are shown by pneumoencephalography to be large, are usually unsuitable for surgery because of the catastrophic results from sudden hypothalamic decompression[743, 58]. For these, x-ray therapy is most suitable and it is fortunate that most pituitary adenomas, especially the acidophilic tumors[239, 59], are radiosensitive[235]. Improvement begins in one or two weeks after radiation therapy and may continue for a year or more[235, 1090]. In any case correlative care must be taken of the endocrine status, for many of these patients are in marginal pituitary balance and surgery can precipitate a fatal hypoadrenal crisis.

2. Craniopharyngioma

Craniopharyngioma is one of several names for benign epithelial tumors or cysts derived from vestiges of the hypophyseal stalk. Other names are hypophyseal stalk tumors, Rathke pouch cysts, epidermoid cysts, cholesteatomas (when they are filled with cholesterol and sebaceous material) and adamantinomas (when they contain anlage of teeth). They may arise anywhere along the hypophyseal stalk and present in the third ventricle (suprasellar cysts), or within the sella (intrasellar cysts), or commonly in both suprasellar and intrasellar regions. While the differentiation of epidermoid cysts from cranio-pharyngiomas is warranted embryologically, they have idential neurologic manifestations and are here considered together.

Being congenital, they become manifest most frequently in child-hood[1100, 723] (unlike pituitary adenomas and meningiomas which predominate in adults), but it is not uncommon to have them first give rise to symptoms in later life[1575] or even in old age[1135, 1570, 1576, 342, 1435, 1253].

The visual symptoms produced by craniopharyngiomas may be the same as those of pituitary adenomas—bitemporal hemianopia, blindness in one eye and temporal hemianopia in the other eye, and central or paracentral scotomas[1505]—but owing to their posterior position, craniopharyngiomas are more likely to be associated with homonymous hemianopia of tract origin than are the pituitary adenomas. They are also more apt to produce papilledema (especially in younger patients[761, 207]) accompanied by vomiting and severe headaches with increase in intracranial pressure. Elevated intracranial pressure is usually an ominous sign since it indicates the tumor is blocking the aqueduct and is in a position that is unfavorable for eradication[1292].

Three non-ocular signs suggestive of craniopharyngioma are diabetes insipidus (which is rare with pituitary tumors[1524]), infantilism of the hypopituitary variety, and calcification in the hypophyseal-pituitary region (Figure 142). Hypopituitarism is particularly suggestive of craniopharyngioma when it occurs in a child or adolescent since pituitary tumors are almost non-existent in the first decade and rare in the second decade. Thus most cases of pituitary dwarfs, hypogeni-talism, and many cases of Frölich's syndrome are due to cranio-

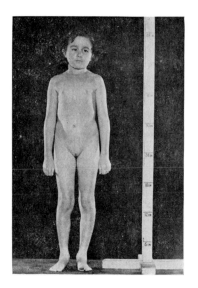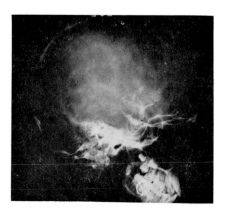

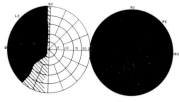

FIGURE 142. Dwarfism and hypogenitalism in a twelve year old girl with a calcified craniopharyngioma in and above the sella turcica. The patient's presenting symptom was growth deficiency. Examination of the visual system showed blindness in the right eye with incomplete temporal hemianopia in the other eye. Craniotomy disclosed a solid tumor mass extending up into the third ventricle.

pharyngiomas. Other non-ocular symptoms are hypoglycemia, circulatory collapse on exertion, postural hypotension[1430] and behavior problems. With craniopharyngiomas of older persons, and with excessively large craniopharyngiomas at any age[1558], mental changes simulating those of senility are conspicuous symptoms[1435].

Craniopharyngiomas are usually slow growing, but acute symptoms may develop at any time with a sudden worsening of the visual symptoms (or blindness[985, 119]), a precipitous development of ophthalmoplegia, convulsions, and collapse with meningitic signs Although not well documented, these crises are thought to result from rupture of the cysts and, in some cases, from inundation of the adjacent structures and cerebrospinal fluid with the irritative contents of the cysts. Following an acute exacerbation, the symptoms may improve spontaneously suggesting that the cyst has decompressed itself.

Skull x-rays and pneumoencephalograms are frequently diagnostic[67, 1292]. Intrasellar craniopharyngiomas produce a ballooning of the sella and extension into the sphenoid sinus exactly as do pituitary adenomas but in children they also frequently reveal a characteristic rim of calcification corresponding to the cyst. This, together with other compatible symptoms, is pathognomonic of craniopharyngioma. Suprasellar craniopharyngiomas may also reveal the characteristic calcification, but, in contrast to the intrasellar tumors, there is usually only slight flattening of the sella and variable erosion of the clinoids; at other times the x-rays may be entirely negative. Pneumoencephalography is usually necessary to determine the size of the tumor (Figure 143) and is particularly important with posteriorly situated craniopharyngiomas.

A rare and curious syndrome occurring with craniopharyngiomas and other lesions causing bitemporal hemianopia is that of see-saw nystagmus[989, 964]. Because of its rarity it is little more than a curiosity at present but it may be the presenting complaint.

The pathology of craniopharyngiomas is that of any congenital epithelial remnant. The tumor may consist of a solid mass (Figure 144) of mature cells with differentiation into ducts or it may consist of a cyst filled with epithelial detritus and lipid material. The reason for its growth and particularly for its occasionally delayed appearance is unknown. Of some theoretical and much practical importance is the suggestive evidence that pregnancy[418] or growth hormone, given therapeutically, may cause a reversible expansion of the tumor and result in a worsening of the symptoms.

The differential diagnosis of craniopharyngiomas has much in common with that of pituitary adenomas. Those craniopharyngiomas which produce only visual symptoms (including the chiasmic group[894]) may be erroneously diagnosed as retrobulbar neuritis or chiasmic arachnoiditis. Perhaps this error is more common with craniopharyngiomas than with pituitary adenomas because of the greater

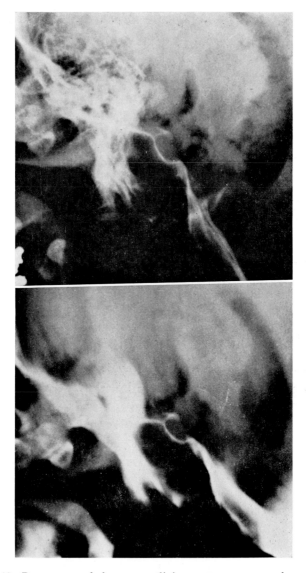

FIGURE 143. Pneumoencephalogram outlining a tumor mass above the sella turcica. The upper picture is a standard lateral PEG taken with the patient in a brow-up position. The lower picture is an autotomogram that permits sharp localization of a mass above the sella turcica.

The patient was a thirty-six year old woman whose chief complaint was blurring of vision. Visual fields revealed a bitemporal hemianopia and craniotomy disclosed a craniopharyngioma.

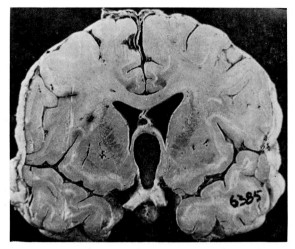

FIGURE 144. Craniopharyngioma presenting as a dark mass filling the third ventricle and pressing on the dorsal surface of the chiasm.

The patient was a forty-five year old woman whose chief clinical symptoms were progressive moroseness and change in personality. She recently had developed headaches and vomiting concomitant with increase in intracranial pressure. The patient died following a frontal craniotomy.

tendency for intermittency of symptoms with the former. In many of these cases diagnosed as retrobulbar neuritis, roentgenograms would have prevented the mistake. Intrasellar craniopharyngiomas and pituitary adenomas may be indistinguishable[1302] but youth of a patient or presence of calcification points to the former. Optic atrophy is said to be less frequent with craniopharyngiomas than with pituitary adenomas[1292] and the discs frequently show less pallor than would be expected from the visual loss. Calcification is a particularly valuable sign of craniopharyngioma[67] (Figure 145) but even this may be simulated at times by aneurysm or occasionally by chordomas, osteomas, and sclerotic carotid arteries.

Elevation of the intracranial pressure with its attendant nausea, vomiting, severe headache, and papilledema favors craniopharygioma as opposed to pituitary adenoma but, or course, does not rule out other space occupying lesions. Pinealomas may simulate craniopharyngiomas by giving rise to intermittently elevated intracranial pressure (as well as to diencephalic signs) but can usually be differentiated by palsy of upward gaze and pupillary areflexia

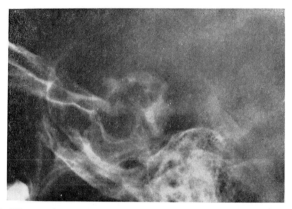

FIGURE 145. X-rays (autotomogram) illustrating extensive calcification above the sella turcica in a patient with a craniopharyngioma.

(Parinaud's syndrome) and by the absence of chiasmic signs.

Treatment of craniopharyngiomas consists of substitution therapy for the hormonal deficits (notably pitressin for the diabetes insipidus, steroids for the adrenal insufficiency and growth hormone for the dwarfism) and surgery for the tumor when the visual or other symptoms warrant it. Tumors that are situated within the sella exclusively may be approached by the transphenoidal route[653]. Those within the third ventricle are precariously situated[1575] and difficult to approach. Not only is this a territory fraught with surgical hazard but the tumors are frequently bound to major vessels and brain stem structures that make attempts at complete removal dangerous. Frequently the best that can be done is to by-pass an obstruction by a prosthetic shunt. Craniopharyngiomas also have an occasional way of evading the neurosurgeon; even those which produce bitemporal hemianopia can be hidden from view despite what is thought at the time to be adequate exposure of the chiasm. Nevertheless, most craniopharyngiomas are accessible to surgery and some may be completely removed [211, 1001]. In others, sufficient removal to relieve the pressure on the chiasm will often result in dramatic return of vision, but recurrences in these cases are the rule. The availability of cortisone and other hormones has greatly reduced the operative mortality[722,1455, 786, 761].

3. Meningiomas

Although meningiomas of the sphenoid or olfactory groove may involve the chiasm, it is the meningiomas of the tuberculum sellæ that most characteristically produce the chiasmic syndrome. Since sphenoidal and olfactory meningiomas have been discussed in connection with optic nerve lesions, the present section will be limited to those of the tuberculum sellæ with the assumption that other meningiomas may on occasion present a similar clinical appearance.

The tuberculum sellæ, lying between the anterior clinoid processes, is the anterior rim of the sella turcica, and forms the basis for a dural fold connecting the cavernous sinuses on either side and forming a roof or diaphragm of the sella turcica.

The tuberculum sellæ is a favorite site for meningiomas of the base of the brain. These tumors occur usually in women in middle or late life. They are slowly progressive like meningiomas elsewhere, and usually benign. Those rare meningiomas which do occur in childhood are prone to undergo sarcomatous degeneration[1417].

The chiasm usually lies just above the diaphragma sellæ and is therefore just superior and posterior to the tuberculum. With meningiomas of the tuberculum the chiasm is pushed upward and backward over the tumor. Depending on the particular anatomic structure of the chiasm in a given case and on the direction of growth of the tumor, meningiomas of the tuberculum sellæ would be expected to produce either a chiasmic or an optic nerve lesion or a combination of chiasmic and nerve lesions.

Visual symptoms are the conspicuous, and frequently sole, manifestation of these suprasellar meningiomas[576, 739] (Figure 146). They may produce a typical bitemporal hemianopia while being of such a small size as to produce no other evidence of compression on contiguous structures and little or no roentgenologic abnormality. Frequently they present with a central scotoma (due to involvement of the prechiasmic

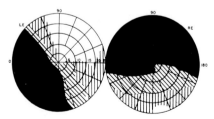

FIGURE 146. Bizarre field defects in a patient with a meningioma of the tuberculum sellae. The sole clinical symptom was gradual loss of vision over an eight month period. Routine roentgenograms were interpreted as normal but pneumoencephalography revealed a suprasellar mass. Following craniotomy and removal of a meningioma the patient showed dramatic recovery of vision.

region[1041]) or with paracentral hemianopic defects (due to involvement of the postchiasmic region). One eye is often involved for a long period of time before the other[576]. Although the characteristic course is one of slow progression of the visual defect, the symptoms sometimes develop with unexplained rapidity and fluctuation; they may then lead to the false impression of retrobulbar neuritis[1282, 576, 1249]. As in all parachiasmic tumors, optic atrophy is a variable sign but by the time the patient comes to medical attention atrophy is more common with meningiomas than with pituitary adenomas or craniopharyngiomas. Papilledema on the other hand is rarely seen with suprasellar meningiomas[576].

The paucity of non-visual symptoms accounts for the great number of erroneous diagnoses with meningiomas of the tuberculum sellæ. Nevertheless headaches occur frequently and are generally more severe than those associated with pituitary adenomas although less severe than those associated with increased intracranial pressure. Expect for amenorrhea, endocrine symptoms are rarely present[576]. Endocrinopathy is in any case hard to evaluate because the patients are frequently of an age group when involutional changes might be expected. Ophthalmoplegia follows extension of the tumor into the cavernous sinus but this is also unusual.

X-rays, arteriography and pneumoencephalography are often crucial. Routine skull films may show either osteoporosis or hyperostosis of the tuberculum with thinning of the clinoids[131] but the sella turcica is often normal[15] and other abnormalities may be so slight as to be non-diagnostic[324, 576, 1249]. Arteriography on the other hand is usually most helpful. Not only are the major arteries (especially the carotid siphon and the anterior cerebral artery), displaced upward, but the vessels in the meningioma itself form, during the venous phase, a compact "blush" of radio-opaque material that is frequently diagnostic[1007, 1292]. Pneumoencephalography is also serviceable in outlining the presence and extent of a large suprasellar tumor (Figure 147), but as a rule arteriography is more useful with meningiomas whereas pneumoencephalography is more useful with craniopharyngiomas.

Histologically, meningiomas of the tuberculum sellæ are like meningiomas elsewhere. They are made up of compact masses of mature endothelial cells with little evidence of invasiveness. They are often associated with meningiomas elsewhere in the cranium.

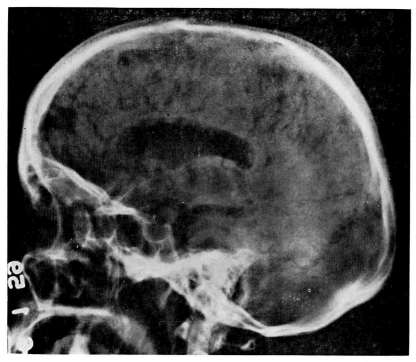

FIGURE 147. Suprasellar meningioma outlined in a pneumoencephalogram. The patient was a thirty-five year old woman who had noted an insidious loss of vision in the right eye for several months. Examination showed almost complete blindness in the right eye and a paracentral defect in the temporal field of the left eye. Routine skull x-rays were interpreted as normal but the pneumoencephalogram showed a mass extending upward from the sella turcica into the third ventricle. Craniotomy revealed an unusually bulky suprasellar meningioma.

The differential diagnosis of suprasellar meningiomas is most important. Of all tumors in the region of the chiasm, meningiomas offer the greatest difficulty in diagnosis. The majority of patients with meningiomas come first to ophthalmologists because of blurred vision and headaches. Those who present central scotomas are often diagnosed as having retrobulbar neuritis[1282, 754, 576] or toxic amblyopia[1250]. In contrast to retrobulbar neuritis, however, the central scotomas of suprasellar meningiomas are less symmetric[1070] and often associated with a peripheral field defect[1282]; moreover, they occur in an older age group of patients (although one case has been reported in a two year old infant[1417]) and are usually of insidious onset.

Those patients with bitemporal hemianopia or junctional scotomas suggest either pituitary adenoma, craniopharyngioma, sphenoid or olfactory groove meningioma or aneurysm. The negative x-ray and absence of endocrinopathy favor suprasellar meningioma, but these are not entirely diagnostic. At times it is impossible to differentiate a suprasellar meningioma from a pituitary adenoma (which has developed extrasellarly) or from a craniopharyngioma unless the latter is calcified. Differentiation of suprasellar meningiomas from other meningiomas may be suggested by other signs and symptoms. Anosmia favors olfactory groove meningiomas. Extensive hyperostosis and exophthalmos favor sphenoidal ridge meningiomas. But the absence of these signs and symptoms is not as meaningful. Patients with bizarre field defects may also be mistaken for those having chiasmic arachnoiditis, syphilis, or gliomas of the chiasm. Probably the most important differential procedure in all of these entities is arteriography[662, 755].

Treatment of suprasellar meningiomas is surgical excision. Fortunately the tumors are relatively small by the time they come to surgery and their position does not invoke the hazards customarily associated with surgery of large pituitary adenomas and craniopharyngiomas. And like these latter, vision may be recovered dramatically after removal of the compression. The most important consideration for treatment is early recognition, for the prognosis is good with surgery of small tumors but may be catastrophic with large tumors[739].

4. Other Tumors of the Chiasmic Region

In addition to pituitary adenomas, craniopharyngiomas, and suprasellar meningiomas, a variety of other tumors may give rise to chiasmic symptoms. These should be considered in any differential diagnosis of chiasmic syndromes but their infrequency warrants little more than identification by name and a few outstanding characteristics.

Nasopharyngeal carcinomas, arising in the sphenoid or ethmoid sinuses, may extend into the chiasmic and parachiasmic region. Along with visual disturbances due to involvement of the optic nerves and chiasm, they frequently produce ophthalmoplegia, pain, numbness (due to trigeminal involvement), and sympathetic paralysis[1037]. Nose bleeds are a significant symptom and enlargement of the cervical nodes is a common finding[457]; other evidence pointing to the nasopharynx may be lacking.

Gliomas of the chiasm occur in association with gliomas of the optic nerve or with those of the third ventricle and frontal lobe[175] which extend through the leptomeninges[745]. Those associated with gliomas of the optic nerve have already been discussed (see p. 191). Involvement of the chiasm is suggested by visual field changes together with x-ray evidence of enlarged optic foramina or of a special pear-shaped or J-shaped excavation of the sella turcica[615, 676] (Figure 148). Sometimes tomography will reveal a characteristic deformity that is not apparent in routine x-ray films[172]. Carotid angiography is often negative but pneumoencephalography frequently reveals obliteration of the basilar cisterns and upward deflection of the frontal horns of the lateral ventricles[676].

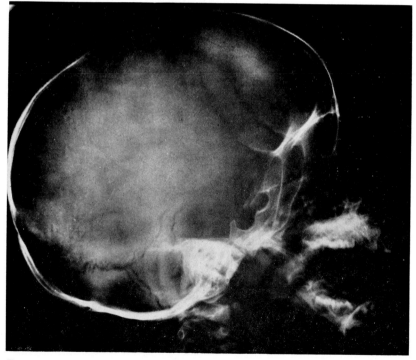

FIGURE 148. Curious deformation of the sella turcica in a three year old child with von Recklinghausen's neurofibromatosis. X-rays revealed bilaterally enlarged optic foramina and the J shaped excavation about the sella turcica typical of glioma of the chiasm.

Ganglioneuromas[281], *ependymomas,* and a hybrid called *infundibuloma* may also occur in the neighboring neural tissue (thalamus and third ventricle) and involve the chiasm secondarily[746]. Such cases are rarely diagnosed preoperatively.

Chordomas are infrequent tumors arising from vestiges of the notochord within the base of the skull. These tumors are highly invasive and may extend into the sella turcica to give the x-ray appearance of pituitary tumors[400]. They may also extend into the nasopharynx or into the orbit[1224, 37, 1600].

Osteochondroma. These tumors occurring preferentially at the base of the skull[918] may, on occasion, cause chiasmic syndromes[899, 792, 1201].

Ectopic pinealomas produce a parachiasmic syndrome with central or junctional scotomas. Such tumors are usually situated anterior and lateral to the chiasm and give rise to symptoms in childhood or early adulthood (Figure 149). Aside from the visual symptoms, sometimes confused with retrobulbar neuritis, they regularly induce diabetes insipidus, hypopituitarism[760] and lymphorrhagia in the spinal fluid.

Metastatic carcinomas in adults and *undifferentiated sarcomas* in children may on occasion occur in the sellar region and give rise to blindness, topical symptoms (diabetes insipidus; panhypopituitarism), and pain.

5. Pseudotumors of the Chiasmic Region

While pseudotumor is not an adequate diagnosis—indeed not a diagnosis at all—it is a useful category for entities which mimic tumors and which must be considered in all atypical cases.

First in importance are *aneurysms.* In their unruptured state, saccular aneurysms may produce compression of the chiasm to yield a clinical syndrome simulating that of tumor (see p. 222). Aneurysms occur most commonly at the site of the major branching of the internal carotid artery and therefore tend to produce lateral chiasmic and ophthalmoplegic signs[1557]. They may, however, extend into the sella turcica and produce the same radiologic and endocrine abnormality as intrasellar chromophobic adenomas or craniopharyngiomas. Symptoms suggestive of an aneurysm are abrupt onset, sudden and severe headache, supraorbital pain, and ophthalmoplegia. The value of arteriography in such cases is obvious.

Calcification of the internal carotid arteries is occasionally mistaken for that of a craniopharyngioma but is easily differentiated by the lateral position of the shadow.

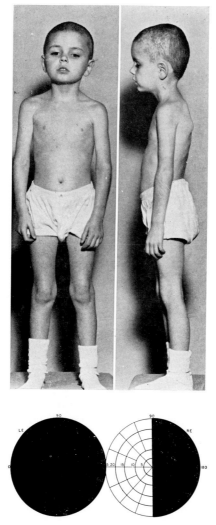

FIGURE 149. Ectopic pinealoma. Five year old girl who presented with the multiple symptoms of retardation of growth, progressive loss of vision, convulsions, and diabetes insipidus. The visual fields showed complete blindness in the left eye and temporal hemianopia in the right eye. Craniotomy revealed a tumor subsequently shown to be a pinealoma, on the left side of the chiasm.

Increased intracranial pressure and *hydrocephalus* with consequent dilatation of the third ventricle will be sufficient at times to cause chiasmic symptoms with optic atrophy and erosion of the clinoids suggesting a suprasellar tumor[873, 523]. Such an x-ray finding in patients with long standing elevation of intracranial pressure thus has no localizing signficance.

Chiasmic arachnoiditis is frequently mistaken for tumor because of its progressive course without evident cause. The failure to outline a tumor in an otherwise satisfactory pneumoencephalogram would favor arachnoiditis but in doubtful cases surgery is indicated. It is better to operate and find only arachnoiditis than not to operate and have a patient blinded unnecessarily by tumor.

Functional enlargement of the pituitary occurs in the last few weeks of pregnancy and probably in other physiologic states. Occasionally it is said to produce a bitemporal hemianopic constriction of the field[445, 748], but it is rarely confused with a true adenoma.

SUMMARY

Occlusive vascular lesions of the chiasm have been infrequently documented. On the other hand aneurysmal involvement of the chiasm is not uncommon, with symptoms that simulate those of tumors.

Injury to the chiasm with bitemporal hemianopia occurs with fractures of the base of the skull. It is accompanied by anosmia and other evidence of damage to the parachiasmic region.

Tumors in the vicinity of the chiasm are particularly important because they are relatively frequent and the visual effects may be the only symptoms. Early recognition is of prime therapeutic importance. The most common tumors are pituitary adenomas, craniopharyngiomas, and suprasellar meningiomas.

The chromophobic adenoma is the most frequent pituitary tumor which presents with visual symptoms but amenorrhea and impotence may also be early symptoms. With eosinophilic adenomas the endocrinologic manifestations (gigantism in youth and acromegaly in adults) are conspicuous and precede visual symptoms. With basophilic adenomas the symptoms of hyperadrenalism (Cushing's syndrome) predominate and the tumors rarely attain sufficient size to involve the chiasm.

The most important diagnostic sign of pituitary tumor is enlargement of the sella turcica. This is easily recognizable in routine lateral roentgenograms of the skull but pneumoencephalography is necessary to delineate the extent of the tumor.

Craniopharyngiomas are epithelial remnants of the embryonic cranio-esophageal stalk and are found most frequently indenting the third ventricle. Bitemporal hemianopia or other fields defects due to involvement of the chiasm from craniopharyngiomas are common. Associated symptoms are diabetes insipidus from lesions of the hypothalamus and increased intracranial pressure from obstruction of the aqueduct. Although craniopharyngiomas are congenital in origin and give rise to symptoms most frequently in childhood they may not become manifest until adulthood. The most characteristic x-ray finding is suprasellar calcification, but, as was the case with pituitary tumors, pneumoencephalography is necessary to determine the limits of the mass.

Meningiomas are the most subtle of the three types of tumors affecting the chiasm. The meningioma may arise from the olfactory groove, the sphenoidal bone or from the tuberculum sellæ. The latter, called the suprasellar meningioma, is the one which gives rise to visual symptoms only and the one most commonly overlooked. Routine x-rays with these meningiomas may show some changes in the tuberculum sellæ and in the clinoids but the findings are often equivocal. Arteriography, however, frequently reveals a characteristic blush of radio-opaque material at the site of the tumor.

Less common tumors in the region of the chiasm are the nasopharyngeal carcinomas, gliomas of the chiasm, chordomas from the base of the skull, osteochondromas, ectopic pinealomas and metastatic carcinomas. The name pseudotumors of the chiasm is used to designate those non-neoplastic lesions which produce symptoms that simulate those of tumors: saccular aneurysms, calcified internal carotid arteries, distended third ventricle, and chiasmic arachnoiditis.

CHAPTER XIII

OPTIC TRACT – LATERAL GENICULATE BODY – GENICULOCALCARINE RADIATION – CORPUS CALLOSUM

A. OPTIC TRACT: Anatomy

THE OPTIC TRACT is that portion of the visual conduction system which extends from the chiasm anteriorly to the lateral geniculate bodies posteriorly. It forms a V-shaped area that incorporates the pituitary stalk at its apex and embraces the cerebral peduncles within its diverging arms.

The optic tracts are made up of visual and pupillary afferent fibers that arise in the retina and, in the case of the visual system, terminate in the lateral geniculate bodies. Some fibers are said to pass directly to the cortex[401] without going through the lateral geniculate body[1608] but this has yet to be confirmed. Fibers arising in corresponding portions of the two retinas gradually approach each other so as to insert on adjacent laminæ in the two geniculate bodies. Coursing with the optic tracts in some species are the accessory bundles of nerve fibers called the tracts of Meynert and Gudden which extend from one side of the mid-brain to the other and probably have nothing to do with the visual system.

The central or macular fibers lie on the medial surface of the optic tract as they emerge from the chiasm but in their course posteriorward they come to have a dorsal position. It is as though the optic tracts rotated through 90° before inserting in the geniculate bodies. Not only do the macular fibers come to assume a dorsal position, but the fibers from the inferior quadrants of the retina come to be situated medially while those from the superior quadrants come to be situated laterally in the optic tracts.

The pupillary fibers on the other hand are deflected at the anteromedial portion of the lateral geniculate body to course in the brachium of the superior colliculus to the pre-tectal region. It seems

[248]

unlikely that the large number of deflected fibers (estimated at 20-30% of those in the optic tract[113]) are concerned exclusively with pupillary movements[178], but no other function has been convincingly attributed to them in human beings. In lower animals, however, most of the deflected fibers terminate systematically in the superior colliculi which are true visual centers[34].

B. OPTIC TRACT: Lesions

Being continuations of the optic nerves and chiasm, the optic tracts are susceptible to the same types of pathologic processes that affect these structures. The differences are those resulting from the more posterior position of the tracts.

The signs and symptoms of optic tract involvement comprise hemianopia, optic atrophy, and pupillary changes. The hemianopia is homonymous and central visual acuity is normal unless there is simultaneous involvement of the chiasm. The optic atrophy, when present, is important in distinguishing the hemianopia of tract origin from that due to lesions in the optic radiation. It is, however, not manfest for several weeks after an acute lesion. The pupillary abnormalities consist of a slightly larger pupil on the side opposite the lesion (Behr's sign) and a hyperreactivity of the light reflex when the stimulus comes from the hemianopic field. This hemianopic pupillary areflexia (Wernicke's sign) should be a valuable aid in differentiating tract from cerebral lesions but, unfortunately, there are no wholly reliable means for testing it. The slit-lamp beam with alternate illumination from either side is perhaps the most readily accessible but even with this there is sufficient intraocular scatter to lead to equivocal responses.

An abnormal optokinetic response may be of service in diffler-entiating a tract from a cerebral hemianopia (see p. 266). The optokinetic response is elicited by having the patient view a series of moving objects such as the stripes on a rotating drum. Normally the resultant nystagmus is symmetric to the two sides. It is also symmetric with tract hemianopias but it is characteristically asymmetric with cerebral hemianopias in which the parietal lobe is involved. Thus an abnormal (asymmetric) optokinetic response suggests a cerebral basis for the hemianopia whereas a normal (symmetric) response has little diagnostic value.

Being close to the diencephalon, midbrain and cerebral peduncles, lesions of the optic tract are often accompanied by autonomic disturbances, loss of consciousness, diabetes insipidus, contralateral pyramidal tract signs and endocrinopathy in addition to the hemianopia. Because of their proximity to the vital centers of the diencephalon, lesions of the optic tract entail, in general, a greater surgical liability than do those involving the chiasm or prechiasmic area.

1. Aneurysms

Saccular aneurysms arising from the internal carotid artery or from the posterior communicating artery may result in pressure on the optic tract. These usually give rise to symptoms simulating neoplasm and are diagnosed by arteriography. Rarely, the optic tracts are involved in rupture of an aneurysm with hemorrhage into the tract.

2. Tumors

Pituitary adenomas and especially craniopharyngiomas involve the tracts as they do the chiasm. The optic atrophy occurs late and the hemianopia is for a long time reversible. Tumors less commonly affecting the optic tracts are nasopharyngeal carcinomas, chordomas, infundibulomas and gliomas[1336]. Diagnosis is usually made by x-rays, arteriography and pneumoencephalography.

3. Demyelinative Diseases

Although much less common than retrobulbar neuritis[944], optic tract lesions do occur with multiple sclerosis[239, 1471, 146], Schilder's disease and other demyelinative processes. The symptoms are often of sudden onset, simulating a vascular lesion. The diagnosis is made by exclusion and by the the association of signs and symptoms pointing to demyelinative involvement of other parts of the nervous system.

4. Trauma

The optic tracts may be injured with fractures of the skull or by direct passage of foreign bodies through the orbit[1356].

C. LATERAL GENICULATE BODY

The lateral geniculate body constituting the termination of the optic nerve and the optic tract fibers is a distinctive portion of the thalamus. As a neuronal relay station it transmits visual impulses to the geniculocalcarine radiation destined for the occipital cortex just as the rest of the thalamus transmits somesthetic impulses to other sensory radiations in the parietal cortex—or just as the medial geniculate bodies relay impulses to the auditory radiations in the temporal cortex.

Situated at the posterior-inferior portion of the thalamus, each lateral geniculate body has the triangular shape of a Napoleonic hat, with afferent optic tract fibers entering its antero-ventral surface and efferent optic radiation fibers leaving its dorsal surface (Figure 150). Within each lateral geniculate body are six laminæ of cells: the four dorsal layers of small cells (parvocellular layers) and the two ventral layers of large cells (magnocellular layers). This lamination, developed most conspicuously in species with binocular vision, is arranged so that layers 1, 4 and 6 represent the opposite eye while layers 2, 3 and 5 represent the homolateral eye. Each retinal point is represented in several laminæ[232, 844].

Evidence for the separate representation of each eye in the dif-

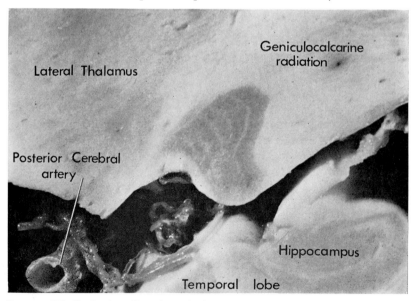

FIGURE 150. Sagittal section through the lateral geniculate body and adjacent structures. Noteworthy is the lamination that is characteristic of this body.

ferent layers of the lateral geniculate bodies is found in the curiously transneuronal atrophy of cells following removal of one eye[1161]. The atrophy is apparent within ten days after the eye is removed[544] or after the optic nerve is sectioned, and is still evident many years later[552]. This trans-synaptic degeneration[257] also occurs in the cerebello-olivary system but is infrequent in the nervous system elsewhere and its significance for the visual system is not understood.

The crown of the Napoleonic hat represents macular or central vision and occupies a large part of the geniculate body[1229, 1230, 1029, 844]. The lateral and medial portions of the geniculate body represent the inferior and superior quadrants of the retina respectively. The two ventral, large-cell layers are believed by some to represent the temporal or monocular fields of each eye[184, 1162, 513], while by others they are believed to represent rod or nocturnal vision[636, 1520].

The significance of lamination, which is characteristic of the visual system but particularly characteristic of the lateral geniculate body, is an enigma. Having no internuncial neurones, there is no anatomic evidence for integration between the layers in the geniculate bodies[544]. One suggestion is that the lamination in man actually serves no useful purpose and is merely a relic of a former primitive visual brain[1520]. This seems unlikely since the lamination is most highly developed in man. Another suggestion based on electrical recordings is that the lamination serves for integration of the two eyes through physiologic spread of impulses between adjacent laminæ[127, 440]. Still other suggestions are that the laminar pattern, three layers representing each eye, serves trichromatic color perception[885], or converts the visual impulses into a code more readily analyzable by the cerebral cortex[178].

Adding to this list of guesses one might also suggest that it is at the level of the lateral geniculate bodies where the remarkable phenomenon of suppression occurs. It is well known that the visual image arriving in consciousness consists not of an additive fusion of the two eyes but of a mosaic for which individual points are selected from each eye[1481]. This process called unification (a name preferable to fusion[1481]) selects points according to their attention value and is capable of rapid alternation of corresponding points, groups of points, or of the entire image of each eye. The attention values will depend not only on the relative optical imagery but also on the physiologic state of the retina and of the activity of the rest of the brain. Thus the entire visual function may be suppressed. The act of "day dreaming," for instance, must depend on the domination of the visual imagery by toning influences from the rest of the brain. The "shouting of the visual impulses," as Brindley calls it[178], is suppressed by competitive impulses from non-visual spheres. The anatomy of the lateral geniculate body lends itself to such an interpretation. The lateral geniculate bodies receive afferent impulses from other portions of the brain and especially the reticular system[1355, 1393]; also the equal[1391] or somewhat greater number of cells within the geniculate bodies than of incoming visual fibers[256, 246] indicates synthetic rather than convergence functions (as occurs at the retinal level)[178].

Lesions of the lateral geniculate bodies resulting in clinical syndromes have been infrequently documented[636], and further data are needed before firm conclusions are justified. A hemianopic defect of the visual fields would be anticipated having predominant involvement of the upper field with lateral lesions, of the lower field with medial lesions, and of the paracentral field with dorsal lesions. One would also expect a dysesthesia (with or without pain) referred to the opposite side of the body owing to contiguous involvement of the thalamus[955]. The degree of hemiplegia varies with the amount of associated involvement of the internal capsule; and the presence of stupor depends on extension of the lesion to the nearby tegmentum in the midbrain and subthalamus[2].

D. GENICULO-CALCARINE RADIATION AND CORPUS CALLOSUM

Traversing the posterior end of the internal capsule as the optic peduncle, the geniculo-calcarine radiation fans out to circumvent the lateral ventricle (Frontispiece). The posterior medial portion of the emergent tract, that which represents fibers from the upper retina, passes directly to the supracalcarine region of the occipital cortex. In so doing its dorsal border rises just above the temporoparietal boundary. The anterolateral portion of the optic peduncle, representing fibers from the lower retina, is deflected anteriorly to pass over the temporal horn of the lateral ventricle before turning backward. Then, the fibers, here called the external sagittal stratum, pass through the substance of the temporal lobe, lateral and ventral to the lateral ventricle, to insert in the infracalcarine portion of the occipital cortex and associated areas[1469]. The most anterior portion of this radiation is called Meyer's loop commemorating the man who first showed these fibers to have a visual function[1015]. Present evidence would indicate that Meyer's loop does not extend as far forward in the temporal lobe as sometimes stated[128] since amputation of much of the tip (6 cms) causes little or no field defect[1059, 195, 707,1552]. The name external sagittal stratum, originally applied to an intracerebral association tract, now distinguishes these fibers from other fibers, most particularly from the internal sagittal stratum, lying in apposition to the ventricles and thought to represent cortico-efferent fibers.

The region just posterior and lateral to the internal capsule is called the *temporal isthmus* (Figure 151). Here there is a conjugation of visual, somesthetic and some motor fibers in an area no more than 1.5 cm in diameter and closely contiguous to the speech area and intracerebral association pathways[14]. A relatively small lesion here, such as results from an occlusion of the anterior choroidal artery, usually [390] (but not always[1046, 484]) gives rise to hemianopia in association with numbness in the opposite extremities and motor signs affecting preferentially the leg. Therapeutic stereotactic lesions in this region may also be expected to cause symptoms of this

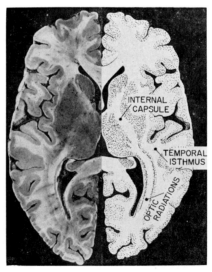

FIGURE 151. Horizontal section of brain through the temporal isthmus.

nature[1351]. Aphasia will be a prominent symptom with lesions of the dominant side whereas loss of body recognition (failure to recognize one's arms and legs as one's own) will occur with lesions of the temporal isthmus on the non-dominant side[1078].

While the dorsal portions of the radiations represent upper retinal functions and the ventral portions of the radiations represent lower retinal functions, the large intermediate portions represent macular functions[96]. There is, however, considerable overlap of the fibers representing peripheral and central vision[1422].

So far as is known all these fibers terminate in the homolateral occipital cortex. The incoming fibers insert in the granular layer (or layer IV) of the cortex similar to the insertion of sensory afferents elsewhere in the cerebrum. In the case of the occipital cortex, however, this granular layer is split by a myelinated intracortical tract, the line of Gennari, which probably serves for association of corresponding points of the two eyes.

In the process of phylogenetic encephalization the occipital lobes have progressively taken over the visual functions from the lower centers but only in man has this become complete. The cat and dog maintain, for instance, considerable visual discriminative ability after occipital lobectomy. Even the monkey responds to moving objects and retains visual placing reactions after removal of the area striata and complete degeneration of the lateral geniculate body[358].

But man is completely blind and retains only pupillary reactions after destruction of the occipital lobes. This contrasts with other sensory modalities which preserve considerable discrimination at subcortical levels. Thus, after removal of the somesthetic areas of the cortex in the post-rolandic areas, a crude touch, pain, and temperature sense is preserved.

There is no convincing evidence for bilateral macular representation as has been suggested to occur from division of the centrally directed fibers. Rather, each macular area is represented homolaterally in a point to point fashion. The macular fibers appear to be represented in the posterior end of the calcarine fissure and at the posterior poles of the occiput while the peripheral retinal fibers are represented anteriorly.

The blood supply to the geniculo-calcarine radiation can best be appreciated by reference to a diagram (Figure 152). It is obvious that the radiation receives arteries from both the carotid and vertebral systems and is thus susceptible to vascular accidents in both systems. The anterior portion of the geniculo-calcarine radiation derives its blood supply from the anterior choroidal artery; the intermediate portion from the middle cerebral artery; and the posterior portion along with the visual cortex from the posterior cerebral artery[485]. But there are considerable anatomic variations and anastomoses between the arteries. Indeed cases have been recorded in which the anterior choroidal artery has been ligated without producing field defects[484].

The prime symptoms of lesions of the geniculo-calcarine pathway are homonymous hemianopic defects. These will be predominantly in the lower visual field with dorsal lesions and in the upper visual field

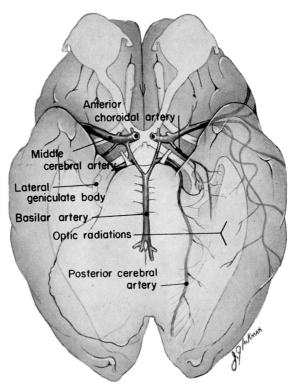

FIGURE 152. Diagram of blood supply to the geniculo-calcarine radiation.

with ventral lesions. The fact that upper and lower quadrants are separated by the extensive fanning out of macular fibers permits a fairly sharply demarcated quadranopia.

The character of the visual field defect is often suggestive of the site of the lesion but topical localization depends greatly on associated involvement of adjacent structures. Hence further discussion of the clinical aspects will be postponed until subsequent sections.

The *corpus callosum* is the major pathway connecting the two halves of the brain. Its posterior portion, designated the splenium, is concerned with integration of opposite halves of the visual field. It is on this commissure that we must depend for much of our depth perception (integration of non-corresponding points on opposite halves of the retinas) and on the transmission of visual experiences from one half of the visual field to the other half. Animals with bitemporal hemianopia (from section of the chiasm) can transfer visual learning from one hemisphere to the other hemisphere only if their commissure is intact[1060, 1061, 384]. The commissure thus establishes a unity of the visual field giving to the brain a single "cyclopean eye"[249].

Despite its obvious importance for integration of the visual system, no syndrome in the visual sphere has been conclusively associated with lesions of the commissure and patients show surprisingly little deficit from its surgical transection[174, 8]. Alexia[998], apraxia and agnosia have been suggested[1077] but not confirmed[8, 174]. Lesions of the corpus callosum have been recognized pathologically as occurring with tumors, vascular accidents, congenital defects, and sometimes surgical transection[8] but few cases have been subjected to a battery of crucial visual tests.

Simultaneous involvement of the splenium and the dominant occipital lobe has, however, been associated (through inconstantly[9]) with the syndrome of alexia without agraphia[1447, 998, 531]. This occasionally results from a vascular accident since both the occipital lobe and the hind portion of the commissure are supplied by the posterior cerebral artery. The basis for this syndrome will become evident after discussion of functional representation in the parietal lobe (see p. 272).

SUMMARY

The optic tracts are continuations of the axones that began in the retinas, extended along the optic nerves, partially decussated in the chiasm and terminated in the lateral geniculate bodies (visual fibers) and in the pretectal nuclei of the midbrain (pupillary fibers). They conduct impulses from homonymous halves of both retinas. Lesions of the optic tracts cause homonymous hemianopia (with variations dependent on the coincidental involvement of the chiasm), optic atrophy, and hemianopic pupillary reactions. The more common lesions of the chiasm are aneurysms, tumors (especially cranio-pharyngiomas and pituitary adenomas), demyelinative diseases and trauma.

The lateral geniculate bodies are modified portions of the thalami wherein the visual impulses from the optic tracts are relayed by an extraordinarily laminated series of neurones to form the calcarine radiation. The clinical symptomatology of lesions of the lateral genicu-late bodies has been infrequently documented. One would expect hemianopia, hemianesthesia, and some hemiplegia (predominantly of the leg) due to involvement of the contiguous thalamus and internal capsule.

The geniculo-calcarine radiation passes first through the most posterior part of the internal capsule, an area called the temporal isthmus, to fan out over and lateral to the large cerebral ventricles. Each radiation terminates exclusively in the occipital cortex of the homolateral side. The prime symptom of lesions of the geniculo-calcarine radiation is a homonymous hemianopia; this hemianopia becomes progressively more symmetric the farther posterior the lesion.

The corpus callosum is the major commissural tract connecting the two hemispheres. The chief visual function is served by its integration of the two occipital lobes for the function of stereopsis, unification and other binocular acts.

CHAPTER XIV

PARIETO-TEMPORAL LOBES

A. ANATOMY AND FUNCTION

THE PARIETAL LOBE is that division of the brain bounded anteriorly by the rolandic fissure, posteriorly by the occipital lobe (from which it is separated by no anatomic landmark), and inferiorly by the sylvian fissure and the temporal lobe (Figure 153). The temporal lobe is that portion occupying most of the inferolateral portion of the brain bounded superiorly by the sylvian fissure and by the parietal lobe, and posteriorly by the occipital lobe.

Noteworthy structures on the lateral surface of the parieto-temporal lobes are the supramarginal gyrus at the termination of the Sylvian fissure and the angular gyrus at the posterior end of the superior temporal sulcus. The angular gyrus and possibly the supramarginal gyrus serve important visual functions. Noteworthy on the infero-medial surface of the temporal lobe is that medial gyrus named the hippocampus, having a characteristic hook, or uncus, at its antero-inferior tip.

The parietal lobe represents discriminative somesthetic sensations. Lesions of it induce such clinical disturbances as deficient two-point discrimination, faulty recognition of forms and shapes of objects placed in the hand (astereognosia), and loss of position sense—all of these on the side of the body opposite to the lesion. The parietal lobes also represent some motor functions and minor motor signs of a hemiplegic nature occur with parietal lesions.

The angular gyri of the parietal lobes are especially associated with visual cognitive functions. Lesions of the angular gyrus in the dominant hemisphere cause loss of visual word recognition (alexia) and inability to write (agraphia). This may be a failure to recognize whole words (verbal alexia), letters (literal alexia), or pictures, faces, objects, or any visual symbols. These defects are collectively known as visual agnosia and will be discussed in connection with lesions of the dominant hemisphere (see p. 271).

[259]

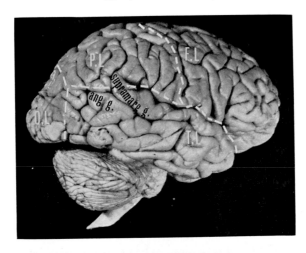

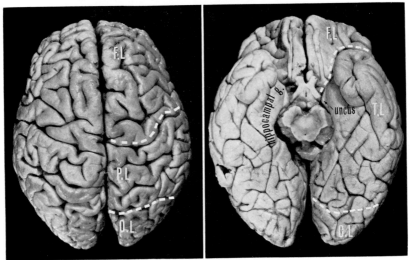

FIGURE 153. A. Lateral view of normal brain. B. Dorsal view of normal brain.
C. Ventral view of normal brain.

FL, frontal lobe; PL, parietal lobe; TL, temporal lobe; OL, occipital lobe.
Supramarginal gyrus; angular gyrus; uncus; hippocampal gyrus.

Visual agnosia is defined by Bender[102] as "a specific difficulty of
visual recognition for objects in the absence of elementary visuosensory deficits, aphasia, and mental deterioration. Agnosia is thus
interpreted as a perceptual disorder in patients with unimpaired
sensory functions."

While visual agnosia is an infrequent symptom in neurologic disease—or infrequently recognized—it causes the same behavior as is commonly seen in the blind, in babies and in animals which lack the visual clues for orientation. Thus, like the visual agnostics, blind persons depend on touch and sound for identification of objects and persons. Babies, during the first few months of life must feel and mouth all objects to learn their nature. And animals with poor visual acuity rely on sound and scent rather than vision to differentiate friend and foe (as all dog owners know). These do not have visual agnosia (which by definition requires normal perceptive mechanisms) but they show many of the same outward manifestations as visual agnostics.

The temporal lobe is concerned with basic auditory, olfactory, and perhaps equilibratory functions. It also represents complex functions of an integrative nature having to do with memory and visual pattern discrimination[814, 1032, 1172, 1301, 1133]. Lesions of the temporal lobe induce vertigo, confusion, loss of memory and often dream-like states[433]. Excitatory lesions cause characteristic auras of odors and tastes (uncinate fits). In addition, the temporal lobe of the dominant hemisphere represents sensory and motor functions concerned with speech. The speech area borders on the junction between frontal, parietal and temporal lobes (Broca's area). Lesions of Broca's area result in an inability to express appropriate words (motor aphasia) whereas lesions in the parieto-temporal area posterior to Broca's area result in failure to comprehend the spoken word (sensory aphasia).

Deep within the parieto-temporal lobes are the basal ganglia and thalami. In addition to the upper quadrantanopia due to involvement of the anterior portion of the visual radiation, or the complete hemianopia when the entire radiation is involved, lesions of the thalami and basal ganglia produce crossed hemihypesthesia, hemi-astereognosia, sometimes choreoathetotic movements, hemiataxia, and hemiparesis.

The arterial supply to the parieto-temporal area comes almost entirely from the middle cerebral artery (Figure 154). This area is thus involved in occlusion of the internal carotid system and with aneurysms at the bifurcation of the middle cerebral and posterior communicating arteries. The temporal isthmus, including its con-tained bundle of the geniculo-striate radiation, is believed to be

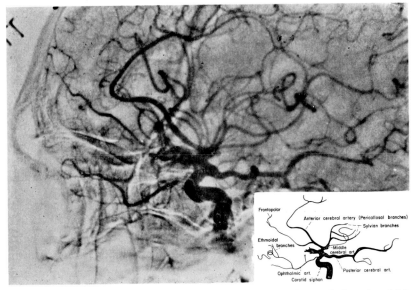

Figure 154. Normal arteriogram obtained by the subtraction technique in which the bony skull is faded out and the blood vessels stand out as dark silhouettes.

supplied in most persons by the anterior choroidal artery, and hemianopia (along with hemiplegia and hemianesthesia) has been reported from its occlusion (syndrome of the anterior choroidal artery)[461]. On the other hand this artery has been ligated in a number of persons (for choreoathetosis) without causing visual impairment[1046, 483, 390].

B. CHARACTER OF THE HEMIANOPIA

The most important symptom of parieto-temporal lobe lesions is hemianopia just as hemiplegia is the most important symptom of frontal lobe lesions. It is perhaps worth emphasizing, however, that the value of hemianopia as a localizing sign depends on the ability of the patient to make reliable observations and on the capacity of the examiner to make valid interpretations. With patients having parieto-temporal lobe lesions cooperation is often less than desirable.

No one criterion invariably distinguishes hemianopia of cerebral origin from that of tract origin, but the combination of associated signs and symptoms is usually sufficient to make differentiation possible. Optic atrophy points to a lesion of the tracts. Correlative reduction in visual acuity also suggests involvement of the tracts and chiasm, for hemianopia, even when complete, will not significantly reduce visual acuity if the lesion is unilateral and well behind the chiasm. Wernicke's hemianopic pupillary reaction is theoretically a sound means of differentiating a tract from a cerebral hemianopia but the problems involved in the intraocular scatter of light have, so far, prevented the widespread use of this as a practical test.

Hemianopias resulting from lesions in the parietal lobe are homonymous and usually symmetrical. They begin in the lower quadrants of the visual fields on the side opposite to the lesion. The field area about the point of fixation is usually spared. For a time the field defect may be that of an inferior quadranopia. Progression of the lesion is manifest by extension of the field defect into the upper quadrants and progression toward the point of fixation so that ultimately there is complete hemianopia with "splitting of the macula."

With lesions in the temporal lobe, on the other hand, the hemianopic defect begins in the upper quadrants[910, 832, 686, 834, 403]; it is often asymmetric[321, 1564, 686, 1445, 1163, 610] but similarly extends progressively throughout the rest of the field to result in complete hemianopia. The field defects with temporal lobe lesions, in comparison with those of the parietal lobe, are more apt to be sharply limited to one quadrant and to extend to the point of fixation[1552]. It should further be noted that insofar as the visual radiation (Meyer's loop) does not extend to the anteromost tip of the temporal lobe, there may be extensive involvement or even resection of this portion of the temporal lobe without causing a field defect[1267, 403, 707, 424]. Lesions of the anterior portion of Meyer's loop are said to cause the earliest visual field defects in the periphery adjacent to the vertical meridian[1552, 424, 497].

The significance of asymmetry in field defects for differentiating temporal lobe lesions from occipital lobe lesions has been both affirmed[610] and denied[1233, 403, 404, 424, 1552]. When asymmetrical the more extensive field defect may be in either eye[267] but is usually greater in the eye opposite the side of the lesion[546]. It is thought by many to be due to coincidental involvement of the optic tract[497]; unreliability of a patient's observation may also be a not inconsiderable factor[1565, 1163].

The degree to which a hemianopia is reversible can be ascertained with some degree of reliability (for partial hemianopias at least) by testing the edge of the defect with different sized test objects. The edge is said to be shallow, and inferred to be reversible, when different sized test objects reveal a considerable difference in the extent of the field defects. On the other hand, the edge is steep and irreversible when the field defect is approximately the same for all sizes of test objects. For this quantitative perimetry and campimetry it is necessary to control not only the size of the test object but the rate of its movement as well since the speed of oscillation will significantly influence the size of the field[427].

The question of "macular sparing" is a hardy perennial which has assumed, by the force of repetition, a prominence out of proportion to its actual importance. By macular sparing is meant the relative absence of hemianopic defects in the central and paracentral areas. The proposition that this sparing depends on bilateral representation of the maculæ through decussation of the corticopetal fibers in the chiasm or corpus callosum is without anatomic[1174, 46] or experimental[968] foundation. More tenable are the explanations that it is an artifact of testing[1482] or a relative sparing due to higher thresholds of visibility in the central region. Favoring the latter explanation is the abundant evidence that the sparing progressively decreases and eventually disappears completely with advance of the lesion. Whatever the explanation, sparing is most frequently seen with parietal or parieto-occipital lesions. It is less common with temporal lobe[1267] and occipital lobe lesions and is characteristically absent with the paracentral scotomas from lesions in the occipital pole.

Visual acuity, as tested by conventional means, is not affected by hemianopia. The resolving power of one half the macula is as good as that of the entire macula. Thus, when the acuity falls there is reason to suspect more than simple hemianopia. In such a case the lesion may be bilateral, if it is situated in the cerebrum, or it may involve both crossed and uncrossed fibers if it is situated in the region of the chiasm. On the other hand, of course, decrease in acuity may be due to some local ocular factor (such as papilledema) independent of the hemianopia.

Although hemianopias are sharply demarcated by the vertical meridian of the visual field, a curious tilting of the midline occasionally occurs. This has been reported after hemispheric injuries and is unexplained[1423].

One might expect that the simultaneous testing of corresponding points in the visual field would occasionally reveal an "extinction" field. Such is the case with other modalities of sensation; thus, simultaneous testing of touch on corresponding points of opposite sides of the body may extinguish the tactile sensation on the affected side in the presence of some parietal lobe lesions. A comparable repression of visual sensations on bilateral stimulation has been observed with geniculo-calcarine lesions[94] and has been claimed in the presence of frontal lobe lesions[1426, 603]; it also has its counterpart of "visual inattention" in monkeys subjected to unilateral frontal lobe ablation[779].

The phenomenon of extinction has been called pseudo-hemianopia[1325] and is characterized by lack of responsiveness on the affected side when corresponding portions of both visual fields are tested simultaneously. It is not a true hemianopia since each half of the field is full when tested separately.

> The analogy between touch and vision should, however, not be pushed too far since the tactile sensation is represented to some extent in both hemispheres whereas visual sensation is strictly unilateral. Thus the phenomenon of tactile extinction may simply mean a process which is occurring in one hemisphere whereas visual extinction may be a quite different process. Moreover, many cases which have been interpreted as visual extinction or pseudo-hemianopia might equally well have been instances of hemi-amblyopia.

C. SYMPTOMS RESULTING FROM HEMIANOPIA PER SE

The symptoms resulting from the hemianopia vary considerably. The patient may be quite unaware of the blind field. He may even deny his blindness when it is pointed out to him (see Anton's syndrome, p. 292).

The most common complaint of patients with hemianopia, aside from collision with objects on the blind side, is the difficulty in reading; the manner of this difficulty varies according to whether the hemianopia is on the right or left side. With hemianopias on the right side and a field defect that extends to the point of fixation, the patient is incapacitatingly slow in reading. He cannot see the words to the right of his point of fixation. On the other hand, patients with a left hemianopia, can read across a line with ease but have difficulty in finding the next line of print. Consequently they complain of skipping lines and getting mixed up in their reading.

Patients with hemianopia often observe, and sometimes complain, that they have a persistence of an after-image in the blind half of the field[98]. Thus, they will say that an arm drawn into the blind field continues to be visible even when the subsequent evidence indicates it was not there. This may give rise to the impression of multiple images[89]. The suggestion has even been made that this is analogous to perseveration in other spheres of neurologic diseases, but in this case called paliopsia[310] or palinopia[1423, 97]. A more likely explanation is that the patient receives no counter impression that the object has been withdrawn from the blind field and therefore "fills in" with what information is obtained from the seeing field just as the normal person fills in the blind spot[1534]. In other words, when the object of regard, such as the arm, is known to move into the blind field or, more likely, when the patient's eyes are moved so that an object is in the blind field, the patient continues to infer that the object is still present and calls it an after-image when he discovers that it is no longer present. Actually, no after-image is induced, as the original image is not visualized.

D. ASSOCIATED SIGNS AND SYMPTOMS

Some of the associated signs and symptoms occurring in patients with parieto-temporal lesions occur regardless of the side of the lesion; other signs and symptoms are specifically related to whether the lesion is in the dominant or non-dominant hemisphere.

1. Symptoms Common to Involvement of Either Hemisphere

(a) *Opticokinetic response.* This appears to be specifically defective with parietal lobe lesions and is manifest by a diminished or absent response with rotation of the objects of regard *toward* the side of the lesion whereas rotation of the objects toward the opposite side elicits a normal response. When this sign is positive, that is asymmetrical to the two sides, it often indicates a parietal lobe lesion[280, 1348] and may be usefully employed in differentiating a hemianopia of cerebral origin from one of tract origin.

While the parietal lobe appears to be the higher cerebral center associated with opticokinetic reflexes, lesions of the efferent pathways from the parietum to the pons will similarly decrease or eliminate the response. Thus, asymmetry of the opticokinetic reflex is found with lesions of the thalamus[1348] and an obliteration of the response to both sides is found with lesions of the pons.

The abnormal opticokinetic response does not depend on the hemianopia. As noted previously it is unaffected by hemianopia of tract origin and conversely, it may be positive, that is abnormal, with dorsal parietal lesions even when there is no involvement of the visual radiation. The defective response is presumably due, therefore, to interruption of parieto-efferent fibers innervating the conjugate motor mechanism.

(b) *Conjugate deviation of the eyes with forced closure of the lids.* This also is a sign pointing often to parietal lobe disease. It is elicited by asking the patient to forcibly close his lids while the examiner tries to open them. Patients with parietal lobe lesions show a deviation of the eyes to the side opposite the lesion instead of the usual Bell's phenomenon. Although this sign is a useful adjunctive bit of evidence for parietal localization, its value is somewhat lessened by the fact that it also occurs with some brain stem lesions and in a small number of normal persons.

(c) *Astereognosia, metamorphopsia and other sensory changes.* Astereognosia is a descriptive term denoting selective inability to recognize objects by the tactile sense. It is most easily detected by asking the patient to recognize coins or other objects (comb, pencil, keys) placed in his hands in such a way that he does not see them. Astereognosia is said to be present when there is a consistent difference in the two sides; it is characteristic of parietal lobe lesions to have a deficiency on the side opposite the lesion. Similarly vibration sense, two point discrimination, and position sense are often lost or diminished with parieto-temporal lesions, especially when the lesions are of acute onset and situated deep in the brain substance. Pain and temperature sense are, by comparison, less commonly affected but when they are involved the lesion is presumably deep.

Patients with astereognosia not only fail to recognize objects in their hands but are often unaware that they are holding an object. Thus the first symptom of a lesion in the deep parietal area is not infrequently an inadvertent dropping of an object such as a glass of water or a coin.

Metamorphopsia has also been described as a symptom of parietal disease[166, 167, 533]. Metamorphopsia is a general term to designate subjective distortion of objects. It is a common symptom of macular disease but may occur occasionally with parietal lesions. Its characteristic manifestations with cerebral diseases have, however, never been critically examined.

Patients with parietal lesions have been described as experiencing a tilting of vertical and horizontal lines[893, 95] and of seeing objects as though they were abnormally near or far off (teleopsia). These symptoms are linked with abnormal interpretations of size of objects, micropsia or macropsia[100, 101, 602,289, 1287]. Nevertheless too few observations have been documented to have, as yet, topographic significance other than to suggest a group of visuospatial symptoms resulting predominantly from parietal lobe lesions.

(d) *Confusion and lack of visual attention.* A sense of unreality, or derealization as it has been called, is a symptom common to lesions in many portions of the brain. However, a specific defect in attention to visual objects appears to be particularly common with parietotemporal lesions. This becomes apparent, and often frustrating, in doing visual fields, for the patient seems to be unable to fixate on one object while responding to another. It has been claimed that this is especially characteristic of lesions in the non-dominant hemisphere[679, 1117].

(e) *Photopsias, hallucinations, and illusions.* Photopsias, consisting of subjective flashes of light, are frequent accompaniments of lesions in the parietotemporal region. So are recurrent hallucinations, often reenacting a scene in the past life of the patient, phenomena which Penfield calls experiential responses associated with lesions of the temporal lobe[1131]. As visual counterparts of Jacksonian convulsions in the motor system, they are especially frequent with glial scars but also occur with tumors, especially those which are calcified. They may occur with vascular anomalies but are unusual in occlusive vascular accidents.

Hallucinations are frequently associated with hemianopia and it is often stated that in the brain posterior foci induce unformed flashes of light while anterior foci induce formed figures such as those of persons or objects[684, 1134, 697]. Exceptions to this generalization are common. The type of hallucination (and particularly the reaction of the patient to it) appear to be determined as much by the personality and experience of the individual[875] as by the site of origin[515]. Thus lesions of the parieto-temporal region may give rise to unformed flashes of light and simple designs, such as triangles, or they may give rise to complex figures such as familiar persons or specific scenes that trigger off illusions or paranoid ideas.

Loss of normal visual orientation is a major factor in the occurrence of visual hallucinations and illusions. Elderly persons, for instance, often develop major hallucinations or illusions on having their eyes blind-folded (as after an eye operation). Patients with genuine blindness are similarly susceptible to psychic disorders owing to their lack of visual orientation.

Suggestion often has a significant influence on the type of hallucination or illusion a blind or partially blind person may have. Thus one of our patients with hemianopia complained of seeing Santa Claus in his blind field; this was at Christmas time. He also thought he saw several washing machines while he was in a laundry when in fact there was only one. Another patient who was in a naval gunnery school when he developed symptoms from a porencephalic cyst interpreted his visual stimuli as "tracer bullets." These are what Penfield terms the interpretive responses (in contrast to experiential hallucinations)[1131].

It is important to differentiate hallucinations resulting from irritative foci which occur episodically and follow a stereotype pattern from the illusory visualization of objects resulting from either a misinterpretation of an organic stimulus or a psychogenic "filling in" of a blind field. In the case of most hallucinations resulting from irritative foci the visual phenomena are spontaneous occurrences and the objects visualized reproduce essentially the same patterns with little relation to the immediate environment. With illusory phenomena, on the other hand, there tends to be a projection of those objects or parts of objects into the blind field which are present in the seeing field. Thus illusions bear on the particular background of the time.

The hallucinations of the irritative variety are characteristically moving. The direction of the movement is usually from the blind side toward the seeing side. Some patients assert that the hemianopia clears up while they are hallucinating.

One form of hallucination that has distinct localizing value is the so-called uncinate fit. This points to a lesion of the inferomedial portion of the temporal lobe with involvement of the uncus. It is characterized by strong and often unpleasant odors, with chewing movements and a dazed expression.

Another form is called peduncular hallucinosis because it occurs with lesions at the base of the brain in the region of the peduncles; it occurs with lesions of the midbrain in the vicinity of the medial aspects of the temporal lobes[904, 1245, 1327]. The hallucinations consist of geometric patterns and designs, often brightly colored, moving continuously in kaleidoscopic fashion. They occur independent of the patient's will and cannot be modified. They are not associated with fear or anxiety and sometimes amuse the patient. They usually occur at the time of sleep (vesperal hallucinations) and have been likened to dreams with involvement of the sleep center. Peduncular hallucinosis may result from vascular, neoplastic, or inflammatory lesions; the hallucinations with some sedatives (barbituates) may also fall into this category[1245].

(f) *Convulsive episodes.* As with cortical lesions anywhere in the cerebrum those in the parieto-temporal region may induce seizures. They are usually ushered in with deviation of the eyes to the side opposite the lesion. Often this is associated with subjective visual phenomena projected in the area toward which the eyes are turned. Of course seizures that are generalized from the onset have no focal significance. Seizures frequently result from glial scars (especially when calcified) and sometimes from tumors (especially benign tumors[101]) but occasionally result from vascular accidents (Figure 155).

(g) *Brain stem compression and herniation.* Any expansive lesion of the supratentorial region may cause herniation of the hippocampus through the tentorium with consequent compression of the brain stem. The most common signs of brain stem compression are decreasing levels of consciousness, mydriasis, nystagmus, internuclear ophthalmoplegia, oculomotor palsy, dysarthria, respiratory

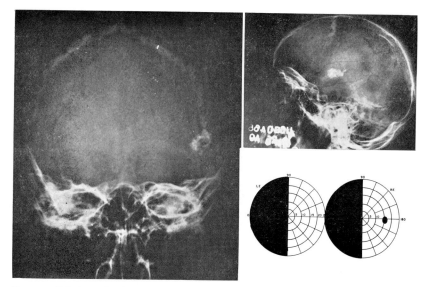

FIGURE 155 A & B. Calcified mass of the right parieto-temporal area and left homonymous hemianopia in a patient with convulsions. The lesion was presumed to be a calcified hematoma.

distress and blindness (when the posterior cerebral arteries are compressed). These symptoms may divert the examiner's attention away from the responsible lesions in the cerebral hemispheres[691, 1089].

Mydriasis is a particularly significant sign (sometimes the only sign) of direct pressure from masses in the temporal lobe or from tentorial herniation[1192]. This sign is particularly valuable with herniations due to subdural hematomas; the mydriasis is usually, but not always, on the side of the lesion[956, 1143].

2. Signs and Symptoms Associated with Lesions of the Dominant Hemisphere

Along with other forms of aphasia resulting from lesions in the dominant parietal lobe, the visual cognitive functions are often specifically impaired[1209, 421]. Most common is the loss of comprehension of the written word and consequent inability to read (Figure 156). This defect, called *alexia,* varies in degree and often shows curious paradoxes whereby understanding of simple words is lost but that for complex words is retained. Sometimes the patient is able to write on dictation but is then unable to read what he has written[753]. To

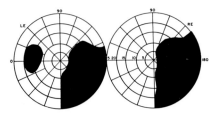

Figure 156. Incomplete right homonymous hemianopia resulting from an infiltrative glioma in the left parieto-temporal region. The patient was a forty-six year old school teacher whose initial symptom was inability to think of the correct word for objects that had been familiar to her (sensory aphasia). This was followed by loss of interpretation of the written word (alexia) and loss of ability to write (agraphia) although she could copy letters or charts adequately. Her auditory comprehension was normal.

manifest pure alexia the patient must have normal recognition for the spoken word and of course must have sufficiently good visual acuity to see what he is trying to read. This latter may be proved by having the patient copy words and letters even though he may not understand their meaning. With progressive alexia the loss of comprehension of words is followed by the loss of recognition of letters (literal alexia) and eventually of numbers (numeral alexia). Alexia is often but not always associated with loss of ability to write (agraphia); and sometimes loss of color perception[1380, 106, 1535]. Failure to recognize faces (prosopagnosia[137]) also occurs as a separate and unique symptom[431, 962, 245]. Alexia generally results from lesions in the region of the angular gyrus and it is one of the most sharply localizable of cerebral symptoms (Figures 157 and 158).

It should be noted that the term dyslexia has come to have a meaning distinct from alexia. Whereas alexia is a specific form of agnosia, dyslexia covers a variety of reading disabilities that may be either perceptual or motor (or even functional) in origin[1117]. It is a less specific term than alexia (for discussion of dyslexia see p. 312).

Alexia without agraphia occurs in patients who have an intact angular gyrus but who have a unilateral occipital lobe lesion in the dominant hemisphere and an associated lesion of the splenium (usually due to posterior cerebral artery occlusion). Such patients retain their ideational visualization of words (owing to the intact angular gyrus) and therefore can write, but words that are seen in the non-dominant visual field do not have access to the interpretive

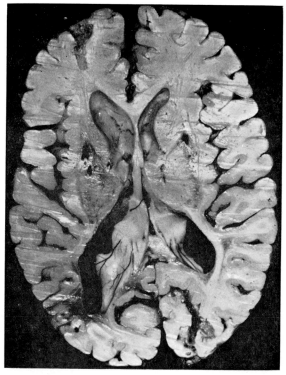

FIGURE 157. Scar formation in left parieto-occipital area resulting from vascular occlusive disease. The patient was a sixty-six year old teacher whose outstanding symptoms and signs had been alexia, dressing apraxia, and right sided homonymous hemianopia.

centers in the dominant hemisphere (owing to the interruption in the splenium) and are therefore meaningless[352, 531]. This comprises a syndrome of alexia without agraphia. It is always vascular in origin but a less complete form of the syndrome may be demonstrated in patients from sectioning the corpus callosum and limiting test words to the left visual field[1447, 998].

A "tactile alexia" consisting of inability to recognize forms of letters presented to the palm of one's left hand results from sectioning the anterior part of the corpus callosum[532]. Bilateral parietal or dominant parietal lesions have been similarly found to underlie the dyslexia in Braille readers[313].

A neurologic syndrome allied to alexia and often associated with

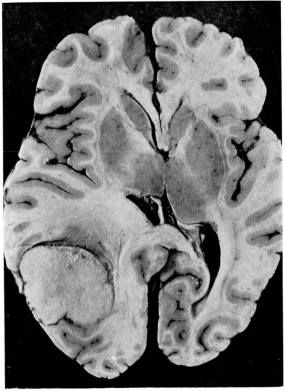

FIGURE 158. Meningioma causing severe compression of the left parieto-occipital region. The patient was a sixty-two year old woman who had had intermittent alexia for several weeks. On examination she was found to comprehend letters but not simple words. Other noteworthy findings were a right homonymous hemianopia and bilateral papilledema. While being prepared for surgery she suddenly developed brain-stem herniation and expired. Autopsy revealed a circumscribed meningioma.

it and with homonymous hemianopia is Gerstman's syndrome[528, 529, 530]. This syndrome, also due to lesions in the region of the dominant angular gyrus[640, 311], consists of inability to write (agraphia), inability to do serial number problems (acalculia), failure to recognize the "belongingness" of one's fingers lesion (finger agnosia[530]), and confusion between right and left sides[31, 1005]. These are, however, significant symptoms only when there is relatively good preservation of other intellectual spheres of activity; they should not be confounded with a generalized stupor or global (massive) aphasia.

Other neurologic symptoms often associated with alexia and characteristic of lesions of the dominant hemisphere are sensory and motor aphasia. The former, characterized by lack of comprehension of appropriate words, is due to parietal involvement while the latter, characterized by loss of ability to use the appropriate word in the presence of intact comprehension, is due to involvement of Broca's area on the dorsal lip of the sylvian fissure.

3. Signs and Symptoms Associated with Lesions of the Non-dominant Hemisphere

Lesions in the region of the angular gyrus of the non-dominant hemisphere induce a different type of visual disorientation. These may be termed forms of topographic agnosia or atopognosia in which the patient loses recognition of what had been familiar territory[1278, 1181, 166, 311, 625, 422] or loses his ability either to reconstruct geographic and geometric diagrams from the abstract[365, 951, 373] or to synthesize parts of a diagram into a whole pattern[620, 1117]. The parietal area is necessary for the "synthesis" or "summation" of spatial dimensions into formed perception[359]. Lesions of it result in disturbances of visuo-spatial cognition[951]. It is as though lesions of the non-dominant parietal area disrupted a person's relationship to his environment whereas comparable lesions in the dominant hemisphere, by contrast, caused a disorientation within his own anatomic relationships[530].

Thus a patient with a lesion in the non-dominant parieto-temporal area will become lost in commuting between two points with which he was formerly familiar; he may lose his way about his house or become confused in the positional arrangements of knobs on the dashboard of his car or buttons on his clothing. Occasionally he will become oriented if someone turns him in the proper direction, but he loses his ability to orient himself.

Although some authors state that topographic agnosia as here described is characteristic of bilateral lesions[1563, 678, 680, 1159] or lesions of the dominant occipital lobe[397, 73] it is most common with lesions of the parietal lobe in the non-dominant hemisphere.

In many of our male patients over the age of sixteen who had a lesion in the non-dominant parietotemporal area, one of the earliest indications was an auto accident. This was not the case with patients having a comparable lesion in the opposite hemisphere or in patients with tract lesions on the same side. Hence the incidence of auto accidents does not seem to be due to the hemianopia per se but rather to a defective judgment of relative distances or spatial relationships.

Associated with topographic agnosia is the loss or impairment of the ability to construct a diagram[952, 373]. Thus diagramming what was a familiar floor plan becomes an impossibility and the patient's diagram of a clock or the petals of a daisy is accompanied by characteristic disarray of the left side of the drawing (Figure 159).

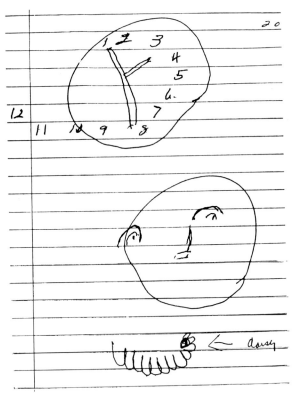

FIGURE 159. Constructional apraxia in a patient with a vascular lesion in the non-dominant parieto-occipital area. Attempts to draw the face of a clock or the face of a person showed primarily a neglect of the left side.

The patient was a sixty-six year old man who suddenly developed a "blackout" with loss of his way (spatial disorientation). His symptoms subsided within a few hours but subsequent examination disclosed a complete left homonymous hemianopia and constructional apraxia.

The numbers on the left side of the clock may be streamed out away from the face of the clock and the petals on the left side of the daisy may be lacking altogether. The patient is often unable to arrange match sticks to accord with a prescribed pattern[893, 95, 906, 101]. One of our patients persistently held her reading matter upside down without being aware of the irregularity. Other cases of inversion of vision have been described[1568, 661, 1136, 812]. Assembling a puzzle may be especially difficult. Attempts at bisecting a line or cutting a strip of paper in two result in a characteristic shortening of the left side. Setting a table may result in a regular tilting of the knives and forks to one side[951]. These defects are collectively called *constructional apraxia* or constructive disability[1117]. This was first described by Kleist[800] in war injuries but has been documented many times since[1546, 1005]. Insight into the deficiency is generally poor and it is a matter of semantics whether these symptoms fall into the category of agnosias or true apraxias.

Commonly associated with these lesions of the non-dominant hemisphere is a difficulty in dressing[166, 623, 1118, 1242, 951]. The patient has particular difficulty in getting clothes on to the left side of his body. He does not seem to be able to tell which is the left arm or leg hole; which way is up; or to differentiate between front and back. The total difficulty is called *dressing apraxia*. A variant of this was demonstrated in one of our patients who, along with dressing apraxia, was particularly distressed that he could not properly place his dental bridge in his mouth.

Failure to recognize faces (prosopagnosia) is a symptom occurring occasionally in conjunction with spatial agnosia in patients with lesions of the non-dominant hemisphere[1107, 1144, 624, 245].

While no concerted effort has been made to measure stereopsis, incidental observations have indicated that a deficiency in stereopsis or faulty projection is present with either bilateral parietal lesions[678, 430] or parietal lesions in the non-dominant hemisphere[1206, 1004, 1117, 430, 289] (Figure 160). Many patients relate that they miss objects reached for, have difficulty in lighting a cigarette, cannot judge the distance of the test chart or pour coffee into a cup. Other symptoms are teleopsia wherein objects seem abnormally far away, as though looking through the wrong end of a telescope, and micropsia wherein objects are interpreted as being abnormally small.

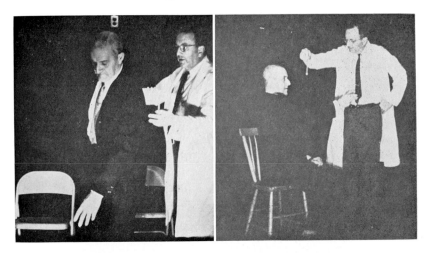

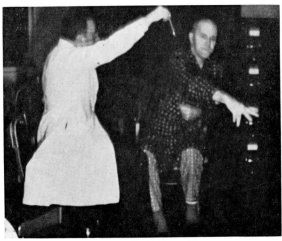

FIGURE 160. Faulty spatial perception manifested by a patient with metastatic carcinoma in the parietal regions. Although able to see the chair in front of him the patient was unable to localize it in space or to grasp a pencil held up before him.

An occasional symptom with lesions of the non-dominant pareito-temporal region is that which has been called *neglect of the left side*[762, 1117, 951, 422]. Patients may leave food on the left side of their plate or, as previously mentioned, leave the left half of drawings incomplete. This might be thought to be due to the hemianopia but is probably more subtle than this since it is not so apparent with lesions in the dominant hemisphere; nor does it occur with hemianopias of tract origin. Moreover it can be demonstrated that patients see the object when the stimulus is presented in that field only but fail to see it when there is simultaneous stimulation of a corresponding point in the opposite field[1117].

Thus while lesions of the parietal area in the dominant hemisphere cause primarily language disturbances, those in the non-dominant hemisphere cause topographic agnosias[373, 629]. The former may be more conspicuous, but the subtle disturbances with lesions of the non-dominant hemisphere may be more incapacitating. A comparison of the higher visual functions in the right and left halves of the brain has indicated that patients with spatial disturbances were more refractory to rehabilitation[763] and had greater difficulty in identification of unfamiliar objects[1592].

4. Signs and Symptoms with Bilateral Lesions of the Parieto-temporal Area

Bilateral hemispheric lesions will generally result in more profound and more lasting symptoms than do unilateral lesions. Many visual interpretive functions have bilateral representation. This bilaterality varies, as does handedness, among different persons so that lesions of one hemisphere produce variably severe deficits but lesions of corresponding areas in both hemispheres always result in severe and relatively uncompensatable symptoms.

From an historical point of view the case of Valerie Clem reported in 1888 by the French ophthalmologist, Jules Badal[53], has interest in being the first recorded patient with (presumably) bilateral parietal lobe disease[106]. Valerie was a thirty-one-year-old woman who developed septic lesions of both parietal areas following pregnancy. She had all the symptoms attributable to lesions of the dominant hemisphere now known as Gerstman's syndrome (alexia, agraphia, right-left confusion, dyscalculia) and those other symptoms now attributable to lesions of the non-dominant hemisphere (inability to find her way about familiar surroundings, constructional apraxia, difficulty in dressing, and faulty stereopsis). In addition there were bilateral defects in the visual fields.

Some syndromes have been associated only with bilateral lesions.

One of these is a complex of visual perceptive defects and ocular motor disturbance known as *Balint's syndrome*[61] believed to be due to biparietal lesions. Patients with this syndrome are unaware of objects and persons in their environment which would be noticed by a normal person[1269]. They also lack full voluntary control of their eye movements while having normal random movements, a phenomenon termed ocular motor apraxia[268].

Bitemporal lobectomy in monkeys results in what appears to be loss of visual attentiveness, as occurs in the Klüver-Bucy syndrome[814, 1031, 1028, 10]. The animals no longer show the excitement and aggressive reaction to visual threats as they did prior to the operation. The same effect may be produced with unilateral temporal lobectomy if the animal views the objects or persons in the corresponding visual field[384].

Global visual agnosia in otherwise alert patients may occur with bilateral lesions deep in the parieto-temporal lobes. An impressive instance of this occurred in one of our patients who had stereotactic electrodes implanted in both amygdaloid areas to localize the trigger zone of psychomotor epilepsy. As soon as she could be tested after surgery she was found unable to identify objects (tooth brush, mirror, magazine) except by touch and was unable to recognize persons who should have been familiar to her (members of her family and physicians who repeatedly visited her) except by the sound of their voices. When asked to identify the door in her room she gazed at the window for a moment and then at the door saying "that is it because I hear through it the nurses' voices in the corridor outside."

E. ETIOLOGY OF PARIETO-TEMPORAL LESIONS

Static examination of the visual functions gives ordinarily little information as to the etiology of the lesions but the course of the disease is often most suggestive. Sudden onset is presumptive evidence of a vascular lesion (Figure 161) (see "Apoplexy Aphorisms," p. 299). Thromboses may give premonitory symptoms with periods of improvement and worsening occurring over a period of several days[3]. When associated with unilateral blackouts in one eye and hemiplegic and hemianopic signs on the opposite side of the body, an underlying carotid occlusion is suspect and ophthalmodynamometry is indicated

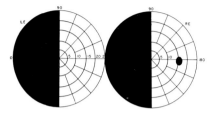

FIGURE 161. Hematoma in the non-dominant *(right)* parietal area. The patient was a fifty-three year old man who suddenly developed severe pain in his head and spatial disorientation. Examination showed complete homonymous hemianopia on the left side.

(see p. 36). On the other hand, sudden and complete hemianopia and hemiplegia with collapse at the onset point especially to hemorrhage in the region of the internal capsule. Embolism is suggested by symptoms occurring suddenly in a person with cardiac or pulmonary disease (rheumatic or arteriosclerotic heart disease, bacterial endocarditis, myocardial infarction or septic focus in the lungs). A sudden onset, however, is not necessarily indicative of a simple vascular accident, for tumors sometimes give rise to abrupt symptoms.

Much of the visual radiation in the parieto-temporal region is supplied by the middle cerebral artery. Aside from the visual and somesthetic effects resulting from occlusion of this artery, one often has hemiplegic signs as well. Occlusion of the middle cerebral artery leads to predominant involvement of the arm and face (whereas occlusion of the anterior cerebral artery leads to predominant involvement of the leg).

Subdural hematomas follow a head injury with fracture of the skull but they may occasionally occur spontaneously. They localize preferentially over the convexity of the hemispheres and produce headache, hemianopia, confusion and coma[971, 569]. In such cases angiography reveals an avascular space adjacent to the cranial vault. The traumatic etiology of subdural hematomas is often obscured by the trivial nature of the injury and by the occasionally long period (weeks) between the injury and onset of symptoms. Sometimes the brain stem signs predominate with little evidence pointing to the cerebral hemispheres[1089]. In such cases the uncus and hippocampus presumably herniate through the tentorium cerebelli.

Whereas subdural hematomas result from venous bleeding with

tears of the bridging veins entering the dural sinuses and usually require days for their evolution, epidural hematomas result from arterial bleeding, most often from fractures involving the middle meningeal artery, and produce symptoms within a matter of minutes or a few hours. The epidural hematomas occur most often in children (especially after bicycle injuries) and cause prompt hemiplegia, coma, and dilatation of the homolateral pupil.

Less well recognized are the vascular accidents resulting from occlusion of the parieto-occipital veins. These vessels leave the convexity of the cerebral hemispheres and enter the superior saggital sinus[1092]. They become thrombosed in the course of various diseases characterized by an increased tendency for blood clotting, and produce unilateral or bilateral field defects in association with parietal lobe signs. The field defects are reversible even after complete surgical transection of the veins[1548].

Gradual onset of symptoms is suggestive of neoplastic origin. Neoplasm is especially likely when the symptoms include headache, increased spinal fluid pressure and elevated spinal fluid protein. Papilledema is presumptive evidence of a tumor but it may also result from bleeding into the subarachnoid or subdural space or from simple obstructive hydrocephalus and meningeal hydrops. Scintillating scotomas with parietal lesions and formed hallucinations with temporal lesions are not common occurrences with tumors but they are more frequent with tumors than with vascular accidents.

Temporal lobe tumors are prone to give rise to third nerve palsy, midbrain signs and occasionally hypothalamic signs. Thus ptosis, anisocoria, palsies of vertical gaze, and drowsiness are frequent. Moreover, temporal lobe tumors are particularly prone to cause acute and serious compression of the brain stem by herniation through the tentorium[1192]. Lumbar punctures and ventriculograms have been known to precipitate such a catastrophe.

Tumors affecting the parieto-temporal region are those common to the central nervous system. These are predominantly the intrinsic astrocytomas and glioblastomas and the extrinsic meningiomas. Metastases, by way of the lungs, also occur. The astrocytomas are slow growing, localized tumors which give rise to focal symptoms of either an irritative or paralytic variety. The glioblastomas are more diffuse and infiltrative (Figure 162); although they give rise to localized symptoms they are found at post-mortem to be much more

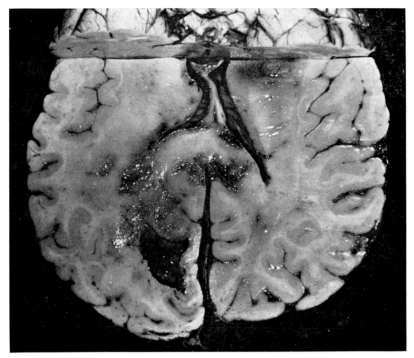

FIGURE 162. Glioblastoma multiforme in non-dominant *(right)* parietal area. Brain is viewed from ventral surface. The patient was a fifty year old woman whose presenting symptoms were erratic driving, loss of way in a previously familiar neighborhood, and a feeling of unreality about her household furniture. Examination showed a complete homonymous hemanopia on the left side.

widespread than might have been anticipated on the basis of the symptoms. The patient with glioblastoma is apt to be stuporous and to show more of a general depression of mentation than is the patient with a more circumscribed glioma.

Meningiomas affecting the parieto-temporal region have sites of predilection for either the sylvian fissure causing temporal lobe symptoms, or the parasagittal regions causing bilateral parietal lobe symptoms. More than other tumors of the parieto-temporal area, meningiomas are apt to cause convulsions. Since they are slow growing and the brain can adjust considerably to their size, they may attain massive dimensions before giving rise to significant symptoms. Papilledema may thus be the presenting sign while visual defects may be absent or slight[811].

Hemangiomas, arteriovenous anomalies, and aneurysms often make themselves manifest first by hemorrhage; they may then simulate strokes. An angioma is always suspect when a young person develops the signs and symptoms of a cerebrovascular accident or subarachnoid hemorrhage. In the case of parieto-temporal lobe lesions, vascular accidents are characterized by sudden headache and loss of consciousness followed by hemianopia, hemiplegia, and other focal signs. On the other hand these vascular lesions may cause symptoms by direct pressure or by cerebral ischemia and present with convulsions or migrainoid attacks[417] (Figure 163).

While diagnosis of a tumor affecting the parieto-temporal region may be inferred from the course, associated signs and symptoms, and

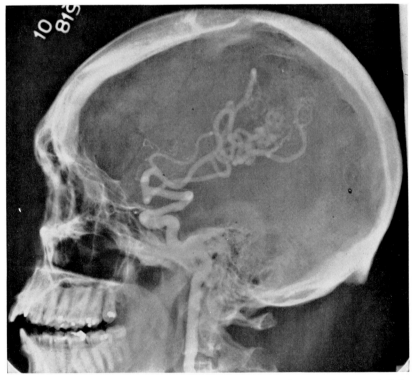

FIGURE 163. Anomalous vascular plexus in the left parietal region revealed by arteriography. The patient was a thirty-two year old man who had had intermittent convulsions, right sided paresthesias, and garbled speech for several years. Prior to these attacks he had had subjective flashes of light. The visual fields were full.

findings in the cerebrospinal fluid, the more definitive tests are x-rays, electroencephalography, and radioactive scanning procedures. Routine skull x-rays may reveal the bony changes associated with meningiomas but x-rays are ordinarily less informative with gliomatous tumors. An exception is the oligodendroglioma which is often calcified. Shift of the pineal gland, which is evident normally by reason of its calcification, is always suggestive of a lateralized mass. Most helpful are air studies and arteriograms which may reveal deformation of the injected air mass or injected opaque material. Electroencephalography and radioactive scanning procedures are helpful but discussion of them is beyond the scope of this text.

Demyelinative lesions in the parieto-temporal lobe usually induce hemianopia and general confusion with a paucity of other symptoms referable to this area. Multiple sclerosis is often accompanied by internuclear ophthalmoplegia or other manifestations of brain stem and cord lesions. Schilder's disease and other forms of diffuse sclerosis may begin with homonymous hemianopia or develop it early in the course of the disease. The symptoms associated with widespread loss of white matter progress over a period of months or at the most a few years, resulting in cerebral blindness and dementia (Figure 164). Optic atrophy is often present but incomplete and the blindness is usually greater than can be accounted for on the basis of involvement of these lower visual pathways alone.

The diffuse demyelinative disease which may cause lesions in the parieto-temporal (and occipital) regions may be divided into the following types.

1. *Schilder's type.* This is acute, like multiple sclerosis, and is characterized by conspicuous accumulation of sudanophilic lipids in the brain. In comparison with multiple sclerosis, however, it is more steadily progressive and causes various degrees of blindness and dementia[1401]; it usually leads to death within a few years. Although occurring predominently in children it is not generally familial; many of the familial cases recorded in the earlier literature were subsequently found to be instances of metachromatic leucodystrophy.

2. *Pelizaeus-Merzbacher type.* This is a slowly progressive disease beginning in early childhood and leading to spasticity, epilepsy, and sometimes hemianopia but is more apt to induce symptoms referable to the spinal cord and brain stem (nystagmus, head

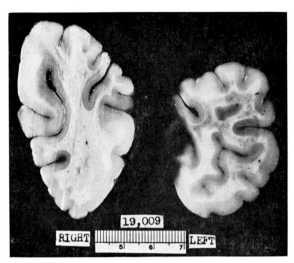

FIGURE 164. Diffuse loss of white matter with Schilder's disease. The patient was a fifteen year old boy who had initially complained of blurred vision and bumping into objects on his left side. Objects seemed far away and indistinct. Examination disclosed a complete left homonymous hemianopia. Over the subsequent weeks the patient became progressively demented with particular sensory impairment on the left side. The patient died following exploratory craniotomy.

nodding, and ataxia). Pathologically there is loss of white matter but little demonstrable lipid (presumably because of its chronicity).

3. *Krabbe type*[829]. This also begins usually in childhood, is familial, and characterized by widespread loss of white matter from the cerebral hemispheres. Its most distinctive characteristic is the histologic finding of globoid cells in the brain containing a non-sudanophilic lipid[327].

4. *Metachromatic leucoencephalopathy (sulfatidosis*[48]*)*. This appears to be a primary disease of the white matter with widespread involvement elsewhere in the body, but loss of vision is a relatively late manifestation (for retinal and optic nerve involvement see p. 163).

5. *Progressive multifocal leucoencephalopathy*. This fifth type has come to be recognized in the past few years as an infrequent complication of lymphatic leukemia, Hodgkin's disease and sarcoidosis[44, 1344, 374, 1320]. The pathologic process consists of patchy lesions of the white matter. Unlike multiple sclerosis but like certain viral infections of animals these lesions are not perivascular[1507].

6. *Spongy degeneration of the brain* (thought to be an edema

from faulty hemato-encephalic barrier[145, 1016]) also causes spasticity, blindness and dementia but the visual defects are usually subordinate to the vast involvement of the entire nervous system[1016,129]. In this condition there may, however, be papilledema from increased intracranial pressure.

Hemianopia or blindness occuring from demyelinative lesions in the cerebrum are of serious portent. On occasion they may clear up spontaneously but more commonly than with demyelinative plaques elsewhere the visual symptoms are prodromal of a progressive process that culminates in death within a matter of months.

SUMMARY

The parietotemporal region is that portion of the cerebral hemispheres bounded anteriorly and inferiorly by the rolandic and sylvian fissures and posteriorly by the occipital lobe. Aside from containing some of the most dorsal fibers of the visual radiation the parietal lobe represents certain visual cognitive functions. Interpretation of the written language and probably other visual symbols are represented in the area of the angular and supramarginal gyri of the dominant hemisphere whereas interpretation of visuospatial relationships are represented in the corresponding parts of the non-dominant hemisphere.

Hemianopia is, when present, an important symptom of lesions in the parieto-temporal region. In contrast to the hemianopia with lesions of the pregeniculate pathways, that due to lesions in the hemispheres is not accompanied by optic atrophy, reduced visual acuity, or pupillary abnormality. Lesions of the parietal lobe cause initially a visual defect in the lower fields while those in the temporal lobe cause a defect in the upper fields. Despite the normal visual acuity a hemianopia that comes to the point of fixation causes particular difficulty in reading. A person with complete right sided hemianopia stumbles in his reading because he cannot anticipate ensuing words whereas a person with left sided hemianopia loses his place in jumping from one line to the next.

The associated signs and symptoms are most important in evaluating a hemianopia of parieto-temporal origin. The opticokinetic response is characteristically impaired with parietal disease as the objects in the visual field are moved toward the side of the lesion. Deviation of the eyes to the contralateral side with forced closure of the lids is also a characteristic sign of parietal disease. Unilateral astereognosia is a standard symptom with lesions in the opposite parietal lobe. Photopsia, hallucinations, and illusions occur occasionally as the visual counterpart of epileptic discharges, but they have little topical significance. True convulsive deviations of the eye also occur occasionally with parieto-temporal lesions; these are frequently premonitory of convulsive movements of the hand on the side toward which the gaze is directed and sometimes of generalized convulsions. Brain stem compression and herniation through the tentorium are especially frequent with masses of the temporal lobe.

Lesions of the parieto-temporal region on the dominant side cause characteristically alexia, other forms of aphasia and particularly an assembly of symptoms known as Gerstman's syndrome: agraphia, acalculia, lack of recognition of one's own anatomic parts, and a confusion of right-left sidedness. Lesions of the non-dominant hemisphere cause particularly a form of visual disorientation that has been termed topographic agnosia. This is manifest by a significant loss of one's way, a failure to construct simple abstract patterns and a difficulty in dressing.

All forms of visual agnosia are more profound and more lasting when the parieto-temporal lesions are bilateral. In addition some disturbances, such as is seen in Balint's syndrome, occur only in the presence of bilateral disease. These patients lack both visual recognition and voluntary control of eye movements.

Parieto-temporal lesions may be vascular (either obstruction of the middle cerebral artery, aneurysm or subdural hemorrhage), neoplastic (especially glioma, meningioma and vascular anomalies) or demyelinative (diffuse sclerosis is more characteristic than multiple sclerosis).

CHAPTER XV

OCCIPITAL LOBES

A. ANATOMY AND FUNCTION

THE OCCIPITAL LOBES comprise the posterior portions of the cerebral hemispheres (Figures 128 and 153). Demarcated on their medial surfaces by the parieto-occipital fissures, each occipital lobe merges into the parietal and temporal lobe on the lateral surface of the brain without distinct anatomic landmarks.

Each occipital lobe is divided into three areas, numbered by Brodman's schema 17, 18 and 19 according to the cellular organization of the cortex. Area 17, also called the striate area, is situated at the posterior pole but extends forward to border on the calcarine fissure. It represents the terminus of the visual radiation and cut sections of its cortex reveal the myelinated tract of association fibers, the line of Gennari, from which it gets the name, striate cortex. Area 18, called the parastriate portion, lies just outside Area 17 while Area 19, the peristriate portion, separates Area 18 from the parietal and temporal lobes.

Some functions may be ascribed to these primarily anatomic divisions with a fair degree of confidence. Other functions have been ascribed to them on a speculative basis. Area 17 is obviously concerned with reception of the primary visual stimulus. Unilateral removal of this area causes degeneration of all cells in the homolateral geniculate body[1179]. The intracortical association tract, which is more conspicuous here than elsewhere in the brain, presumably serves to associate corresponding and non-corresponding points in the retinas of the two eyes[1163]. It offers the first evidence of anatomic correlation between the two eyes for stereopsis, retinal rivalry, and other aspects of binocular coordination[801, 1228]. Area 18 is believed to synthesize the visual impressions, received in Area 17, and has abundant commissural connections with corresponding areas in the opposite hemisphere[1062] but only limited direct connections outside the occipital lobes. Area 19, on the other hand, is involved with the rest of the brain[1132] and integrates visual impressions with hearing, speech, and other functions of the sensorium as well as serving for visual memory[719]. In addition to fiber connections within the cerebrum the visual cortex has efferent fiber connections with the thalami, superior colliculi and pons[108].

Area 17 may thus be considered a visual perceptive portion of the brain whereas Areas 18 and 19, collectively designated as the prestriate area[872], are concerned with visual patterns[5], visual associations[719] and possibly with visual motor functions[1573]. Evidence in the monkey, presumably applicable to man, suggests, however, that these occipital areas are not concerned with perception of color or visuospatial orientation[872].

The calcarine fissures (Figure 128) are convenient landmarks on the medial surface of the hemispheres separating upper from lower portions of the visual field. The occiput has a point to point representation with the retina in which the calcarine fissure corresponds to the horizontal raphé of the retina[1163, 1561]. Central visual functions, represented in the maculas occupy the posterior poles of the occipital lobes but extend anteriorly along the calcarine fissure. The peripheral visual functions occupy the zone between the calcarine gyri and the parastriate area[1362]. Noteworthy are the large areas in the cerebral hemispheres representing central visual functions as compared with the small areas in the retinas representing central visual functions.

Blood supply to the occiput is derived almost entirely from the paired posterior cerebral arteries which are the terminal branches of the basilar artery. These posterior cerebral arteries arise at the anterior end of the pons and give off branches to some internal structures of the cerebrum (the posterior choroidal artery) and connect through the posterior communicating artery with the circle of Willis.

B. SYMPTOMS

The one and only reliable sign of occipital disease is hemianopia. This is homonymous and meticulously symmetrical in the two eyes[637, 1565, 1163] (although it is said to be asymmetrical in some traumatic cases[1422]). Characteristic of posterior lesions is involvement of the point of fixation[697]; this is the opposite of macular sparing. Indeed, homonymous paracentral scotomas with apices at the points of fixation are pathognomonic of occipital pole disease[93] (Figure 165). Equally characteristic of occipital lesions is absence of neurologic and neuro-ophthalmic symptoms other than visual (although pain in the homo-lateral eye occurs with some vascular accidents). The opticokinetic response is symmetrical, unless the parietal lobe is involved, and there is no deviation of the eyes with forced closure of the lids. Nor has a difference in the symptomatology been associated with sidedness of the lesion, except for the lateralization of the hemianopia. Anterior lesions that also involve the parietal area may, of course, cause alexia when situated on the dominant side or topographic agnosia when situated on the non-dominant side but these always indicate extension of the lesion beyond the confines of the occiput.

Although true hallucinations are infrequent with occipital lesions, flashes of light occur occasionally and are said to be present in approximately 5 per cent of all epileptics prior to a convulsion[720]. One of the regular characteristics of these subjective phenomena is that they are moving, either toward or away from the point of fixation, whence they are frequently likened to kaleidoscopes or shooting stars. Occasionally they are colored. Certain types of lesions are especially apt to be accompanied by these subjective phenomena: they are common with glial scars, occasional with vascular anomalies, but rarely seen with tumors. At times they may be associated with in-voluntary deviation of the eyes toward the site of the projected photopsia and occasionally they constitute aura preceding a Jacksonian convulsion.

A characteristic zig-zag or picket-fence flashing is seen prior to a migraine hemianopia. This is generally attributed to arterial spasm in the occipital lobe and may be accompanied by brain stem[120, 292]

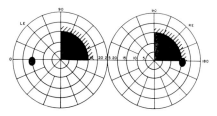

FIGURE 165. Homonymous paracentral scotomas characteristic of a lesion of the occipital pole. The patient was a fifty-two year old woman whose presenting complaint was "cannot read fast." Surgery disclosed a metastatic tumor.

or other focal[1305] signs, but it is curious that no similar phenomenon is commonly associated with non-migrainous lesions of the occiput. Yet migrainoid symptoms, followed by prolonged and sometime permanent[1200] hemianopia, do occasionally occur with arteriovenous anomalies[1194, 369], less commonly with aneurysms[493, 398, 1239], and sometimes after trauma[1423] and angiography[618]. These differ from true migraine by always occurring on the same side[954, 883] and sometimes by having blood in the spinal fluid and are apt to be accompanied by ophthalmoplegia.

Aside from the popular notion of migraine as being caused by arterial spasm and subsequent vasodilatation, other proposals have been herniation of the brain stem through the tentorium[611] and narrowing of the carotid artery in the cavernous sinus[1532]. It is curious that this most common malady involving the visual system in the brain is the one we know the least about.

With bilateral lesions of the occipital lobes the patient may be completely blind. (This is often called cortical blindness even when the lesion involves primarily white matter.) The normal pupillary responses and absence of optic atrophy differentiate occipital blindness from that due to lesions of the optic nerves.

Blindness of cerebral origin, whether it be due to occipital or parieto-occipital lesions, is often accompanied by denial of the blindness (Anton's syndrome[31, 1182]). Hemianopia may also be denied (although this is less paradoxic than is the presence of total blindness). Like the denial of hemiplegia, or the denial of illness in general, the failure to recognize visual defects is not so much a characteristic of the lesion as of an associated intellectual deterioration[1182, 1545, 547]. It thus occurs in persons having widespread neurologic disease, especially with other vascular lesions, in addition to the lesion responsible for the visual defect. When confronted with their paradoxical behavior, patients with Anton's syndrome resort to various alibis exactly as do patients with Korsakoff's psychosis. Patients with Anton's syndrome are also apt to hallucinate and then present behavior problems since the blindness shuts off visual clues which might permit differentiation between hallucinosis and reality. Moreover, the sudden onset of blindness in a person who denies it can be confusing to an examiner not familiar with the entity. In consequence, the uninformed examiner interprets the paradoxic behavior of such patients as hysterical.

In addition to the blindness from involvement of the perceptual centers in the occiput, subtle disturbances of vision occur with involvement of the visual interpretive centers in the peristriate and neighboring parieto-temporal regions. Such patients are unable to cull up visual images from the past (visual irreminiscence[311]); to recognize the significance of objects and persons[431] (visual agnosia) or identify faces (prosopagnosia[660, 1105, 118, 1144]; to recognize colors (achromatopsia); to recognize words or letters (alexia); or to identify the relation of objects in space (topographic agnosia)[1327]. Some of these symptoms will be recognized as signs of parietal disease.

Since other symptoms associated with occipital lesions reflect the types of lesions rather than the sites, they will be discussed under the appropriate etiologic headings.

C. TYPES OF LESIONS

1. Vascular Lesions

Occlusion of one or both posterior cerebral arteries causing homonymous hemianopic defects is a relatively common manifestation of vertebral-basilar artery disease. The lesions may be thrombotic, embolic, or may represent transitory ischemia (called basilar insufficiency[1324]) in the presence of arteriosclerotic stenosis. The basilar artery is that vessel in the body which most frequently shows arteriosclerosis[907] (Figure 166). Less common vascular lesions of the occiput are hemorrhage, arteriovenous anomalies, and occlusions of the parieto-occipital veins.

(a) *Thrombotic occlusion of the posterior cerebral artery.* This is usually due to arteriosclerosis and may induce ischemia of the occipital lobes only, when the posterior cerebral arteries are the responsible vessels, or may also involve the brain stem when the basilar artery is stenotic[773, 306]. Thus, depending on the site of occlusion, the occipital lesions may be associated with brain stem signs due to involvement of pyramidal tracts, cerebellar pathways, cranial nerve nuclei and their interconnections[123, 1323, 1030, 769]. The symptoms often include vertigo, diplopia, facial weakness, dysarthria, dysphagia, ataxia, sensory symptoms, palsies of conjugate gaze, vertical nystagmus, internuclear ophthalmoplegia and perioral numbness. The vertigo may be severe when the internal labyrinthine artery is occluded[1026] and is then often misdiagnosed as labyrinthitis.

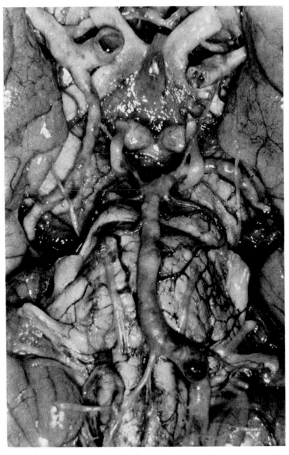

FIGURE 166. Severely atheromatous basilar artery and anomalous circle of Willis. In this patient the right posterior cerebral artery came off the internal carotid rather than the basilar artery.

The onset may be sudden and bilateral, for thrombotic plaques have a preferential localization in the terminal bifurcation of the basilar artery[840, 1403]. More frequently, however, a series of blackouts or transient blurring of vision[452, 693], called "small strokes," precedes the major ischemic event culminating in hemianopia or blindness[1024, 1403, 547,1569]. These crises may be precipitated by some incidental lowering of blood pressure[357], and when repetitive are called visual claudications[508]. They are often so transient as to be ignored by the patient (unless they occur while driving his car, when they may be

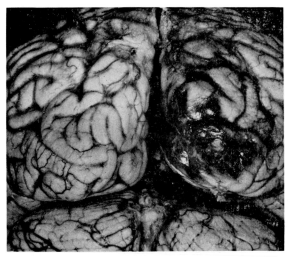

FIGURE 167. Hemorrhagic infarct of the right occipital lobe in a patient whose presenting symptom was left homonymous hemianopia.

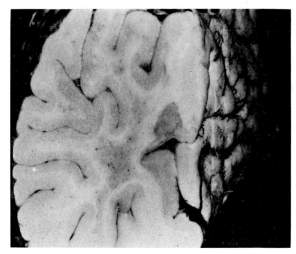

FIGURE 168. Localized infarct of right supracalcarine gyrus in a patient with lupus erythematosus who developed a left sided paracentral scotoma.

alarming)[693]. Many of the thrombotic occlusions occur during sleep and some occur in association with incidental operations involving loss of blood[1586]. A few have come on after giving blood for transfusion[840], several have resulted from cardiac arrest[542, 696, 1542], and some have occurred in association with systemic lupus erythematosus[670, 255], polycythemia[1328] and macroglobulinemia[927].

To produce transient ischemic attacks there must be extensive sclerosis not only of the basilar system but of the collateral channels. It has been estimated that the diameter of the vessels must be reduced by at least 80 per cent before blood flow is sufficiently reduced to cause symptoms[452].

Pain in the homolateral eye is sufficiently often associated with occipital thrombosis to be noteworthy[818]. The pain is presumably referred from the tentorium which has been shown to be richly supplied by branches of the trigeminal nerves that cause ocular pain on stimulation[434].

Scintillating scotomas are surprisingly infrequent during the acute thrombotic episode although they may occur at a later date in association with glial scars. Although infrequent, traces of blood are occasionally present in the spinal fluid following thrombosis.

Hemianopia due to thrombosis usually recedes considerably in the few weeks after the acute episode. The arteriosclerotic variety is, however, characteristically recurrent although it does not necessarily follow the same pattern or even the same artery. Thus quadrantic defects in one area may be followed at intervals of months or years by other homonymous scotomata on the same or opposite side, culminating in blindness (Figure 169). Just as often, however, occlusive thrombotic disease occurs in other portions of the brain or elsewhere in the body, for sclerosis of the basilar and posterior cerebral arteries is merely a local manifestation of generalized sclerotic disease.

In the presence of adequate collateral circulation through the posterior communicating arteries the internal carotid arteries may provide the requisite blood supply to the posterior cerebral arteries despite occlusion of the basilar system. In such a case occipital blindness may occur only when the internal carotid arteries become stenosed.

(b) *Embolic occlusion of the posterior cerebral arteries.* Differentiation of thrombotic from embolic disease of the posterior cerebral arteries is often impossible. Both induce hemianopic defects with characteristically sudden onset. Brain stem signs may be present[307] with emboli although less frequently than with thrombotic lesions. Suggestive of embolic origin is a source for the emboli and the absence

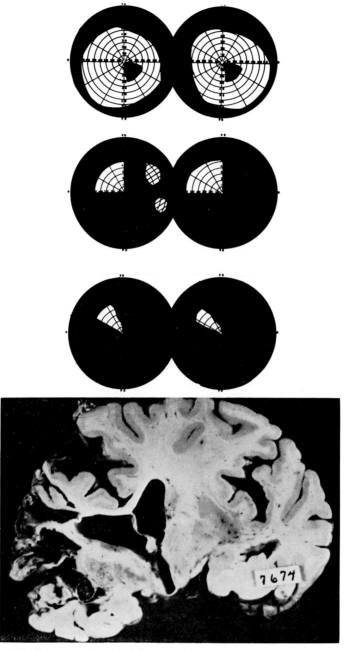

FIGURE 169. Sequence of field defects and brain specimen from a patient who first developed pie-shaped paracentral scotomas and then by stages complete blindness. The patient died ten years after the onset of visual symptoms and was found to have extensive loss of brain substance from both hemispheres but especially from the left parietum and right occiput.

of a history of preceding "small strokes." Emboli may occur with valvular disease of the heart, auricular fibrillation, infectious disease in the lungs or elsewhere and operations such as arterial transplants or mitral valvulotomy[17, 688]. Several instances have resulted from angiography of the vertebral arteries[914, 1189, 1175] or from accidental injection of air into the vertebral arteries[133].

Embolism of the basilar artery is less frequent than is thrombosis but is usually lethal. The few patients who recover sufficiently to permit testing, show hemianopic and brain stem signs (including quadriplegia)[307].

(c) *Other vascular disease.* A few cases have been reported indicating that hemorrhage in the occiput may produce sudden hemianopia or blindness[328] and that obstruction of the venous sinuses may induce transient cortical blindness[561, 1548]. Only a few of these have been documented pathologically.

Supratentorial masses[691, 523] or distension of the brain at the time of ventriculography[1214] may herniate the temporal lobes through the tentorial incisura and cause pressure occlusion of the posterior cerebral arteries. Migraine, which is also thought to cause ischemia in the area of the posterior cerebral arteries, occasionally results in permanent scotomata[398, 1223, 1163].

> Of especial interest is the case of Dr. Frank Mallory who developed a sudden and permanent hemianopic scotoma at the age of forty-seven and directed in his will that his brain should be examined after his death, which occurred at the age of seventy-eight. Dr. Polyak found a discrete lesion of the inferior calcarine gyrus, probably representing an infarct that had occurred thirty-one years previously[1163].

Aneurysms are relatively infrequent in the area of the posterior cerebral artery[369, 69] but arteriovenous anomalies of either a racemose or hemangiomatous type do involve the occipital lobe occasionally[141, 1243, 1194]. Sometimes they are associated with hemangiomas of the face (Sturge-Weber syndrome) and of the choroid. These angiomatous anomalies may induce scintillating scotomata and a hemianopia suggestive of that which occurs with migraine, but differ from migraine in that the attacks are always on the same side[883] and the hemianopia becomes permanent early in the attacks[1259]. With frank rupture of one of the vessels the patient may lose consciousness for a while, subsequently have a stiff neck, and be found to have blood in the spinal fluid. Definitive diagnosis is usually established by vertebral or carotid arteriography[1035].

The "subclavian steal syndrome"[402] results from a reversal of blood flow through the vertebral artery[1195,978] and may have prominent visual symptoms. Stenosis of one subclavian artery proximal to the origin of the vertebral artery will result in blood traveling up the contralateral vertebral artery and down the homolateral vertebral artery to supply blood to the arm. With exercise of the arm, therefore, blood will be "stolen" from the basilar system with consequent brain stem and occipital signs[1088]. The diagnosis can usually be suspected whenever the history indicates blackouts with exercise of one arm and examination discloses a relatively lower blood pressure in that arm. Digital compression of the radial arteries or sphygmomanometry should be a mandatory procedure in all patients with vertebral basilar insufficiency. Definitive diagnosis can be made during life by vertebral angiography.

Tangentially related to cerebrovascular lesions and sometimes identified with them is anoxic encephalopathy. Thus hemianopia occurring at a high altitude has been attributed to infarction. More common is the anoxia of cardiac arrest. This may result in selective visual deficits although the visual involvement is frequently associated with symptoms of widespread cerebral disease. In general the visual and motor areas of the brain are especially vulnerable while the brain stem and spinal cord are relatively resistant[1543]. Nevertheless, vision may recover to a surprising extent several weeks or months after the arrest[696,1542].

In the differentiation of the various causes for vascular diseases of the brain several "Apoplexy Aphorisms" have been found useful (though not invariably reliable) in neurology[3]. Some of these are:

Sudden onset of headache with confusion leading to deep coma with bloody spinal fluid is indicative of cerebral hemorrhage.

Brain embolism can be diagnosed only when there is an obvious source.

Sudden onset of severe suboccipital headache, stiff neck, nausea and vomiting without lateralizing signs is usually caused by subarachnoid hemorrhage from a ruptured saccular aneurysm.

More than five episodes of spontaneous subarachnoid hemorrhage are indicative of hemangioma rather than of saccular aneurysms.

Increasing headaches, drowsiness, confusion, hemianopia and hemiparesis over a period of a few weeks suggest chronic subdural hematoma whatever the cerebrospinal fluid shows. Symptoms progressing over a longer period suggest tumor.

Repeated convulsions may result from tumor, syphilis, or trauma but rarely from vascular disease.

Hypertensive encephalopathy produces seizures and stupor but, in contrast to a stroke, it does not ordinarily cause focal neurologic signs.

2. Tumors

Tumors of the occiput might be expected to induce a slowly progressive hemianopia. This is usually the case but sudden onset of symptoms, simulating a vascular crisis, is also frequent[593]. Fortifying the impression of a vascular lesion the hemianopia may even show partial resolution. The eventual advance of the symptoms, however, with involvement of the adjacent parieto-temporal areas which, unlike the onset, causes progressive symptoms, makes the diagnosis of tumor suspect[1113]. Headache is a variable symptom but, since tumors arising in the occiput are less apt to cause increased intracranial pressure than are those elsewhere in the cerebrum, headache is less common with occipital tumors. Scintillating scotomas and hallucinations are infrequent. Positive evidence of tumor is increased protein in the spinal fluid and deformation of the posterior ventricles on ventriculography.

The types of tumors occurring in the occiput are the same as those found elsewhere in the cerebrum: the relatively localized astrocytoma, the infiltrative glioblastoma multiforme, the metastatic tumor, and the meningioma. The first two are intrinsic tumors which, when they arise in the occiput, may produce hemianopia as the sole symptom. Metastatic tumors of the occiput also produce a unilateral hemianopia but because of multiplicity of foci they often produce signs and symptoms referable to other sites of the central nervous system in addition to the occiput. Meningiomas constitute a special case: they not only grow slowly but, by reason of being extrinsic and often parasagittal, they frequently produce bilateral hemianopic defects.

3. Demyelinative Diseases

Although not common, hemianopia from loss of white matter in the occipital lobes may be the presenting symptom of multiple sclerosis, Schilder's disease, or other leucoencephalopathies (Figure 170) (see p. 285). Usually, however, the occipital lobe involvement is only part of the nervous system disease and other manifestations suggest the diagnosis. Such other manifestations are intermittent internuclear ophthalmoplegia, optic neuropathy, nystagmus, and ataxia in the case of multiple sclerosis, and progressive brain disease with mental deterioration in the case of Schilder's disease. Less common are the patchy necrosis of the white matter occurring with Hodgkin's

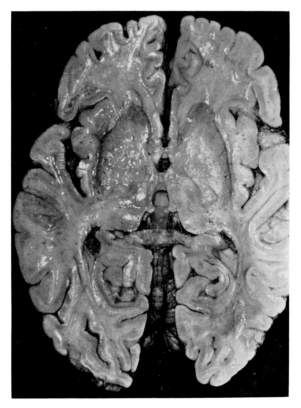

FIGURE 170. Brain of a patient with diffuse demyelinative encephalopathy showing extensive loss of white matter.

At the age of thirty years the patient lost all vision in the left eye and had pain on movement of eyes. The disc was elevated and showed peripapillary hemorrhages. A diagnosis was made of papillitis. Subsequently the patient developed hemianopia and progresive paralysis of her limbs, aphasia, and dementia with death two and one-half years after the onset.

disease or with other systemic diseases[1202] and the loss of white matter occurring with familial metachromatic leucoencephalopathy.

4. Trauma and Poisons

Injury may cause direct laceration or compression of the occipital lobes or it may impair occipital function indirectly by edema or ischemia. In either case the result will be a varying degree of either hemianopia or blindness, depending on the involvement of one or both lobes, with a remarkable tendency for recovery of some visual function in the subsequent days or weeks. Since the signs and symptoms differ with direct and indirect injury, they will be discussed under separate headings and the special case of traumatic blindness in infants will be discussed in a subsequent section (see p. 304).

(a) *Direct injury.* Penetrating missiles and depressed bone fragments from fractures of the skull are the common causes of injury to the occipital lobes. These induce, of course, immediate loss of vision. Transection of both occipital lobes will cause complete blindness; injuries limited to the occipital poles may cause central or paracentral scotomas; injuries farther forward cause peripheral constriction with sparing of the macula. Injuries to both supracalcarine areas cause inferior altitudinal hemianopia. Although it is theoretically possible to have superior altitudinal hemianopia from injuries to both infracalcarine areas, this is rarely seen because the associated injury to the nearby venous sinuses prevents survival of the patient[813].

Much of our knowledge of cerebral representation of vision comes from the classic studies of injuries in World War I by Holmes and Lister[681], and Riddoch[1205] in England, Marie and Chatelin[986] in France, and Poppelreuter[1165] in Germany. It is to these studies that we are indebted for knowledge of macular representation at the posterior poles and peripheral representation in the anterior parts. Similar studies of injuries from World War II and the Korean War by Teuber, Battersby, and Bender[1423] have confirmed most of the earlier concepts although the asymmetry in their fields cast doubt on the precise congruence of representation of the two eyes in the occiput.

Injuries to the back of the head produce visual defects with no other neurologic deficit. In fact, cases have been recorded in which a missile penetrating the skull has caused the victim to ask for a bandage for his eyes, thinking his visual loss was of ocular origin; or the visual defect may be so ill-defined as to hide the source of injury until the victim takes off his helmet and finds a hole in it. Nevertheless, some visual disturbance is always apparent to the patient; traumatic cases do not show the denial of blindness seen with Anton's syndrome[1423].

Recovery of some visual function occurs almost invariably in the day or weeks following the injury. The amount of recovery is, of course variable, but it is surprisingly complete in comparison with injuries to the optic nerve and chiasmal area. After months or years, however, the scar tissue may result in trigger points for paroxysmic episodes of visual aura, migrainoid attacks or convulsions. These visual experiences consist of feelings of unreality of objects, changes in apparent size (micropsia and macropsia) or of distance (teleopsia). Sometimes they are described as flickering lights and moving lights (whence they are likened to migraine) but actual formed hallucinations are rare.

The causes of injury to the occiput are manifold. Most thoroughly documented are, as previously noted, the war injuries. Automobile accidents are a common cause but unlike the missile injuries they are usually associated with general skull trauma and are therefore first detected when a patient recovers from a state of unconsciousness.

A benign form of injury is that resulting from ventriculography[1189, 932], especially when the needle passes too close to the mid-line and entails excessive probing. Although the resultant hemianopic defect is alarming to the patient (and to the doctor), the post-ventriculography disturbances clear up usually in the course of a few days[999].

(b) **Indirect injury.** Indirect injuries do not present primarily visual problems which the direct injuries may do since there is usually widespread central nervous system involvement and the visual aspect is of less significance.

Transient blindness may be part of a general concussion syndrome. Although the pathogenesis of this may be cerebral edema, as generally postulated, there has been little opportunity for documentation of specific cases. A few of those which have come to autopsy, have shown a conspicuous cerebellar pressure cone suggesting that the blindness may be due to compression of the posterior cerebral arteries with ischemia of the occipital lobes[691].

(c) **Poisons.** Some poisons appear to have a predilection for the occipital area. Carbon monoxide induces necrotic foci in the occipital lobes and survivors of carbon monoxide poisoning have lasting homonymous field defects[337] or blindness[1538, 443].

Some drugs appear to affect the higher visual centers preferentially, although the sites of this effect are unknown. Toxic doses of digitalis cause a subjective yellowness (xanthopsia) or whiteness, like snow, of the visual field[214, 538, 1452, 492, 1458]. (Santonin also causes a yellow vision but this is thought to result from alterations in the optic nerve or retina rather than the cerebrum[578].) Mescal, opium, and lysergic acid characteristically cause visual hallucinations of a dream-like quality; these drugs presumably owe their effect to alteration in cerebral function although they are also accompanied by changes in the electroretinogram[35].

D. INFANTILE CEREBRAL BLINDNESS

The diagnosis of a cerebral origin for blindness in the infant depends, as in the adult, on an intact pupillary response and on the absence of optic atrophy. These criteria are, however, not as clear-cut in the infant, for the pupils are normally so miotic as to make their further constriction to light unimpressive and the nerve heads are normally so pale as to suggest optic atrophy to those unaccustomed to the normal infant's fundus. Thus the cerebral origin for some infantile blindness is masked by spurious signs suggesting optic nerve lesions. A further point of difference in the blindness of the infant as compared with that in the adult is that congenital absence of occipital function in the infant is still compatible with retained light perception whereas destruction of the occiput in the adult causes complete blindness. Thus the infant with no occipital lobes, or, for that matter, with no suprathalamic brain at all, will show a blepharospasm and startle-reaction when exposed to a flash of light[646].

Blindness dating from birth is usually not detected until several months of age. A blind infant shows little departure from the normal pattern of behavior during the first few weeks of neonatal life. Then the mother usually notices either a failure to fix on an object or a "searching" type of nystagmus. With complete blindness, however, the nystagmus may not be as striking as when blindness is incomplete. Nystagmus is therefore generally less conspicuous with cerebral lesions, in which the blindness is usually complete, than with the blindness resulting from ocular lesions, in which the blindness is usually partial.

The causes of infantile cerebral blindness are manifold. Most frequent is cerebral agenesis in which the blindness is associated with varying degrees of dementia. Meningoencephalitis is an occasional cause of infantile cerebral blindness and, as with cerebral agenesis, it is nearly always associated with some degree of mental retardation.

Trauma presents a special problem in infants. Subdural hematomas are relatively frequent prior to the age of two years and may result from trivial injuries. In comparison with intracranial hematomas of adults, those in infants are apt to be bilateral and produce complete blindness. Infants are also more apt to have blood in the subarachnoid fluid, to show retinal and peretinal hemorrhage[671] and to have convulsions[569]. These deviations from the manifestations of subdural hematomas in the adult are presumably due to the delicateness of the arachnoid membranes separating the meningeal compartments in the infant[569]. Infants are also prone to have transient blindness from cerebral edema of traumatic origin. This clears up with dramatic rapidity in one to two days after the injury[1147] often while plans are being made to do subdural taps. Cortical blindness, also of a transient variety, is prone to follow cardiac arrest in infants[1542].

Progressive cerebral degenerations of infancy and childhood commonly involve the occipital lobes and may cause blindness along with apathy, mental deterioration, epilepsy, and pyramidal tract signs. Several types of degeneration can now be diagnosed by specific tests: galactosemia by finding reducing substances in the urine; metachromatic leucoencephalopathy by finding metachromatic bodies in renal cells in the urine; phenylpyruvic oligophrenia by a color reaction with ferric chloride in the acidified urine; and Tay-Sachs disease by finding excess gangliosides in autonomic ganglia obtained by rectal biopsy. Infantile or intrauterine infections with toxoplasma and the virus of cytomegalic inclusion disease may involve the occiput and are suggested by the ophthalmoscopic finding of chorioretinal lesions and the roentgenographic evidence of calcification within the cranium. Infantile cerebral softening from vascular occlusions at birth commonly causes hemianopia and sometimes blindness and spastic palsy of the new born. Porencephaly is also frequently associated with hemianopia or blindness. This disease, characterized by communicating fistulas between the cerebral ventricles and the subarachnoid space, is best diagnosed by pneumoencephalography[20].

A rare but discrete form of infantile cerebral disease in which blindness is a prominent symptom is that which goes by the pathologic designation of spongy degeneration of the brain[145, 129]. The infants appear normal at birth but are obviously blind and demented within the first few months of life. Optic atrophy is commonly present but the pupils are reactive and the cause of blindness is cerebral rather than peripheral. These infants are often deaf, or become so, and develop bilateral pyramidal tract signs. At death, which usually occurs by the second year of life, the white matter of the brain is contracted and gelatinous in appearance and in microscopic sections is seen to consist of a meshwork of glial elements with large tissue spaces. In contrast to the demyelinative processes of most diffuse scleroses, there is no evidence of lipid storage nor phagocytosis. The process seems to be one of faulty myelination rather than active demyelination.

Another rare and only recently recognized cause of cerebral blindness and dementia is infantile neuraxonal dystrophy[303]. This disease is familial as is spongy degeneration and runs a similar clinical course except that the affected children live somewhat longer. The distinguishing feature is the pathologic finding of swollen nerve fibers, called "spheroids," in the central nervous system. These spheroids are histologically like individual cystoid spaces in the retina (although no such lesions are found in the retina with this disease). Optic atrophy is usually present but the pupils are reactive and the blindness is greater than can be accounted for by the optic nerve lesion.

But the largest intracranial cause of blindness in infants and children is hydrocephalus. Here there may be ample reason to think that the occipital lobes and visual pathways are involved but there is almost invariably evidence that the optic nerves are sufficiently damaged to also account for the blindness.

SUMMARY

The occipital lobes, constituting the posterior portions of the cerebral hemispheres, are arbitrarily subdivided into Areas 17, 18, and 19 (Brodman's classification). Area 17, surrounding the calcarine fissure on the medial surface of the brain and overlapping onto the lateral surfaces at the posterior poles, is primarily the receptive center for the geniculo-calcarine (visual) radiation. Area 18 is believed to serve primarily for integration of impulses within the visual sphere, whereas Area 19 is believed to coordinate vision with other sensory and motor activities.

Hemianopia or hemianopic defects are the only regular symptoms of occipital lesions. They are congruous in corresponding fields of the two eyes. Less frequent symptoms are photopsia, visual hallucinations and occasionally pain in the homolateral eye or forehead. When both occipital lobes are involved, as is frequently the case since they are supplied by the posterior cerebral arteries which come off a common basilar artery, the patient is completely blind. Despite this blindness the pupils are normally reactive. In the presence of associated intellectual deterioration the patient may deny the blindness (Anton's syndrome) and be led into extravagant confabulations to account for his erratic behavior.

The prime cause of occipital lobe lesions is vascular disease. Thrombotic and embolic occlusions of the posterior cerebral arteries are relatively common. The lesion is frequently situated at the site of bifurcation of the basilar artery and is associated with various lesions of the mid-brain and brain stem such as diplopia, nystagmus, vertigo, internuclear ophthalmoplegia, confusion and coma.

Less frequent vascular lesions of the occipital lobes are hemorrhage, occlusion of the venous sinuses, compression of the posterior cerebral arteries by herniation of the brain through the incisura of the tentorium, arteriovenous anomalies, ischemia from cardiac arrest, and a curious bypass in the vertebral arteries (known as the subclavian steal syndrome) due to stenosis of the subclavian artery.

Tumors of the occiput produce a hemianopia that is usually insidious in onset but may be abrupt. The types of tumors include astrocytomas, glioblastomas, metastatic tumors, and meningiomas. Diagnosis is suggested by significant elevation of the protein in the spinal fluid but definitive diagnosis requires ventriculography and craniotomy. Demyelinative diseases and leucodystrophies also produce lesions in the occipital lobe but these are part of widespread disease of white matter which gives other evidence of the diagnosis.

Because of their position in the posterior portion of the skull, the occipital lobes are frequent sites of isolated injury. Lesions of the occipital pole cause hemianopic scotomas (occasionally bilateral) in the central area, whereas anterior and incomplete lesions cause peripheral constrictions with sparing of the central field. Coincidental lesions of the supratentorial venous sinuses adjacent to the lower occipital pole often cause death; hence superior altitudinal defects in the visual field are found less frequently after injury to the occipital lobes than are inferior altitudinal defects. Indirect injuries to the occipital lobes result from blunt blows to the head. The ensuing blindness may be due to cerebral edema or to interference with the blood supply; in any case, the visual defect is merely part of a widespread cerebral deficit.

Certain poisons may cause organic or functional disease of the occipital lobes. Carbon monoxide may cause specific necrotic foci. Digitalis produces a yellow vision thought to be due to an action on the occipital lobe, whereas mescal and opium notoriously produce visual hallucinations.

Infantile cerebral blindness requires special consideration. In the first place it is not always easy to diagnose blindness in a non-responsive infant. Secondly there are special conditions which produce blindness in an infant: cerebral agenesis, meningo-encephalitis, subdural hematoma, cerebral edema, and several types of inflammation and cerebral dystrophy. Vascular lesions thought to account for many cases of spastic palsy also commonly have hemianopic or amaurotic accompaniments. But the most common cause of infantile cerebral blindness is probably hydrocephalus.

CHAPTER XVI

FUNCTIONAL ABNORMALITIES OF VISION

Visual disturbances of a functional nature include quasipatho-
logic syndromes such as hysteria, quasiphysiologic syndromes
such as suppressive amblyopia, and voluntary deceptions such as
malingering. The major clinical manifestations may be grouped into
the following headings.

1. Tubular Fields

The name tubular fields connotes generalized constriction in which
linear dimensions of the central seeing area are the same for all
distances of testing; that is, they are cylindric. Differing thus from
organically induced constrictions in which the field increases linearly
with distance (cone shaped), tubular fields are thought to be
pathognomonic of hysteria and probably are its most frequent ocular
manifestation.

But there are other noteworthy features of the hysterical constriction aside from the tubular aspect. Patients rarely present the
field constriction as one of their complaints; rather it is usually picked
up during a routine examination for some other symptom. Nor do the
patients show the visual incapacity which one might expect with a
field reduction such as the test would indicate[977]. Thus, in comparison
with the patients having constricted fields of organic origin, patients
with tubular fields show no difficulty in walking about or avoiding
objects. Rather, their normal visual activity seems to belie their visual
field defects.

Because of the discrepancy between the function and field,
hysterical patients are assumed to see in their "blind" field. That
this paradox may have another explanation, bound up in the nature
of hysteria, is suggested by the following observation. If, instead of
testing the field at greater distances, one tests it at the same distance
but with increasingly larger background screens one frequently
finds a corresponding enlargement of the central seeing area. Thus

a field tested on a 2 meter screen will show twice as large a central seeing area as on a 1 meter screen. When the screen is removed entirely and one uses the entire room as a background, the field defect will often disappear entirely. Thus an hysterical constriction is a function of the size of the background. It is, in other words, an artifact of testing in which the hysterical patient correlates the test object with the background on which he projects it. The act of testing creates an artificial field defect. It is thus not surprising that the patients do not present the field constriction as one of their complaints nor that the constriction should have, when the same size screen is used, a tubular type of defect.

Another characteristic of the hysterical field is its apparently sharp border. Unlike most organic lesions, at least those characterized by general constriction, the boundary is approximately the same for all sized test objects.

Tubular fields are usually demonstrable in both eyes, although occasionally present in one eye only, and they are often permanent. Their prognosis, however, is of no major concern since they present no symptoms to the patient. As a matter of fact, tubular fields are more important to the physician, who must rule out other causes for constricted fields, than they are to the patient. Especially difficult is the question of a possible relationship of the hysterical manifestation to alleged trauma.

Several artifacts in the testing of tubular fields should be noted lest false constrictions be obtained. Thus patients with constricted fields should be reminded that they are to respond when they first perceive an object in the periphery: some patients show an artifactitious constriction under the impression that they should respond only when they see the object clearly. Similar artifacts are found in patients with diffuse opacities of their ocular media; a generalized constriction may result from the fact that the object is not seen until it approaches the point of fixation. Both these artifacts may be avoided by using a sufficiently large test object; indeed, it may be said that a generalized constriction present for small test objects only is not a consequence of hysteria.

2. Amblyopia and Amaurosis

Amblyopia means reduction in vision whereas amaurosis means complete blindness. Amblyopia ex anopsia is the reduction in vision occurring in an eye with strabismus. The term comes from the early supposition that lack of use of an eye causes the vision to deteriorate; it seems more likely that the amblyopia develops as a positive suppressive, and useful, role to prevent diplopia. In any case the ease with which it develops is a function of age; the younger the patient the easier it is for amblyopia to develop. An adult who develops strabismus may never learn to suppress one eye and a troublesome diplopia persists throughout life.

Amblyopia ex anopsia has its counterpart in kittens which have had one eye continuously occluded early in life. The occluded eye can be shown to be functionally blind and recordings from the occipital cortex reveal only those cells associated with activity of the opposite eye[696a]. Surprisingly, the amblyopia is not reversed after a three month period of occlusion. No comparable amblyopia occurs in adult cats which are similarly occluded.

Functional amblyopia in *both* eyes is not so well recognized. Nevertheless it appears to be a genuine entity, most common in children, and brought to light by school-testing programs. The acuity may be 20/70 or less and identical in the two eyes. It is a matter of concern to the teacher and to the parents but, unlike amblyopia of organic origin, it causes little handicap to the patient who is able to carry on his or her school work with no unusual difficulty. The possibility of this being hysteria is suggested whenever there are associated tubular fields, blepharospasm or other symptoms suggestive of such a diagnosis. There is also always the possibility of an uncorrected ametropia which should be ruled out by appropriate refractive examination.

Functional amaurosis, meaning denial of all vision in one or both eyes, is infrequent. However, transient blackouts do occur for which no organic basis is found and in which an associated apprehensiveness suggests a functional origin[265]. Prolonged amaurosis also occurs on functional grounds but it is almost impossible to disassociate hysteria from malingering as a cause. The diagnosis of functional amaurosis is based on the subjective testimony of the patient that he cannot see despite objective evidence of an intact opticokinetic response and other behavioral evidence of a normal visual mechanism[1594].

Less common functional visual disturbances falling into the category of amblyopia-amaurosis are: the blurring of vision which occurs with spasm of the near reflex[270]; the day-dreaming blur which may become so habitual as to constitute a genuine symptom[1457]; the blurring of vision with narcolepsy[775]; and sensations of "heat waves" and "oil slicks" that suggest migraine equivalents.

3. Reading Difficulties (dyslexia)

Whereas alexia is an inability to recognize written words or letters and is generally attributable to lesions of the dominant angular gyrus (see p. 271), dyslexia is a more comprehensive term spanning difficulties in reading that range from the functional to the organic. It is a diagnosis that requires cautious interpretation.

On the functional side are the natively slow readers who exasperate teachers and parents during the first few years of the child's schooling. Under the American school system all children are expected to develop equivalent intellectual and adaptive facilities at approximately the same age. If a child lags during the first few years of school where an inordinate premium is put on understanding the printed word, he is labelled a reading problem. The majority of such slow readers develop passable facility in reading after the first few years of school and have no further difficulties. It is not clear whether they become better readers or find their outlets in subjects more suitable for their talents. In any case, such children have a benign and usually self curative problem.

A somewhat more difficult problem in reading comprises the left handed or ambidextrous person who, in mimicking their right handed elders, develop mirror reading[312, 563], a syndrome known as *strephosymbolia*[1103] (and thought to be due to mixed cerebral dominance). These children, mostly boys[423], have a real handicap in the first few years of school and the majority never do become facile readers. They too, however, become better adjusted in the later years of school where the literal arts are emphasized less. Many excel in mathematics since Arabic numbers usually offer no difficulty[1330]; many top scientists, it is said, presented reading problems in their elementary school days.

The most devastating, but fortunately rare, form of reading difficulty is that in which the angular gyrus region on the dominant side of the brain is injured (or that in which both angular gyri fail to develop[531]). The EEG often points to a lesion in the parietotemporal region[551].

Such persons may never be educatable in the world of letters. One such patient with whom I've had close contact could never learn more than five letters of the alphabet despite eight years of schooling. Yet he is a person of more than average intelligence and at the age of twenty-seven he is a master mechanic. His brain lesion resulted from a blow on the head in childhood. On the other hand extensive lesions of either hemisphere may be compatible with learning adequate reading skills provided the lesion was unilateral and occurred early in life (up to the age of six years)[1036].

A still more rare but serious form of dyslexia is that secondary to ocular movement disorders. Most poor readers have normal ocular motor coordination[1074, 590], but those with paretic horizontal movements, represented most strikingly in ocular motor apraxia[262], are unable to read across a line adequately and are in consequence severely handicapped. Nor does any amount of exercise rehabilitate them.

Reading epilepsy is a curious form of so-called reflex epilepsy which may be precipitated by any of many stimuli related to reading[121, 314, 77, 867, 1085]. Often the conditions of reading are highly specific, sometimes associated only with casual reading and sometimes only with concentrated reading. The epilepsy frequently begins with jaw clicking or eye blinking and may consist simply of a few myoclonic jerks or may go on to a generalized convulsion. The primary type occurs only with reading and constitutes an idopathic form of epilepsy in which no brain lesions have been demonstrated; the secondary type develops convulsions from various triggers of which reading is only one. Brain lesions have been demonstrated in this latter type.

4. Photopsia and Hallucinations

Whereas ill defined flashes of light (photopsia) result from focal lesions, formed images (hallucinations) appear to result from functional disturbances of the brain as a whole. These latter occur especially often in blind persons, or in persons who have their eyes covered (as after an eye operation) and probably depend on loss of the normal criteria for visual orientation; e.g., they can be induced experimentally by general sensory deprivation[370, 901, 887]. Hallucinations not based on recognized organic lesions also occur with some psychoses (notably schizophrenia) and with some drugs (mescaline, cannabis, and lysergic acid)[839]. The hallucinogenic properties of

atropine and scopolamine are of particular concern to the ophthalmologist because hallucinations along with confusion and excitement
occur occasionally as the result of topical use of these drugs in the eye.

Traction on the retina is a well recognized cause of photopsia that
occasionally may be confused with excitation of the central nervous
system. Rubbing the sclera through the closed lids will produce a
transient white ring projected to the opposite visual field. A more
disturbing photopsia occurs occasionally in persons of middle age or
over, associated with sudden movements of the eye. A flash of light,
associated with the movement and called Moore's lightening streak,
results from the traction of a partially liquefied vitreous on the
retina[1042, 1483, 1066].

5. Pain and Headache

Merging into one another these two symptoms have a similar significance. That with a sharp stabbing quality is called pain while that
of a dull continuous nature is called headache.

The involvement of the sensory nerves in the meninges is the
common source of pain and headache with intracranial disease, and
these symptoms may therefore have topical significance: lesions in
the region of the superior orbital fissure or cavernous sinus project
symptoms to the homolateral eye or supraorbital region; lesions in
the region of the sella turcica project pain to the bitemporal region;
lesions in the temporo-parieto-occipital area project pain to the
overlying region of the scalp but are not sharply localized. Lesions
of the thalamus and of the tentorium frequently project uncomfortable
sensations and pain to the homolateral eye.

Excitation of the sensory centers within the brain and peripheral
nerves constitutes the other source of pain with intracranial lesions.
The periodic pain of trigeminal neuralgia is possibly the most common. Arising in the gasserian ganglion or its central representation,
the stabbing pain is frequently projected to the eye or to its environs.
Such pain may signify a paratrigeminal lesion (meningioma, aneurysm,
carcinoma) or may result from contact with the internal carotid
artery[787]. Usually, however, the pain must be labelled cryptogenic
as no cause is found.

Periodic pain may also result from lesions within the somesthetic
portion of the brain. It then has the same topical significance as do

motor signs in Jacksonian epilepsy; that is, the pain will project to the site of representation in the brain. Pain, however, is much less frequent as a symptom of neural discharge than are paresthesias or numbness.

Cluster headaches (variously known as Ræder's syndrome, Horton's headaches, and histaminic cephalagia) are characteristically unilateral, occur predominantly in males, and are accompanied by lacrimation and congestion of the homolateral eye and sometimes by Horner's syndrome (Figure 171). They are called "cluster" because of their tendency to recur in groups of attacks separated by asymptomatic intervals. Some of these patients show evidence of a paratrigeminal lesion (trauma, meningioma) but the majority never show an organic lesion; the fact that the symptoms in most cases recur at infrequent intervals over a span of many years points to the absence of a progressive lesion. Some authors believe them to be migraine equivalents[843].

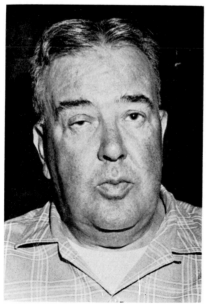

FIGURE 171. Ptosis with cluster headaches (Raeder's syndrome). The patient was a fifty-six year old man who had had intermittent attacks of pain behind the right eye and on the right side of his head for several months. The symptoms occurred most severely in the late afternoon and were associated with right sided lacrimation. Except for the Horner's syndrome the ophthalmic and neurologic examination revealed nothing of note.

Sinus headaches are usually localized over the site of inflammation. Most characteristic of sinus headaches are the local tenderness and congestive signs in the nose. They are recurrent, usually worse in the morning, and accompanied by x-ray evidence of chronic sinusitis.

6. Photogenic Epilepsy

Mention has previously been made to seizures triggered by concentration on reading. In a larger sense epilepsy may be triggered by any of a variety of visual stimuli. Best known is the photic driving in which attacks are precipitated by flashes of light of a specific frequency. Patients have been reported to have had convulsions set off by the rotations of a helicopter blade[750], moving a hand back and forth in front of the eyes[892], viewing Venetian blinds[25] and many by the flickering of a television screen[1110, 132, 1003]. One case together with convincing EEG evidence is reported to have been precipitated by simple viewing of vertical lines[1203].

SUMMARY

Functional abnormalities of vision usually follow one of several patterns. Tubular vision is most common and is generally considered a manifestation of hysteria. Amblyopia or amaurosis may also be of psychogenic origin and then probably serves a useful purpose to replace diplopia in the presence of a strabismus. In contrast to tubular fields, amaurosis is frequently a manifestation of malingering. When complete or nearly complete, the functional nature of this amaurosis can be readily detected by the opticokinetic test.

Reading difficulties (dyslexias) are often functional disturbances of vision. Some are, to be sure, based on organic lesions in the angular gyrus region of the dominant hemisphere but the majority occur in persons who are either natively slow readers or in persons who, having been basically left handed, develop an habitual preference for their right hand. Occasionally the primary fault is an ocular motor abnormality (as in ocular motor apraxia). Although not a true dyslexia a recognized form of reading difficulty is epilepsy triggered by the act of reading.

Photopsia and hallucinations may arise from functional as well as organic disturbances of the brain, but the majority of such visual experiences are illusory in nature arising in blinded persons or persons who are either drugged or are mentally deteriorated, that is persons who have lost their normal capacity for interpretation of adequate visual stimuli. Mechanical stimulation of the retina may also cause photopsia.

Pain in the eye and headache may be referred from lesions of the meninges in the retro-orbital region and tentorium or from lesions of the thalamus and parietal lobe. Trigeminal pain has a characteristically stabbing quality. It may connote a paratrigeminal lesion but is often functional. Intermittent unilateral headaches with congestion of eye and nose (and sometimes Horner's syndrome) are called cluster headaches; they may similarly signify organic or functional disease; some believe they are migraine equivalents.

Photogenic epilepsy is a term generally used to designate convulsions that are set off by visual stimuli. Most common is that produced by flashes of light such as the flickering of a television screen, but the triggers are many and varied.

CHAPTER XVII

NEURO-OPHTHALMIC ABNORMALITIES INVOLVING OCULAR STRUCTURES OTHER THAN THE VISUO-SENSORY AND OCULAR MOTOR SYSTEMS

AFTER CONSIDERING the major ocular motor disturbances in a previous text[263], and the major visual disturbances from lesions of the visual pathways in the present text, several entities of neuro-ophthalmic interest remain to be considered in this final chapter. These might be classified as opacity-producing disturbances and sub-classified according to whether the opacity is in the cornea or the lens. But it seems more expedient to consider them according to the neurologic or systemic disease of which they are a part. Their manifestations in the eye has clinical importance because this is the one place in the body where transparency of the tissues permits the visualization of some of these processes during life. Their ocular localization, significant as it is for diagnostic purposes, should not necessarily imply any specific predilection for the eye.

1. Hepatolenticular Degeneration (Wilson's Disease)

This is a familial disease, transmitted as a Mendelian recessive trait[79], in which a patient develops progressive neurologic symptoms referable to lesions of the basal ganglia (chorea, spasticity, dysarthria, and dysphagia), cirrhosis of the liver, faulty renal function (aminoaciduria and glucosuria) and deposition of a pigment ring in the periphery of the cornea (Kayser-Fleischer ring). Children develop predominantly postural abnormalities (dystonias) whereas adults develop predominantly flapping tremors of the intention type[357a].

The disease is linked to defects in copper metabolism and one of its chief manifestations is the extracellular deposition of copper throughout the body[1461]. Ceruloplasmin is the blood protein that normally binds copper[677]. This binding capacity is significantly reduced in patients with hepatolenticular degeneration[1277, 80, 319] (and sometimes

[318]

in siblings who show no other evidence of the disease[1451, 198]; the excess copper is excreted in the urine. The normal function of ceruloplasmin is not precisely known but it can be shown to be an oxidative enzyme. Current theories as to the pathogenesis of the disease suggest either a failure of ceruloplasmin as an enzyme or else copper intoxication. Therapy consists in lowering the copper intake and giving penicillamine to bind and excrete the copper[1388].

The major ocular manifestation is the presence of a polychromatic zone (Kayser-Fleischer ring) in the periphery of the cornea (Figure 172A). By gross inspection this is predominantly brown but frequently shows an iridescent green or aquamarine hue. By slit lamp microscopy it can be seen to be in Descemet's membrane and gonioscopy shows

A

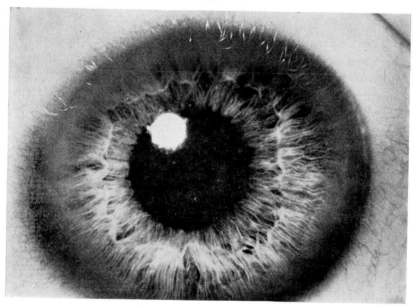

FIGURE 172A. Kayser-Fleischer ring in hepato-lenticular degeneration. The ring consisted of a brown opacification of the peripheral 3 mm of cornea, here represented by masking of the base of the iris. The opacity fades off centrally. (The streaky high-lights in the upper portion of the photograph are reflections of the upper eye lashes.)

The patient was an eighteen year old boy who developed tremor of hands, difficulty in gait, and speech disturbance beginning insidiously two years previously.

B

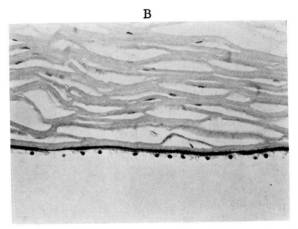

FIGURE 172B. Histologic appearance of the Kayser-Fleischer ring. The section shows a dark lamina in the posterior portion of Descemet's membrane at the periphery of the cornea.

it to have a sharp peripheral edge corresponding to the termination of this membrane. Histologic sections (Figure 172B) show it to consist of dark granules situated in the posterior portion of Descemet's membrane (thereby differing from the lipid deposits with arcus senilis which are deposited anteriorly); these granules give a positive rubeanic acid test for copper[169, 1462]. Electron microscopy suggests (but not too convincingly) that the granules have a laminar distribution that has been likened to the distribution of Liesegang rings[1462]; the lamination has been held responsible for the polychromatic luster. The corneal ring is progressive and may extend several millimeters toward the center of the cornea but it is never sufficient to occlude the pupil or to impair vision.

Less common, but nevertheless definite, is the occasional occurrence of an opacity of the anterior lens capsule[1428]. This has a sun-flower distribution identical with that produced characteristically by copper particles in the eye[1379].

2. Gargoylism (Hurler's Disease[709])

This is a familial disease characterized by widespread deposition of a complex glycolipid throughout the body. Because of the thick tongue and puffy cheeks due to infiltration with this substance, the patients have been likened to gargoyles[411] (Figure 173). The prime

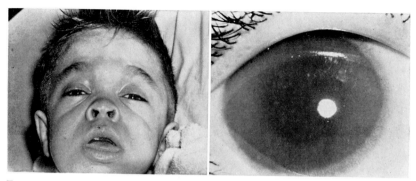

FIGURE 173. Face and eye of a patient with gargoylism. The patient, who was a dwarf and mentally retarded, showed the characteristic puffiness of cheeks, flat bridge of nose, thick tongue, and a diffuse haze of the entire cornea.

clinical symptoms consist of mental retardation, dwarfism, hepato-splenomegaly, excessive secretion of mucus, corneal clouding and occasionally papilledema. The head is also often enlarged, the eyes are set far apart and the bridge of the nose is depressed.

The brain shows cells swollen with a lipid similar to that in some of the amaurotic family idiocies[170, 802]. Hence in neurologic texts the disease is usually classified with the lipidoses. The cornea, like many of the viscera (liver and spleen especially), shows clusters of foam cells situated throughout the stroma. These cells contain material which stains with PAS but is not glycogen[631]. It comprises a complex substance containing lipid, protein, and several polysaccharides[1460]. Curiously, the corneal infiltration is found only in instances which are transmitted as Mendelian recessives and not in those which are transmitted as sex linked traits[1079, 1027].

3. Myotonia Dystrophica

This disease represents a familial disturbance, usually transmitted from parent to offspring as a dominant trait. It is characterized clinically by a myotonia (failure to relax one's grip or to walk rapidly) (Figure 174), muscle atrophy, frontal baldness, endocrinopathy (especially testicular atrophy) and cataracts.

It begins usually in early life and is slowly progressive. The muscle atrophy involves especially the adductors of the thumb, the muscles of the forearm, the sternocleidomastoids, and the facial muscles. The

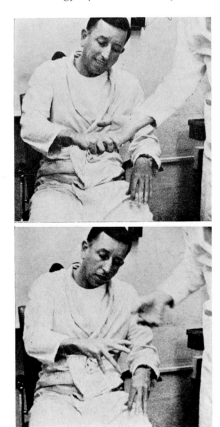

FIGURE 174. Difficulty in relaxing the hand-grip in a patient with myotonia dystrophica.

cataracts appear first as punctate white and polychromatic opacities in the anterior and posterior cortices of the lens[459, 18]. They cause no visual impairment for some time but, as in the case of hypoparathyroid cataracts which they simulate, they may progress to posterior cortical, and eventually to mature, cataracts (Figure 175).

Myotonia is generally classified into the congenital type (also called Thomsen's disease) and the dystrophic type[4], although the distinction is not universally accepted[227]. Cataracts are typically associated with the dystrophic variety[18].

4. Hypoparathyroidism and Pseudohypoparathyroidism

The fact that tetany is such a regular feature of hypoparathyroidism

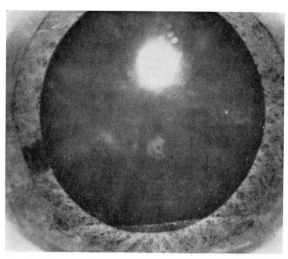

FIGURE 175. Spoke-like opacities of the lens in a patient with myotonia dystrophica. (The bright spot just above the center of the pupil and the dull spot just below it are light reflexes from the flash lamp.)

and pseudohypoparathyroidism lends neuro-ophthalmic interest to these syndromes[469]. Hypoparathyroidism may occur idiopathically or may follow accidental removal of the parathyroids (incidental to thyroidectomy). In either case insufficient formation of parathormone constitutes the underlying pathogenesis. On the other hand, pseudohypoparathyroidism appears to be a genetically determined syndrome the features of which are small stature, short metatarsals and metacarpals (especially the fourth digit), moon face, and a refractoriness to parathormone (which may be secreted in normal amounts)[11]. Both hypoparathyroidism and pseudohypoparathyroidism share the common chemical denominators of low serum calcium (less than 8 mg. %) and elevated serum phosphate (more than 8 mg.%). They also have in common the essential clinical features of tetany and a specific type of cataract[607].

The cataracts of hypoparathyroidism and pseudohypoparathyroidism consist of punctate white and sometimes polychromatic opacities in the cortex. These are at first situated superficially but if the blood calcium is restored by effective treatment the new transparent fibers will displace the opacities to a deeper layer so as to form a lamellar cataract. On the other hand, failure of effective therapy, as reflected by continued tetany, will result in a progressive and eventually mature cataract (Figure 176).

These cataracts are similar to those which occur with myotonia dystrophica. In their minimal manifestation they can be seen only by slit lamp examination. Although they are linked to that of hypocalcemia and thereby to that of tetany[554] their pathogenesis is far from clear.

Also noteworthy are the increase in spinal fluid pressure and papilledema that occasionally accompany hypoparathyroidism. This has been referred to elsewhere (see p. 147). Less frequent and less well recognized is also the predisposition such patients have to monilia infection with consequent keratoconjunctivitis.

The name pseudohypoparathyroidism, suggested by Albright *et al.*[11] who first identified the syndrome, refers of course to the fact that there is no real deficiency in parathyroid hormone. Rather the defect appears to be an inability of the end organ to react to the normal parathormone which is present. It has been likened to the Seabright-Bantam family of chickens in which the tail feathers of the cock undergo no metamorphosis on the injection of testosterone—hence it is sometimes called the Seabright-Bantam syndrome.

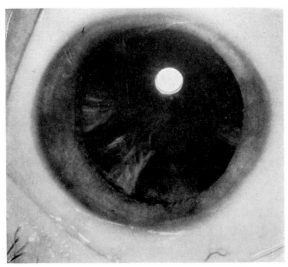

FIGURE 176. Spoke-like opacities of the lens in a patient with hypoparathyroidism. The patient was a fifty-five year old woman who developed tremor of her hands shortly after a thyroidectomy (with incidental parathyroidectomy). Cataracts gradually developed first as punctate dots and later as spoke-like opacities.

The term pseudo-pseudohypoparathyroidism has been applied to the syndrome in which all the anthropologic features of pseudohypoparathyroidism are present (small stature, dwarfed metatarsals, etc.) but in which the serum calcium and phosphate are normal[12]. Pseudopseudohypoparathyroidism has no real neuro-ophthalmic interest because there is neither tetany nor cataracts.

5. Galactosemia

This is a familial disease, transmitted as an autosomal recessive trait, in which galactose and galactose-1-phosphate accumulate in the blood owing to a defective enzyme system that normally converts galactose-1-phosphate to glucose-1-phosphate[727]. It becomes manifest within the first few weeks of life in an infant who presents a feeding problem on a milk diet. Vomiting and apathy are conspicuous initial symptoms. If the milk diet is continued the child is found to be mentally retarded, to have a large liver, and to develop cataracts. Diagnosis is made by the finding of a reducing substance (galactose and protein) in the urine. All of the symptoms clear up dramatically if the milk diet is withdrawn and glucose is substituted for galactose, provided this substitution is made shortly after onset of the symptoms. Later the changes are irreversible.

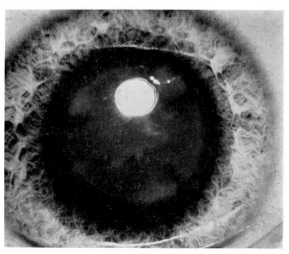

FIGURE 177. Central zonular cataract in galactosemia. The patient was a three year old boy who had been a feeding problem beginning shortly after birth. He developed a cataract before the cause of the condition was recognized.

The cataracts of galactosemia appear first as a sclerosis of the nucleus resulting in the ophthalmoscopic appearance of a large oil drop in the lens. Later the lenses develop a zonular opacity (Figure 177) and in severe cases they become completely opaque. The cataracts may be produced experimentally by giving excessively high galactose in the diets of young animals. The pathogenesis of the cataracts appears to depend on retention of the sugar alcohol and consequent hyperosmolality of the lens fibers[793].

SUMMARY

Several systemic diseases characterized by opacification of the ocular media are of tangential concern to neuro-ophthalmology.

Hepatolenticular degeneration (Wilson's disease) is a syndrome associated with a defect in copper metabolism and is characterized by cirrhosis of the liver, lesions of the basal ganglia (producing choreo-athetosis), faulty renal function (causing amino-aciduria) and a copper deposit in the periphery of Descemet's membrane (Kayser-Fleischer ring) and occasionally in the lens capsule.

Gargoylism (Hurler's disease) consists of a diffuse deposition of an unidentified glycolipid throughout many tissues of the body. Most patients with this entity have stunted growth, large livers and spleens, excessively mucoid secretions, and mental retardation. The ocular signs comprise corneal clouding and occasionally papilledema.

Myotonia dystrophica is a syndrome that includes a certain type of cataract in addition to the muscular and endocrinopathic abnormalities. The cataracts consist initially of punctate white opacities in the cortex similar to those which are found with hypoparathyroidism.

Hypoparathyroidism and pseudohypoparathyroidism are entities characterized by low blood calcium, tetany and cataracts. The cataracts consist first of punctate white spots that are not reversible but are not necessarily progressive if the blood calcium is restored to normal. Hypoparathyroidism may result from surgical or functional (idio-pathic) loss of parathormone whereas pseudohypoparathyroidism is a congenital syndrome consisting of dwarfism, curious abnormalities of the metatarsal and metacarpal bones, and a low blood calcium due apparently to parathormone unresponsiveness.

Galactosemia results from an inborn failure of galactose utilization and is manifest within the first few weeks of life by failure to grow and by reducing sugars in the urine. The chief clinical manifestations later are mental deficiency and cataracts. These latter are primarily nuclear but become total cataracts if the galactosemia is not corrected by dietary control.

REFERENCES

1. ACKERMAN, A. L.: The ocular manifestations of Waldenström's macroglobulinemia and its treatment. *Arch. Ophthal., 67*:701, 1962.
2. ADAMS, R. D.: Concerning certain psychological principles which have been derived from clinico-pathologic study. *Trans. Coll. Physicians Phila., 27*:1, 1959.
3. ADAMS, R. D., AND COHEN, M. E.: Vascular disease of the brain. *Bull. New Engl. Med. Ctr., 9*:180, 222, 261, 1947.
4. ADAMS, R. D., DENNY-BROWN, D., AND PEARSON, C.: *Diseases of Muscle. A Study in Pathology.* London: Cassell, 1953.
5. ADES, H. W., AND RAAB, D. H.: Effect of preoccipital and temporal decortication on learned visual discrimination in monkeys. *J. Neurophysiol., 12*: 101, 1949.
6. ADLER, F. H., AUSTIN, G., AND GRANT, F. C.: Localizing value of visual fields in patients with early chiasmal lesions. *Arch. Ophthal., 40*:579, 1948.
7. ADSON, A .W.: Surgical treatment of vascular diseases altering the function of the eyes. *Amer. J. Ophthal., 25*:824, 1942.
8. AKELAITIS, A. J.: Studies on the corpus callosum. II. The higher visual functions in each homonymous field following complete section of the corpus callosum. *Arch. Neurol. Psychiat., 45*:788, 1941.
9. AKELAITIS, A. J.: Studies on corpus callosum; study of language functions (tactile and visual lexia and graphia) unilaterally following section of corpus collosum. *J. Neuropath. Exper. Neurol., 2*:226, 1943.
10. AKERT, K., GRUESEN, R. A., WOOLSEY, C. N., AND MEYER, D. R.: Klüver-Bucy syndrome in monkey with neocortical ablations of temporal lobe. *Brain, 84*:480, 1961.
11. ALBRIGHT, F., BURNETT, C. H., SMITH, P. H., AND PARSON, W.: Pseudohypoparathyroidism—Example of "Seabright-bantam syndrome"; Report of 3 cases. *Endocrinology, 30*:922, 1942.
12. ALBRIGHT, F., FORBES, A. P., AND HENNEMAN, P. H.: Pseudo-pseudohypoparathyroidism. *Trans. Ass. Amer. Physicians, 65*:337, 1952.
13. ALCALDE, S. O., AND VILLANUEVA, P. U.: Compresion quias matica aguda por hematoma intratumoral en adenoma de la hipófisis. *Rev. Esp. Otoneuroftal., 9*:333, 1950.
14. ALEXANDER, H. B.: Vascular lesions affecting the visual pathways. *Arch. Ophthal., 57*:65, 1957.
15. ALFANO, J. E., ALMEIDA, H. C., AND WHITWORTH, C.: Advanced neuroophthalmologic disorders associated with normal roentgenograms of the skull. *Amer. J. Ophthal., 55*:312, 1963.
16. ALFANO, J. E., AND BERGER, J. P.: Retinitis pigmentosa, ophthalmoplegia, and spastic quadriplegia. *Amer. J. Ophthal., 43*:231, 1957.

[328]

17. ALFANO, J. E., FABRITUS, R. E., AND GARLAND, M. A.: Visual loss following mitral commissurotomy for mitral stenosis. *Amer. J. Ophthal., 44*:213, 1957.
18. ALLEN, J. H., AND BARER, C. G.: Cataract of dystrophia myotonica. *Arch. Ophthal., 24*:867, 1940.
19. ALLEN, R. A., AND STRAATSMA, B. R.: Ocular involvement in leukemia and allied disorders. *Arch. Ophthal., 66*:490, 1961.
20. ALPER, M. G., AND DESSOFF, J.: Porencephaly. *Arch. Ophthal., 54*:541, 1955.
21. ALPERS, B. J., AND WOLMAN, I. J.: Arteriosclerotic disease of the optic nerve. *Arch. Ophthal., 6*:21, 1931.
22. ALSTROM, C. H., AND OLSON, O.: Heredoretinopathia congenitalis. Monohybrida recessive autosomalis. *Hereditas, 43*:1, 1957.
23. ALTENBERGER, S.: [Lesions in the eye fundus in polycythemia rubra vera]. *Klin. Oczna, 30*:3, 1960. (Abst., *Excerpta Med., XII 14*:#1880, 1960.)
24. AMSLER, N.: Earliest symptoms of diseases of the macula. *Brit. J. Ophthal., 37*:521, 1953.
25. ANDERMANN, K., BERMAN, S., COOKE, P. M., DICKSON, J., GASTAUT, H., KENNEDY, A., MARGERISON, J., POND, D. A., TIZARD, J. P., AND WALSH, E. G.: Self-induced epilepsy. A collection of self-induced epilepsy cases compared with some other photoconvulsive cases. *Arch. Neurol., 6*:49, 1962.
26. ANDERSEN, O. C.: Grubenbildungen auf der Papille mit Gesichtsfeldausfällen. *Klin. Mbl. Augenheilk., 122*:159, 1953.
27. ANDERSON, R. G., AND GRAY, E. B.: Spasm of the central retinal artery in Raynaud's disease. Report of a case. *Arch. Ophthal., 17*:662, 1937.
28. ANDERSON, S. R.: Norrie's disease: Congenital bilateral pseudotumor of the retina with recessive x-chromosomal inheritance; Preliminary report. *Arch. Ophthal., 66*:614, 1961.
29. ANDERSSON, B., AND SAMUELSON, A.: Case of hyperglobulinemia with pronounced eye changes and acrocyanosis. *Acta Med. Scand., 117*:248, 1944.
30. ANGELONE, L.: Particolare sindrome di atrofia dell 'ottico pretestata come da colpo di sole. *Boll. Oculist., 35*:769, 1956.
31. ANTON, G.: Ueber die Selbstwahrnehmung der Herderkrankungen des Gehirns durch den Kranken bei Rindentaubheit. *Arch. Psychiat. Nervenkr., 32*:86, 1899.
32. APPELBAUM, A.: An ophthalmoscopic study of patients under treatment with thioridazine. *Arch. Ophthal., 69*:578, 1963.
33. APT, L.: Complications of phenothiazine tranquillizers: Ocular side-effects. *Survey Ophthal., 5*:550, 1960.
34. APTER, J. T.: Projection of retina on superior colliculus of cats. *J. Neurophysiol., 8*:123, 1945.
35. APTER, J. T., AND PFEIFFER, C. C.: The effect of the hallucinogenic drugs LSD-25 and Mescaline on the electroretinogram. *Ann. N.Y. Acad. Sci., 66*:508, 1957.
36. ARDOUIN, M., PECKER, J., STABERT, C., CATROS, A., AND JAVOLET, A.: Méningiome du canal optique chez un enfant de sept ans. *Rev. Otoneuroophtal., 30*:486, 1958.

37. ARGUAD, GORSE, AND CALMETTE: Chordome intraorbitaire chez un enfant de 3 ans. *Ann. Anat. Path., 14*:419, 1937. (Cited by Dyson, ref. 400.)

38. ARMINGTON, J. C., GOURAS, P., TEPAS, D. I., AND GUNKE., R.: Detection of the electroretinogram in retinitis pigmentosa. *Exp. Eye Res., 1*:74, 1961.

39. ARSENI, C., AND OPRESCO, I.: Quelques particularitiés anatomocliniques du retinoblastome. *Ann. Anat. Path. (Bucarest), 4*:129, 1959.

40. ASHTON, N.: Retinal vascularization in health and disease. *Amer. J. Ophthal., 44*:7, 1957.

41. ASHTON, N.: Larval granulomatosis of the retina due to Toxocara. *Brit. J. Ophthal., 44*:129, 1960.

42. ASHTON, N., PEARS, M. A., AND PICKERING, G. W.: Neuroretinopathy following haemorrhage; With a discussion on the nature of cytoid bodies. *Brit. J. Ophthal. 45*:385, 1961.

43. ASK-UPMARK, E.: On the "pulseless disease" outside of Japan. *Acta Med. Scand., 149*:161, 1954.

44. ASTROM, K. E., MANCALL, E. L., AND RICHARDSON, E. P.: Progressive multifocal lenko-encephalopathy; a hitherto unrecognized complication of chronic lymphatic leukaemia and Hodgkin's disease. *Brain, 81*:93, 1958.

45. AUSTEN, F. K., CARMICHAEL, M. W., AND ADAMS, R. D.: Neurologic manifestations of chronic pulmonary insufficiency. *New Engl. J. Med., 257*:579, 1957.

46. AUSTIN, G. M., LEWEY, F. H., AND GRANT, F. C.: Studies on the occipital lobe. I. Significance of small areas of preserved central vision. *Arch. Neurol., 62*:204, 1949.

47. AUSTIN, J. H.: Metachromatic form of diffuse cerebral sclerosis. I. Diagnosis during life by urine sediment examination. *Neurology, 7*:415, 1957.

48. AUSTIN, J. H.: Metachromatic form of diffuse cerebral sclerosis. III. Significance of sulfatide and other lipid abnormalities in white matter and kidney. *Neurology, 10*:470, 1960.

49. BABEL, J.: La pathogénie de la stase papillaire. *Prakis, 37*:925, 1948. (Abst., *Excerpta Med., XII 3*:#1272, 1949.)

50. BABEL, J.: Le rôle de la choriocapillaire dans les affections dégénératives du pole posterieur. *Bull. Soc. Franc. Ophthal., 71*:389, 1958.

51. BABEL, J., AND ZIV, B.: L'action du dithizone sur la rétine du lapin; etude électrophysiologique. *Experientia, 13*:122, 1957.

52. BACHMANN, R.: Schwund markhaltiger Nervenfasern in der Netzhaut nach Embolie der Art. centralis retinae. *Graefe Arch. Ophthal., 17*:10, 1921.

53. BADAL, J.: Contribution à l'étude des cécités psychiques: alexie, agraphie, hémianopsie inférieure, trouble du sens de l'espace. *Arch. ophtal., 8*:97, 1888.

54. BADTKE, G.: Über die Pseudoneuritis und Pseudostauungspapille bei Myopie nebst Bemerkungen zur Genese dieser Veränderungen. *Klin. Mbl. Augenheilk., 126*:546, 1955.

55. BADTKE, G.: Über das Wesen die Genese der sogenannten atypischen Kolobome der inneren Augenhäute und des Sehnerven. *Klin. Mbl. Augenheilk., 131*:1, 1957.

56. VON BAHR, G.: Intraocular vascular proliferations in diabetes mellitus. *Acta Med. Scand. supp. 196*, pp. 24-39, 1947.

57. BAILLIART, P., DAVID, AND SCHIFF-WERTHEIMER: Arachnoidite opto-chiasmatique avec cécité totale. Intervention. Amélioration. *Bull. Soc. Ophtal. Paris,* 1934, p. 293.
58. BAKAY, L.: The results of 300 pituitary adenoma operations. (Prof. Herbert Olivecrona's series.) *J. Neurosurg.,* 7:240, 1950.
59. BAKER, G. S.: Treatment of pituitary adenomas. *Arch. Surg., 81*:842, 1960.
60. BALAKRISHANAN, E.: Bilateral intra-ocular cysticerci. *Brit. J. Ophthal., 45*:150, 1961.
61. BALINT, R.: Seelenlähmung des Schauens, Optische Ataxie, räumliche Storung der Aufmerksamkeit. *Mschr. Psychiat. Neurol., 25*:51, 1909.
62. BALL, S., GOODWIN, T. W., AND MORTON, R. A.: Studies on vitamin A: 5. The preparation of retinene—vitamin A aldehyde. *Biochem. J., 42*:516, 1948.
63. BALLANTYNE, A. J.: The ocular manifestations of spontaneous subarachnoid haemorrhage. *Brit. J. Ophthal., 27*:383, 1943.
64. BARDAWIL, W. A.: Personal communication.
65. BARKMAN, Y.: A clinical study of a central tapetoretinal degeneration. *Acta Ophthal. (Kbh), 39*:663, 1961.
66. BARNARD, R. I., AND SCHOLZ, R. O.: Ophthalmoplegia and retinal degeneration. *Amer. J. Ophthal., 27*:621, 1944.
67. BARNETT, D. J.: Radiologic aspects of craniopharyngiomas. *Radiology, 72*: 14, 1959.
68. BARON, A., GUIMBRETIERE, PASQUIER, AND CHEVANNES: A propos de quelques cas de dysprotéinémies. *Bull. Soc. Ophtal. Franc.,* 1960, p. 293.
69. BARROWS, L. J., KUBIK, C. S., AND RICHARDSON, E. P.: Aneurysms of the basilar and vertebral arteries—A clinico-pathologic study. *Trans. Amer. Neurol. Ass., 81*:181, 1956.
70. BARSKY, D.: Quinine idiosyncracy and optic atrophy. *J. Mich. Med. Soc., 60*:612, 1961.
71. BATTEN, F. E.: Cereberal degeneration with symmetrical changes in the maculae in two members of a family. *Trans. Ophthal. Soc. U.K., 23*:386, 1903.
72. BATTEN, F. E., AND MAYOU, M. S.: Family cerebral degeneration with macular changes. *Proc. Roy. Soc. Med. (Sect. Ophthal.), 8*:70, 1915.
73. BATTERSBY, W. S., BENDER, M. B., POLLACK, M., AND KAHN, R. L.: Unilateral "spatial agnosia" ("inattention") in patients with cerebral lesions. *Brain, 79*:68, 1956.
74. BATTISTINI, A., AND CAFFI, M.: Alterazioni vascolari del nervo ottico nella senilità (Studio istologico). *Ann. Ottal., 85*:715, 1959.
75. BAUER, F.: Über einen Fall von Retinitis exsudativa externa Coats, mit besonderer Rücksicht auf die Histopathologischen Veränderungen. *Graefe Arch. Ophthal., 161*:373, 1959.
76. BAUMANN, C. H. H., AND BUCY, P. C.: Aneurysms on the anterior cerebral artery; Evaluation of surgical and "conservative" treatments. *J.A.M.A., 163*:1448, 1957.
77. BAXTER, D. W., AND BAILEY, A. A.: Primary reading epilepsy. *Neurology, 11*:445, 1961.
78. BEAM, A. D.: Amblyopia due to dietary deficiency. *Amer. J. Ophthal., 30*: 66, 1947.

79. BEARN, A. G.: Genetic and biochemical aspects of Wilson's disease. *Amer. J. Med., 15*:442, 1953.

80. BEARN, A. G., AND KUNKEL, H. G.: Localization of Cu⁶⁴ in serum fractions following oral administration: Alteration in Wilson's disease. *Proc. Soc. Exp. Biol. Med., 85*:44, 1954.

81. BEATTIE, P. H.: Three unusual cases. *Trans. Ophthal. Soc. U.K., 81*:311, 1961.

82. BEAVER, P. C.: Larva migrans. *Exp. Parasit., 5*:587, 1956.

83. BECK, D. J. K.: Upper parietal meningioma showing Foster Kennedy syndrome. *Bristol Med.-Chir. J., 64*:11, 1947.

84. BECKER, B., AND POST, L. T.: Retinal vein occlusion. *Amer. J. Ophthal., 34*:677, 1951.

85. BEDROSSIAN, R. H.: Neuroretinitis following measles. *J. Pediat., 46*:329, 1955.

86. BELICET, H.: Über rezidivierende, aphthöse, durch ein Virus verursachte Geschwüre am mund, am Auge und den Genitalien. *Derm. Wschr., 105*: 1152, 1937.

87. BEHRMAN, S.: Retinal vein obstruction. *Brit. J. Ophthal., 46*:336, 1962.

88. BEIGELMAN, M. N.: Unilateral pigmentary retinitis. *Arch. Ophthal., 6*:254, 1931.

89. BEKENY, G., AND PETER, A.: Über Polyopie und Palinopsie. *Psychiat. Neurol. (Basel), 142*:154, 1961.

90. BELL, J.: The Laurence-Moon syndrome. Part 3, Vol. 5 of *The Treasury of Human Inheritence*, Ed., L. S. Penrose, Cambridge: University Press, 1958.

91. BELLER, A. J., AND TIBERIN, P.: Glioma of the optic nerve: Its relationship to von Recklinghausen's disease. *Harefuah, 59*:197, 1960. (Abst., *Excerpta Med. XII, 15*:#1648, 1961.)

92. BEMBRIDGE, B. A.: The problem of myelination of the central nervous system with special reference to the optic nerve. *Trans. Ophthal. Soc. U.K., 76*:311, 1956.

93. BENDER, M. B., AND BATTERSBY, W. S.: Homonymous macular scotomata in cases of occipital lobe tumor. *Arch. Ophthal., 60*:928, 1958.

94. BENDER, M. B., AND FURLOW, L. T.: Phenomenon of visual extinction in homonymous fields and psychologic principles involved. *Arch. Neurol. Psychiat., 53*:29, 1945.

95. BENDER, M., AND JUNG, R.: Abweichungen der subjektiven optischen Vertikalen und Horizontalen bei Gesunden und Hirnverletzten. *Arch. Psychiat. Nervenkr., 181*:193, 1948.

96. BENDER, M. B., AND KANZER, M. G.: Dynamics of homonymous hemianopias and preservation of central vision. *Brain, 62*:404, 1939.

97. BENDER, M. B., AND SOBIN, A. J.: Polyopia and palinopia in homonymous fields of vision. *Trans. Amer. Neurol. Ass., 88*:56, 1963.

98. BENDER, M. B., AND TEUBER, H. -L.: Phenomena of fluctuation, extinction and completion in visual perception. *Arch. Neurol. Psychiat., 55*:627, 1946.

99. BENDER, M. B., AND TEUBER, H. -L.: Neuro-ophthalmology. In: *Progress in Neurology and Psychiatry*, Ed., E. A. Spiegel. Vol. 2. New York: Grune and Stratton, 1947, p. 163.

100. BENDER, M. B., AND TEUBER, H. -L.: Spatial organization of visual perception following injury to brain. *Arch. Neurol. Psychiat., 58*:721, 1947.
101. BENDER, M. B., AND TEUBER, H. -L.: Spatial organization of visual perception following injury to the brain. II. *Arch. Neurol. Psychiat., 59*:39, 1948.
102. BENDER, M. B., AND TEUBER, H. -L.: Psychopathology of Vision. In: *Progress in Neurology and Psychiatry*, Ed., E. A. Spiegel. Vol. 4. New York: Grune and Stratton, 1949, p. 166.
103. BENEDICT, W. L.: Etiology and treatment of optic neuritis. *Texas State, 45*: 126, 1949.
104. BENHAMOU, E., AND FOISSIN, J.: Streptomycine et nerf optique. *Rev. Otoneuroophtal., 23*:30, 1951.
105. BENNETT, G.: Central serous retinopathy. *Brit. J. Ophthal., 39*:605, 1955.
106. BENTON, A. L., AND MEYERS, R.: An early description of the Gerstmann syndrome. *Neurology, 6*:838, 1956.
107. BENTON, C. D., AND CALHOUN, F. P.: The ocular effects of methyl alcohol poisoning. Report of a catastrophe involving 320 persons. *Amer. J. Ophthal., 36*:1677, 1953.
108. BERESFORD, W. A.: Fibre degeneration following lesions of the visual cortex of the cat. In: *The Visual System: Neurophysiology and Psychophysics*, Ed., R. Jung and H. Hornhuber. Berlin: Springer-Verlag, 1961, p. 247.
109. BERGAUST, B.: Unusual course of internal carotid artery accompanied by bitemporal hemianopia. *Acta Ophthal., 41*:270, 1963.
110. BERGMEISTER, R.: Ueber primäre miliare Tuberkulose der Retina. *Wien. Med. Wschr., 79*:1116, 1929.
111. BERKSON, J.: Pseudo-glaucoma progressing to blindness with calcification of the carotid artery. *Trans. Ophthal. Soc. U.K., 71*:239, 1951.
112. BERLINER, M. L.: Cytologic studies on retina; normal coexistence of oligodendroglia and myelinated nerve fibers. *Arch. Ophthal., 6*:740, 1931.
113. BERNHEIMER, S.: Die Wurzelgebiete der Augennerven, ihre Verbindungen und ihr Anschluss an die Gehirnrinde. In: *Graefe-Saemisch Handbuch der Gesamten Augenheilkunde*, Ed., T. Saemisch. Band I, Kap. VI. Leipzig: Wilhelm Engelmann, 1900, p. 1.
114. BERNOULLI, R.: Über das sogenannte Diktyom-Neuroepithelioma teratoides ciliare. *Ophthalmologica, 141*:386, 1961.
115. BESSIERE, E.: La cécité foudroyante des enfants. *J. Med. Bordeaux 128*:482, 1951. (Abst., *Excerpta Med. XII, 5*:#1989, 1951.)
116. BEST, F.: Die Augenveränderungen bei den organischen nichtentzündlechen Erkrankungen des Zentralnervensystems. In: Kurzes Handbuch der Ophthalmologie, Ed., F. Schieck and A. Brückner. Berlin: Julius Springer, 1931, p. 476.
117. BETETTO, G.: Modificazione istologiche del'arteria centrale della retina nel quadro dell'angiosclerosi sistemica o distrettuale extraoculare. *Ann. Ottal., 84*:337, 1958. (Abst., *Excerpta Med. XII, 14*:#1698, 1960.)
118. BEYN, E. S., AND KNYAZEVA, G. R.:The problem of prosopagnosia. *J. Neurol. Neurosurg. Psychiat., 25*:154, 1962.
119. BHAGWATI, S. N., AND VUCKOVICH, D. M.: Craniopharyngioma presenting with acute blindness, a case report. *Arch. Neurol., 8*:101, 1963.

120. BICKERSTAFF, E. R.: Basilar artery migraine. *Lancet, 1*:15, 1961.

121. BICKFORD, R. G., WHELAN, J. L., KLASS, D. W., AND CORBIN, K. B.: Reading epilepsy: Clinical and electro-encephalographic studies of a new syndrome. *Trans. Amer. Neurol. Ass., 81*:100, 1956.

122. BIEGEL, A.C.: Oguchi's disease: A case report. *Amer. J. Ophthal., 39*:405, 1955.

123. BIEMOND, A.: Thrombosis of basilar artery and vascularization of brain stem. *Brain, 74*:300, 1951.

124. BIEMOND, A.: Nervus Opticus und Chiasma. *Bibl. Ophthal., 36*:79, 1952.

125. BIRD, A.: The lipidoses and the central nervous system. *Brain, 71*:434, 1948.

126. BIRKHEAD, N. C., WAGENER, H. P., AND SHICK, R. M.: Treatment of temporal arteritis with adrenal corticosteroids: Results in 55 cases in which lesion was proved at biopsy. *J.A.M.A., 163*:821, 1957.

127. BISHOP, P. O., AND DAVIS, R.: Bilateral interaction in the lateral geniculate body. *Science, 118*:241, 1953.

128. BJORK, A., AND KUGELBERG, E.: Visual field defects after temporal lobectomy. *Acta Ophthal., 35*:210, 1957.

129. BLACKWOOD, W., AND CUMINGS, J. N.: Histological and chemical study of 3 cases of diffuse cerebral sclerosis. *J. Neurol. Neurosurg. Psychiat., 17*:33, 1954.

130. BLATT, N., AND ATHANASIU, M.: Rélations anatomique entre le canal optique et le sinus sphenoidal. *Ann. Oculist., 190*:241, 1957.

131. BLATT, N., AND ATHANASIU, M.: Les altérations du canal optique dans les tumeurs de la région opto-chiasmatique. *J. Radiol. Electrol., 39*:815, 1958.

132. BLATTNER, R. J.: Photic seizures—television induced. *J. Pediat., 58*:746, 1961.

133. BLEGEN, S. D.: Transient amaurosis following vertebral angiography. *Acta Psychiat. Scand., 32*:181, 1957.

134. BLODI, F. C., AND VAN ALLEN, W.: Retinal artery blood pressure determinations in surgery of the carotid system. Presented before the Midwestern Section of the Association for Research in Ophthalmology, 1957. (Abst., *Amer. J. Ophthal., 43*:779, 1957.)

135. BLODI, F. C., WHINERY, R. D., AND HENDRICKS, C. A.: Lipid-proteinosis (Urbach-Wiethe) involving the lids. *Trans. Amer. Ophthal. Soc., 58*:155, 1960.

136. BLOOM, S. M., SHERZ, E. H., AND TAYLOR, W. W.: Nutritional amblyopia in American prisoners of war liberated from the Japanese. *Amer. J. Ophthal., 29*:1248, 1946.

137. BODAMER, J.: Die Prosop-Agnosie (Die Agnosie des Physiognomieerkennens). *Arch. Psychiat. Nervenkr., 118*:6, 1947.

138. BOHRINGER, H. R.: Opticusschädigungen durch Thalliumvergiftung. *Praxis, 41*:1092, 1952.

139. BOKE, W.: Untersuchungen über die praktische Verwertbarkeit okulärer Symptome bei Heintumoren. *Klin. Mbl. Augenheilk., 118*:113, 1951.

140. BOKE, W., AND JANSSEN, G.: Tierexperimentelle Untersuchungen zur Frage der Sehnervenschädigung durch INH. *Graefe Arch. Ophthal., 158*:334, 1957.

141. BOERI, R.: Ophthalmic hemicrania as a symptom of cerebral angioma. *Riv. Oto-Neuro-Oftal., 34*:126, 1959.

142. BORNER, R.: Über Optikusaffektion beim Herpes zoster ophthalmicus. *Klin. Mbl. Augenheilk., 120*:636, 1952.

143. VAN BOGAERT, L.: Erreur de diagnostic neuromyélite optique aigue, premier stade d'une sclerose en plaques typique. *J. Neurol. Psychiat. Bruxelles, 32*:234, 1932.

144. VAN BOGAERT, L.: Post-infections encephalomyelitis and multiple sclerosis. significance of perivenous encephalomyelitis. *J. Neuropath. Exp. Neurol., 9*:219, 1950.

145. VAN BOGAERT, L., AND BERTRAND, I.: Sur une idiotie familiale avec dégénerescence spongieuse du névraxe (note preliminaire). *Acta Neurol. Belg., 49*:572, 1949.

146. BOLDT, H. A., HAERER, A. F., TOUTELLOTTE, W. W., HENDERSON, J. W., AND DEJONG, R. N.: Retrochiasmal visual field defects from multiple sclerosis. *Arch. Neurol., 8*:565, 1963.

147. BOLES, W. M., NAUGLE, T. C., AND SAMSON, C. L. M.: Glioma of the optic nerve. *Arch. Ophthal., 59*:229, 1958.

148. BOLLACK, J., DAVID, M., AND PUECH, P.: *Les arachnoidites optochiasmatiques.* Paris: Masson & Cie, 1937.

149. BONAMOUR, C., AND RAVAULT, M.: Nervites optiques ourliennes d'apparence primitives. Leur diagnostic. *Ann. Oculist., 192*:640, 1959.

150. BONAMOUR, G., AND RAVAULT, M.: Les manifestations ophthalmologiques de la mononucleose infectieuse. *Gaz. Med. France, 66*:387, 1959.

151. BONYNGE, T. W., AND VON HAZEN, K. O.: Severe optic neuritis in infectious mononucleosis, report of a case. *J.A.M.A., 148*:933, 1952.

152. BORGESON, E. J., AND WAGENER, H. P.: Changes in eye in leukemia. *Amer. J. Med. Sci., 177*:663, 1929.

153. BORIONI, D.: L'atrofia ottica nell'anemia post-emorragica. *Accad. Med. (Genova), 66*:241, 1951. (Abst., *Excerpta Med. XII, 6*:#1887, 1952.)

154. BOROVY: [Atrophy of the optic nerve following intoxication by Aspidium Filix-mas]. *Cesk. Oftal., 6*:301, 1950. (Abst., *Excerpta Med. XII, 5*: #790, 1951.)

155. BOSSI, R., AND PISANI, C.: Collateral cerebral circulation through ophthalmic artery and its efficiency in internal carotid occlusion. *Brit. J. Radiol., 28*:462, 1955.

156. BOUMAN, L.: *Diffuse sclerosis (Encephalitis periaxialis diffusa).* Baltimore: Williams and Wilkins, 1934.

157. BOUMAN, M. A.: Mechanisms in peripheral dark adaption. *J. Optic Soc. Amer., 42*:941, 1952.

158. BOUMAN, M. A., AND VAN DER VELDEN, H. A.: The two-quanta explanation of the dependence of the threshold values and visual acuity on the visual angle and the time of observation. *J. Optic. Soc. Amer., 37*:908, 1947.

159. BOURNE, M. C.: Retinitis pigmentosa in rats. *Trans. Ophthal. Soc. U.K., 58*:234, 1938.

160. BOZSIK, G.: Erweichungen im Rückenmark und im Sehnerv bzw. Chiasma auf vasculärer Basis *Nervenarzt., 24*:229, 1953.

161. TER BRAAK, J. G., AND HERWARDEN, A.: Ophthalmoencephalomyelitis. *Klin. Mbl. Augenheilk., 91*:316, 1933.

162. BRADSHAW, P.: Benign intracranial hypertension. *J. Neurol. Neurosurg. Psychiat., 19*:28, 1956.

163. BRANDLE, K.: Die posttraumatischen Opticusschädigungen (insbesondere die Opticusatrophie). *Confin. Neurol., 15*:169, 1955.

164. BRAENDSTRUP, P.: Central retinal vein thrombosis and hemorrhagic glaucoma. *Acta Ophthal. (Kbh.), Supp. 35*, p. 162, 1950.

165. BRAGA MAGALHAES, P., AND ATTADIA, E. R.: Do estudo crítico das classificacoes oftalmoscópicas. *Rev. Bras. Oftal., 17*:189, 1958. (Abst., *Excerpta Med. XII, 14*:#452, 1960.)

166. BRAIN, R.: Visual disorientation with special reference to lesions of the right cerebral hemisphere. *Brain, 64*:244, 1941.

167. BRAIN, R.: Some observations on visual hallucinations and cerebral metamorphopsia. *Acta Psychiat. Scand., Supp. 46*, p. 28, 1947.

168. BRAIN, W. R.: Critical review: disseminated sclerosis. *Quart. J. Med., 23*: 343, 1930.

169. BRAND, I., AND TAKATS, I.: Histochemische Untersuchung des Kayser-Fleischerschen Hornhautringes. *Graefe Arch. Ophthal., 151*:391, 1951.

170. BRANTE, G.: Gargoylism—mucopolysaccharidosis. *Scand. J. Clin. Lab. Invest., 4*:43, 1952.

171. BREAKEY, A. S.: Ocular findings in cerebral palsy. *Arch. Ophthal., 53*:852, 1955.

172. BREGAET, P., FISCHGOLD, H., AND DAVID, M.: Quelques réflexions sur la radiographie des gliomes du chiasma. *Bull. Soc. Franc. Ophthal., 67*:271, 1954.

173. BRICKNER, R. M., AND FRANKLIN, C. R.: Visible retinal arteriolar spasm associated with multiple sclerosis, preliminary report. *Arch. Neurol. Psychiat., 51*:573, 1944.

174. BRIDGMAN, C. S., AND SMITH, K. U.: Bilateral neural integration in visual perception after section of corpus callosum. *J. Comp. Neurol., 83*:57, 1945.

175. BRIHAVE, M., GRAFF, G., BRIHAYE, J., AND DANIS, P.: Volumineux gliome kystique du chiasma à symptomatologie cérébrale predominante. *Acta Neurol. Belg., 61*:525, 1961.

176. BRIHAYE-VAN GEERTRUYDEN, M.: Retinal lesions in Hodgkin's disease. *Arch. Ophthal., 56*:94, 1956.

177. BRIHAYE,-VAN GEERTRUYDEN, M., DANIS, P., AND TOUSSAINT, C.: Fundus lesions with disseminated lupus erythematosus. *Arch. Ophthal., 51*:799, 1954.

178. BRINDLEY, G. S.: *Physiology of the retina and visual pathway.* London: Edward Arnold, 1960.

179. BROGNOLI, C., AND CITTERIO, M.: La funzionalita epaticà nell'ambliopia alcoolico-tabagico. *Boll. Oculist., 30*:12, 1951.

180. BRONNER, A.: Papillite oedémateuse à évolution rapide vers l'atrophie optique et la cécité définitive après thyroidectomie. *Strasbourg Med., 2*:304, 1951. (Abst., *Excerpta Med. XII, 6*:#752, 1952.)

181. BRONSKY, D., KUSHNER, D. S., DUBIN, A., AND SNAPPER, I.: Idiopathic hypoparathyroidism and pseudohypoparathyroidism: case reports and review of the literature. *Medicine, 37*:317, 1958.

182. BROSNAN, D. W.: Occlusion of a cilioretinal artery with permanent central scotoma. *Amer. J. Ophthal., 53*:687, 1962.

183. BROUGHAM, M., HEUSNER, A. P., AND ADAMS, R. D.: Acute degenerative changes in adenomas of the pituitary body—With special reference to pituitary apoplexy. *J. Neurosurg., 7*:421, 1950.

184. BROUWER, B., AND ZEEMAN, W. P. C.: The projection of the retina in the primary optic neuron in monkeys. *Brain, 49*:1, 1926.

185. BROWN, K. T., AND WATANABE, W.: Isolation and identification of a receptor potential from the pure cone fovea of the monkey retina. *Nature, 193*:958, 1962.

186. BRUCE, G. M.: Temporal arteritis as a cause of blindness. Review of literature and report of a case. *Trans. Amer. Ophthal. Soc., 47*:300, 1949.

187. BRUCE, G. M., DENNING, C. R., AND SPALTER, H. F.: Ocular findings in cystic fibrosis of the pancreas. *Arch. Ophthal., 63*:391, 1960.

188. BRUETSCH, W. L.: Late cerebral sequelae of rheumatic fever. *Arch. Intern. Med., 73*:472, 1944.

189. BRUETSCH, W. L.: Etiology of optochiasmatic arachnoiditis. *Arch. Neurol. Psychiat., 59*:215, 1948.

190. BRUETSCH, W. L.: Syphilitic optic atrophy. Monograph of American Lecture Series, 1953. (Abst., *Excerpta Med. XII, 7*:#1426, 1953.)

191. BREWER, A. J., AND KIERLAND, R. R.: Neurofibromatosis and congenital unilateral pulsating and nonpulsating exophthalmos. *Arch. Ophthal., 53*: 2, 1955.

192. DE BUEN, S., AND GONZALEZ-ANGULO, A.: Diktyoma (embryonal medulloepithelioma). Review of the literature and report of a case. *Amer. J. Ophthal., 49*:606, 1960.

193. BURKI, E.: Ueber den primären Sehnerventumor und seine Beziehungen zur Recklinghausenschen Neurofibromatose. *Bibl. Ophthal. supp. to Ophthalmologica., vol. 30,* 1944.

194. BULLINGTON, S. J., AND WAKSMAN, B. H.: Uveitis in rabbits with experimental allergic encephalomyelitis. Results produced by injection of nervous tissue and adjuvants. *Arch. Ophthal., 59*:435, 1958.

195. VAN BUREN, J. M., AND BALDWIN, M.: The architecture of the optic radiation in the temporal lobe of man. *Brain, 81*:15, 1958.

196. BURIAN, H. M., AND FLETCHER, M. C.: Visual functions in patients with retinal pigmentary degeneration following the use of NP 207. *Arch. Ophthal., 60*:612, 1958.

197. BURNS, R. P.: Cytomegalic inclusion disease uveitis; Report of a case with isolation from aqueous humor of the virus in tissue culture. *Arch. Ophthal., 61*:376, 1959.

198. BUSH, J. A., MAHONEY, J. P., MARKOWITZ, H., GUBLER, C. J., CARTWRIGHT, G. E., AND WINTROBE, M. M.: Studies on copper metabolism. XIV. Radioactive copper studies in normal subjects and in patients with hepatolenticular degeneration. *J. Clin. Invest., 34*:1766, 1955.

199. BUXEDA, R.: Chiasmal optic neuritis. *Arch. Ophthal., 59*:29, 1958.

200. BYRNES, V. A., BROWN, D. V. L., ROSE, H. W., AND CIBIS, P. A.: Retinal burns: New hazard of the atomic bomb. *J.A.M.A., 157*:21, 1955.

201. CACCAMISE, W. C., AND WHITMAN, J. F.: Pulseless disease, a preliminary case report. *Amer. Heart J., 44*:629, 1952.

202. CAGIANUT, B.: Le syndrome oculaire de la macroglobulinemie. (Syndrome de Waldenström). *Ann. Oculist (Par.), 191*:579, 1958.
203. CAGIANUT, B., AND HOFFMAN-EGG, L.: Über Augenhintergrundsveränderungen bei Makroglobulinämien. *Graefe Arch. Ophthal., 153*:391, 1953.
204. CARMETTES, L., DEODATI, F., AND AMALRIC, P.: Deux cas d'arachnoïdite optochiasmatique tuberculeuse. *Arch. Ophthal. (Par.), 16*:615, 1956.
205. CAMP, W. A., AND FRIERSON, J. G.: Sarcoidosis of the central nervous system, a case with postmortem studies. *Arch. Neurol., 7*:432, 1962.
206. CAMPBELL, E. H.: Relationship of sinusitis to optic and retrobulbar neuritis, with special reference to etiology and treatment. *Arch. Ophthal., 16*:236, 1936.
207. CAMPBELL, J. B., AND HUDSON, F. M.: Craniobuccal origin, signs, and treatment of craniopharyngiomas. *Surg. Gynec. Obstet., 111*:183, 1960.
208. CAPOLONGO, G.: Neurite Ottica da Morbillo. *Arch. Ottal., 55*:71, 1951.
209. CARBAJAL, U. M.: Metastasis in retinoblastoma. *Amer. J. Ophthal., 48*:42, 1959.
210. CARDELL, B. S., AND HANLEY, T.: Fatal case of giant-cell or temporal arteritis. *J. Path. Bact., 63*:587, 1951.
211. CAREY, P. C.: Epidermoids of the orbit. Presented at 55th Meeting: Society of British Neurological Surgeons. (Abst., *J. Neurol. Neurosurg. Psychiat., 20*:230, 1957.)
212. CARLBORG, U.: Studies of circulatory disturbances, pulse wave velocity and pressure pulses in larger arteries in cases of pseudoxanthoma elasticum and angioid streaks; contribution to knowledge of function of elastic tissue and smooth muscles in larger arteries. *Acta Med. Scand., supp. 151*, p. 1, 1944.
213. CARROLL, F. D.: "Alcohol" amblyopia, pellagra, polyneuritis. *Arch. Ophthal., 16*:919, 1936.
214. CARROLL, F. D.: Visual symptoms caused by digitalis. *Amer. J. Ophthal., 28*:373, 1945.
215. CARROLL, F. D.: Nutritional retrobulbar neuritis. *Amer. J. Ophthal., 30*:172, 1947.
216. CARROLL, F. D.: Optic neuritis. A 15-year study. *Amer. J. Ophthal., 35*:75, 1952.
217. CARROLL, F. D., AND FRANKLIN, C. R.: Tobacco amblyopia, alcohol amblyopia. *Amer. J. Ophthal., 19*:1070, 1936.
218. CARROLL, F. D., AND GOODHART, R.: Acute alcoholic amaurosis. *Arch. Ophthal., 20*:797, 1938.
219. CARROLL, F. D., AND HAIG, C.: Congenital stationary night blindness without ophthalmoscopic or other abnormalities. *Arch. Ophthal., 50*:35, 1953.
220. CASANOVAS, J., RUBIO, S., AND VILAPLANA, A.: Tuberculoma solitario de la papila, *An. Med. (Espec.), 44*:278, 1958. (Abst., *Excerpta Med. XII, 14*: #987, 1960.)
221. Case Records of the Massachusetts General Hospital: Case 38241. *New Engl. J. Med., 246*:939, 1952.
222. Case Records of the Massachusetts General Hospital: Case 40261. *New Engl. J. Med., 251*:31, 1954.
223. Case Records of the Massachusetts General Hospital: Case 43092. *New Engl. J. Med., 256*:417, 1957.

224. Case Records of the Massachusetts General Hospital: Case 45821. *New Engl. J. Med., 261*:89, 1959.

225. CASELLI, F., AND PONTE, F.: Sindromi otticochiasmatiche ed esame cisternografico. *Riv. Oto-Neuro-Oftal., 33*:26, 1958. (Abst., *Excerpta Med. XII, 14*:#1435, 1960.)

226. CATROS, A., JAVALET, A., LeMENN, G., AND URVOY: La place des étiologies rares dans les cécités unilaterales immediates des traumatismes craniens. *Rev. Otoneurooftal., 32*:57, 1960. (Abst., *Excerpta Med. XII, 15*:#253, 1961.)

227. CAUGHEY, J. E.: Relationship of dystrophia myotonica (myotonic dystrophy) and myotonia congenita (Thomsen's disease). *Neurology, 8*:469, 1958.

228. CELOTTI, M., AND FRERA, C.: Symptomatology of the meningiomas of the olfactory groove. *Ann. Ottal., 85*:14, 1959.

229. CENTANNI, L., AND MORELLO, F.: Alterazioni oculari in alcuni tumori della regione sellare ed iuxtasellare e loro modificazioni dopo radioterapias. *Riv. Oto-Neuro-Oftal., 32*:279, 1957.

230. CERLETTI, A.: Cited by Weekley, R. D. et al., ref. 1539.

231. CHABANIER, H., PUECH, P., LOBO-ONELL, C., AND LELU, E.: Hypophyse et diabète (à propos de l'ablation d'une hypophyse normale dans un cas de diabète grave), *Presse Med., 44*:986, 1936.

232. CHACKO, L. W.: The laminar pattern of the lateral geniculate body in the primates. *J. Neurol. Neurosurg. Psychiat., 11*:211, 1948.

233. CHAMBERS, J. W., and WALSH, F. B.: Hyaline bodies in the optic discs: Report of ten cases exemplifying importance in neurological diagnosis. *Brain, 74*:95, 1951.

234. CHAMLIN, M.: Visual field defects due to optic nerve compression by mass lesions. *Arch. Ophthal., 58*:37, 1957.

235. CHAMLIN, M.: Visual field changes produced by x-ray treatment of pituitary tumours. *Brit. J. Ophthal., 42*:193, 1958.

236. CHAMLIN, M., and BILLET, E.: Ophthalmoplegia and pigmentary degeneration of the retina. *Arch. Ophthal., 43*:217, 1950.

237. CHAMLIN, M., AND DAVIDOFF, L. M.: Drusen of optic nerve simulating papilledma. *J. Neurosurg., 7*:70, 1950.

238. CHAMLIN, M., AND DAVIDOFF, L. M.: Drusen of the optic nervehead; Ophthalmoscopic and histopathologic study. *Amer. J. Ophthal., 35*:1599, 1952.

239. CHAMLIN, M., AND DAVIDOFF, L. M.: Homonymous hemianopia in multiple sclerosis. *Neurology, 4*:429, 1954.

240. CHAMLIN, M., AND DAVIDOFF, L. M.: Ophthalmologic criteria in diagnosis and management of pituitary tumors. *J. Neurosurg., 19*:9, 1962.

241. CHAMLIN, M.; DAVIDOFF, L. M., AND FEIRING, E. H.: Ophthalmologic changes produced by pituitary tumours. *Amer. J. Ophthal., 40*:353, 1955.

242. CHERINGTON, F. J.: Metastatic adenocarcinoma of the optic nerve-head and adjacent retina. *Brit. J. Ophthal., 45*:227, 1961.

243. CH'IN, K. Y.: Histogenesis of glioma retinae: Report of early case with review of literature. *Amer. J. Path., 17*:813, 1941.

244. DI CHIRO, G.: Ophthalmic arteriography. *Radiology, 77*:948, 1961.

245. CHLENOV, L. G., AND BEIN, E. S.: Agnosia for faces. *Zh. Nevropat. Psikhiat. Korsakov., 58*:914, 1958. (Abst., *Excerpta Med. XII 14*:#372, 1960.)

246. CHOW, K-L; BLUM, J. S., AND BLUM, R. A.: Cell ratios in the thalamocortical visual system of Macaca mulatta. *J. Comp. Neurol., 92*:227, 1950.

247. CHRAST, B.: [Late papilledema in subarachnoid hemorrhage]. *Cesk. Nevrol., 20*:118, 1957. (Abst., *Excerpta Med. XII, 12*:#428, 1958.)

248. CHRISPIN, A. R., AND DARKE, C. S.: Papilloedema and polycythoemia. *Brit. Med. J., 1*:989, 1962.

249. CHRISTENSEN, H.: Observationen und Reflektionen über das binokulare Tiefensehen. *Acta Ophthal. (Kbh.), 33*:167, 1955.

250. CHRISTENSEN, L.; BEEMAN, H. W., AND ALLEN, A.: Cytomegalic inclusion disease. *Arch. Ophthal., 57*:90, 1957.

251. CIBIS, P. A.; BROWN, E. B., AND HONG, S.-M.: Ocular effects of systemic siderosis. *Amer. J. Ophthal., 44*:158, 1957.

252. CIBIS, P. A.; CONSTANT, M.; PRIBYL, A., AND BECKER, B.: Ocular lesions produced by iodoacetate. *Arch. Ophthal., 57*:508, 1957.

253. CIBOLDI, A.: Quattro casi di Neuropapillite Ottica in Corso di Pandemia da Virus A/1 Singapore 1957. *Arch. Ottal., 63*:45, 1959.

254. CICCARELLI, E. C.: A new syndrome of tapetal-like fundic reflexes with ring scotoma: Report of two cases. *Arch. Ophthal., 67*:316, 1962.

255. CLARK, E. C., AND BAILEY, A. A.: Neurological and psychiatric signs associated with systemic lupus erythematosus. *J.A.M.A., 160*:455, 1956.

256. CLARK, W. E. L.: Laminar organization and cell content of lateral geniculate body in monkey. *J. Anat., 75*:419, 1941.

257. CLARK, W. E. L., AND PENMAN, G. G.: Projection of retina in lateral geniculate body. *Proc. Roy. Soc. (Biol.) 114*:291, 1934.

258. CLARKE, E.: Ophthalmological complications of multiple myelomatosis. *Brit. J. Ophthal., 39*:233, 1955.

259. CLIFTON, F., AND GREER, C. H.: Ocular changes in acute systemic lupus erythematosus. *Brit. J. Ophthal., 39*:1, 1955.

260. COATS, G.: Thrombosis of the central vein of the retina. *Roy. London Ophthal. Hosp. Rep., 16*:62, 1904.

261. COGAN, D. G.: Pathology in Symposium: Primary chorioretinal aberrations with night blindness. *Trans. Amer. Acad. Ophthal. Otolaryng., 54*:629, 1950.

262. COGAN, D. G.: A type of congenital ocular motor apraxia presenting jerky head movements. *Trans. Amer. Acad. Ophthal. Otolaryng., 56*:853, 1952.

263. COGAN, D. G.: *Neurology of the ocular muscles,* 2nd ed., Springfield, Ill.: Charles C Thomas, Publisher, 1956.

264. COGAN, D. G.: Amaurotic family idiocy, a case for eponyms. *New Engl. J. Med., 258*:1212, 1958.

265. COGAN, D. G.: Blackouts not obviously due to carotid occlusion. *Arch. Ophthal., 66*:180, 1961.

266. COGAN, D. G.: Retinal architecture and pathophysiology. *Amer. J. Ophthal., 54*:347, 1962.

267. COGAN, D. G.: Personal observation.

268. COGAN, D. G., AND ADAMS, R. D.: A type of paralysis of conjugate gaze (ocular motor apraxia). *Arch. Ophthal., 50*:434, 1953.

269. COGAN, D. G., AND FEDERMAN, D. D.: Retinal involvement with reticuloendotheliosis of unclassified type. *Arch. Ophthal., 71*:489, 1964.

270. COGAN, D. G., AND FREESE, C. G.: Spasm of the near reflex. *Arch. Ophthal.,* 54:752, 1955.
271. COGAN, D. G., AND KUWABARA, T.: Some common artifacts in the retina. *J. Histochem. Cytochem.,* 6:290, 1958.
272. COGAN, D. G., AND KUWABARA, T.: Further observations on lipid crystals in tissue. *J. Histochem. Cytochem.,* 7:80, 1959.
273. COGAN, D. G., AND KUWABARA, T.: Histochemistry of the retina in Tay-Sachs disease. *Arch. Ophthal., 61*:414, 1959.
274. COGAN, D. G., AND KUWABARA, T.: Capillary shunts in the pathogenesis of diabetic retinopathy. *Diabetes, 12*:293, 1963.
275. COGAN, D. G., AND KUWABARA, T.: Development and senescence of the human retinal vasculature. *Trans. Ophthal. Soc. U.K., 83*:465, 1963.
276. COGAN, D. G., AND KUWABARA, T.: Ocular pathology of the 13-15 trisomy syndrome. *Arch. Ophthal., 72*:246, 1964.
277. COGAN, D. G.; KUWABARA, T., AND MOSER, H.: Fat emboli in the retina following angiography. *Arch. Ophthal, 71*:308, 1964.
278. COGAN, D. G.; KUWABARA, T.; RICHARDSON, E. P., AND LYON, G.: Histochemistry of the eye in metachromatic leukoencephalopathy. *Arch. Ophthal., 60*:397, 1958.
279. COGAN, D. G.; KUWABARA, T.; YOUNG, G., AND KNOX, D. L.: Herpes simplex retinopathy in an infant. *Arch. Ophthal.* In press.
280. COGAN, D. G., AND LOEB, D. R.: Optokinetic response and intracranial lesions. *Arch. Neurol. Psychiat., 61*:183, 1949.
281. COGAN, D. G.; POPPEN, J. L., AND HICKS, S. P.: Ganglioneuroma of chiasm and optic nerves. *Arch. Ophthal., 65*:481, 1961.
282. COGAN, D. G.; TOUSSAINT, D., AND KUWABARA, T.: Retinal vascular patterns IV. Diabetic retinopathy. *Arch. Ophthal., 66*:366, 1961.
283. COHEN, H., AND DIBLE, J. H.: Pituitary basophilism associated with a basophil carcinoma of the anterior lobe of the pituitary gland. *Brain., 59*:395, 1936.
284. COHEN, J. H., AND MILLER, S.: Eyeball bruits. *New Engl. J. Med., 255*:459, 1956.
285. COHEN, M.: Lesions of the fundus in polycythemia. Report of cases. *Arch. Opthal., 17*:811, 1937.
286. COLAS, COLLET, AND CHEVANNES: Les atteintes du nerf optique dans les traumatismes craniens. *Rev. Otoneuroophtal. 28*:1, 1956.
287. COLBY, M. Y., AND KEARNS, T. P.: Radiation therapy of pituitary adenomas with associated visual impairment. *Proc. Mayo Clin., 37*:15, 1962.
288. COLE, J. G.; COLE, H. G., AND JANOFF, L. A.: A toxic ocular manifestation of chloramphenicol therapy. *Amer. J. Ophthal., 44*:18, 1957.
289. COLE, M.; SCHUTTA, H. S., AND WARRINGTON, E. K.: Visual disorientation in homonymous half-fields. *Neurology, 12*:257, 1962.
290. COLLIER, J., AND GREENFIELD, J. G.: Encephalitis periaxialis of Schilder; a clinical and pathological study, with an account of two cases, one of which was diagnosed during life. *Brain, 47*:489, 1924.
291. CONE, W., AND MACMILLAN, J. A.: The optic nerve and papilla. Section 17, Vol. 2 of *Cytology and Cellular pathology of the nervous system.* Ed., W. Penfield. New York: Paul B. Hoeber, 1932, p. 839.
292. CONNOR, R. C. R.: Complicated migraine: A study of permanent neurological and visual defects caused by migraine. *Lancet., 2*:1072, 1962.

293. CONTRERAS, J. S., FIELD, R. A., HALL, W. A., AND SWEET, W. H.: Ophthalmological observations in hypophyseal stalk section. Report of 8 cases of advancing diabetic retinopathy. *Arch. Ophthal., 64*:428, 1962.

294. COOKE, W. T.; CLOAKE, P. C. P.; GOVAN, A. D. T., AND COLBECK, J. C.: Temporal arteritis; generalized vascular disease. *Quart. J. Med., 15*:47, 1946.

295. COPENHAVER, R. M., AND GOODMAN, G.: The electroretinogram in infantile, late infantile, and juvenile amaurotic family idiocy. *Arch. Ophthal., 63*:559, 1960.

296. CORDES, F. C.: A type of foveo-macular retinitis observed in the U.S. Navy. *Amer. J. Ophthal., 27*:803, 1944.

297. CORDES, F. C.: Optic atrophy in infancy, childhood, and adolescence; A survey of 81 cases. *Trans. Amer. Ophthal. Soc., 49*:365, 1951.

298. CORDES, F. C.: Subhyaloid hemorrhage following subarachnoid hemorrhage. Report of two cases. *Amer. J. Ophthal., 36*:1192, 1953.

299. CORDES, F. C., AND HOGAN, M. J.: Primary malignant melanoma of the optic disc. *Amer. J. Ophthal., 32*:1037, 1949.

300. COSNETT, J. E., AND MACLEOD, I. N.: Retinal haemorrhages in severe anaemias: Their diagnostic significance. *Brit. Med. J., 5158*:1002, 1959.

301. COSTI, C.: Hemianopsia post-hemorragica. *Arch. Soc. oftal. hisp.-amer., 12*:685, 1952.

302. COULONJOU; MORIN; MARC, AND TUSET: Considérations cliniques et thérapeutiques sur un anévrysme cérébral. *Rev. otoneuroophtal., 32*:9, 1960.

303. COWEN, D., AND OLMSTEAD, E. V.: Infantile neuroaxonal dystrophy. *J. Neuropath. Exper. Neurol., 22*:175, 1963.

304. COYLE, J. T.; FRANK, P. E.; LEONARD, A. L., AND WEINER, A.: Macroglobulinemia and its effect upon the eye. *Arch. Ophthal., 65*:75, 1961.

305. CRAIG, W. M., AND LILLIE, W. I.: Chiasmal syndrome produced by chronic local arachnoiditis, report of eight cases. *Arch. Ophthal., 5*:558, 1931.

306. CRAVIOTO, H.; REY-BELLET, J.; PROSE, P. H., AND FEIGIN, I.: Occlusion of the basilar artery; A clinical and pathologic study of 14 autopsied cases. *Neurology, 8*:145, 1958.

307. CRAWFORD, B.: Basilar embolism. *Brit. J. Ophthal., 44*:689, 1960.

308. CREVASSE, L. E., AND LOGUE, R. B.: Carotid artery murmurs; continuous murmur over carotid bulb—new sign of carotid artery insufficiency. *J.A.M.A., 167*:2177, 1958.

309. CRICK, R. P.; HOYLE, C., AND SMELLIE, H.: The eyes in sarcoidosis. *Brit. J. Ophthal., 45*:461, 1961.

310. CRITCHLEY, M.: Types of visual perseveration: "Paliopsia" and "illusory visual spread." *Brain, 74*:267, 1951.

311. CRITCHLEY, M.: *The parietal lobes.* London: Arnold, 1953.

312. CRITCHLEY, M.: Inborn reading disorders of central origin. *Trans. Ophthal Soc. U.K., 81*:459, 1961.

313. CRITCHLEY, M.: Dyslexia in Braille-readers. *Bull. Johns Hopkins Hosp., 111*:83, 1962.

314. CRITCHLEY, M.; COBB, W., AND SEARS, T. A.: On reading epilepsy. *Epilepsia (Amst.), 1*:403, 1960.

315. CROMPTON, M. R.: The visual changes in temporal (giant-cell) arteritis. Report of a case with autopsy findings. *Brain, 82*:377, 1959.

316. CROMPTON, M. R., AND LAYTON, D. D.: Delayed radionecrosis of the brain following therapeutic x-radiation of the pituitary. *Brain, 84*:85, 1961.
317. CROSBY, R. C., AND WADSWORTH, R. C.: Temporal arteritis; Review of literature and report of 5 additional cases. *Arch. Intern. Med., 81*:431, 1948.
318. CULLER, A. M.: Fundus changes in leukemia. *Trans. Amer. Ophthal. Soc., 49*:445, 1951.
319. CUMINGS, J. N.; GOODWIN, H. J., AND EARL, C. J.: Blood copper and its relationship to globulins. *J. Clin. Path., 8*:69, 1955.
320. CUNIER, F.: Médicin Militaire, "Histoire d'une Héméralopie héréditaire depuis deux siècles dans une famille de la commune de Vendémian, près Montpellier." *Ann. de la Soc. Méd. da Gand.,* 1838, pp 383-395.
321. CUSHING, H.: The field defects produced by temporal lobe lesions. *Brain, 44*:341, 1922.
322. CUSHING, H.: The chiasmal syndrome of primary optic atrophy and bitemporal field defects in adults with a normal sella turcica. *Arch. Ophthal., 3*:505 and 704, 1930.
323. CUSHING, H.: Basophil adenomas of pituitary body and their clinical manifestations (pituitary basophilism). *Bull. Johns Hopkins Hosp., 50*:137, 1932.
324. CUSHING, H., AND EISENHARDT, L.: Meningiomas arising from the tuberculum sellae with the syndrome of primary optic atrophy and bitemporal field defects combined with a normal sella turcica in a middle-aged person. *Arch. Ophthal., 1*:1 and 168, 1929.
325. CUSHING, H., AND WALKER, C. B.: Distortions of the visual fields in cases of brain tumor. IV. Chiasmal lesions, with especial reference to bitemporal hemianopsia. *Brain, 37*:341, 1915.
326. CUTLER, W. M., AND BLATT, I. M.: The ocular manifestations of lethal midline granuloma. *Amer. J. Ophthal., 42*:21, 1956.
327. D'AGOSTINO, A. N.; SAYRE, G. P., AND HAYLES, A. B.: Krabbe's disease, globoid cell type of leukodystrophy. *Arch. Neurol., 8*:82, 1963.
328. DAMBSKA, M.: [A case of cortical blindness following bilateral hemorrhage into the occipital lobes]. *Klin. Oczna, 31*:151, 1961. (Abst., *Ophthal. Lit., 15*:#672, 1961.)
329. DANDY, W. E.: *Orbital tumors, results following the transcranial operative attack.* New York: Oskar Piest, 1941.
330. DANIS, P.: Le syndrome chiasmatique d'origine traumatique; A propos de cinq nouvelles observations. *Rev. Otoneuroophtal., 26*:1, 1954.
331. DANIS, P., AND BASTENIE, P.: Les atteintes du nerf optique au course des exophtalmies oedémateuses endocréniennes. *Ophthalmologica, 126*:65, 1953.
332. DANIS, P.; BEGAUX, C., AND DECOCK, G.: Bases ophthalmologiques d'une classification des idioties amaurotiques; sur la valeur relative d'un groupement d'après les âges du début et les durees d'évolution clinique. *J. Genet. Hum., 6*:91, 1957.
333. DANIS, J.; BRAUMAN, J., AND COPPEZ, P.: Les lésions du fond d'oeil au cours de certaines hyperproteinémies, en particulier celles d'origine myelomateuse. *Acta. 17 Conc. Ophthal., 2*:1042, 1955.
334. DANIS, P.; BRAUMAN, J.; AND COPPEZ P.: Les lésions du fond d'oeil au

cours de certaines hyperproteinémies (myélome à cryoglobuline, macroglobulinémie). *Acta Ophthal., 33*:33, 1955.

335. DANIS, P., AND BRIHAYE-VAN GEERTRUYDEN, M.: Névrite optique rétrobulbaire bilaterale par métastases cancéreuses dans les gaines arachnoidiennes. *Acta Neurol. Belg., 52*:345, 1952.

336. DANIS, P., AND VAN EYCK, M.: Volumineux myxo-chondrome du carrefour pterygo-maxillaire à symptomatologie réduite. *Acta Neurol. Belg., 55*:581, 1955.

337. DANIS, P., AND TOUSSAINT, D.: Hémianopsie homonyme après intoxication oxycarbonée. *Acta Neurol. Belg., 55*:1010, 1955.

338. D'ARRIGO, P.: Considerazioni clinico terapeutiche sulla neuro mielite ottica. *Arch. Ottal., 62*:93, 1958.

339. DAVID, M., AND RENARD, G.: Les oedèmes aigus de la partie postérieure du nerf optique. *Bull. Soc. Ophtal. Franc., 3*:436, 1949.

340. DAVID, N. J.; KLINTWORTH, G. K.; FRIEDBERG, S. J., AND DILLON, M.: Fatal atheromatous cerebral embolism associated with bright plaques in the retinal arterioles. *Neurology, 13*:708, 1963.

341. DAVIDOFF, L. M., AND EPSTEIN, B. S.: *The abnormal pneumoencephalogram.* Philadelphia: Lea and Feibiger, 1950.

342. DAVIDOFF, L. M., AND FIERING, E. H.: *Practical neurology.* New York: Landsberger, 1955.

343. DAVIS, F. A.: Primary tumors of the optic nerve (a phenomenon of Recklinghausen's disease), a clinical and pathologic study with a report of five cases and a review of the literature. *Arch. Ophthal., 23*:735 and 957, 1940.

344. DAVIS, L., AND HAVEN, H. A.: A clinico-pathologic study of the intracranial arachnoid membrane. *J. Nerv. Ment. Dis., 73*:129 and 286, 1931.

345. DAWSON, B. H.: The blood vessels of the human optic chiasma and their relation to those of the hypophysis and hypothalamus. *Brian, 81*:207, 1958.

346. DAY, R. M., AND CARROLL, F. D.: Optic nerve involvement associated with thyroid dysfunction. *Arch. Ophthal., 67*:289, 1962.

347. DAYAL, Y., AND RODGER, F. C.: Mutations of the retinal pigment cells in a case of pseudoglioma. *Arch. Ophthal., 62*:785, 1959.

348. DEBES, L. T., LUCAS, J. G. S., AND BARCONS, F. B.: A case of Takayasu's syndrome: The pulseless disease. *Brit. Heart. J., 17*:484, 1955.

349. DEJEAN, C.: Le vrai gliome de la rétine; astrocytome de la rétine adulte. *Arch. Ophtal. (Par.), 51*:257, 1934.

350. DEJEAN, C.: Les oedèmes atypiques de la papille optique. *Bull. Soc. Franc. Ophtal., 69*:23, 1956.

351. DEJEAN, C., AND GASSENE, R.: Note sur la généologie de la famille Nougaret, de Vendemain. *Bull. Soc. Ophtal. Franc., 1*:96, 1949.

352. DEJERINE, J.: Contribution a l'étude anatomo-pathologique et clinique des differentes variétés de cécité verbale. *Mem. Soc. Biologie, 4*:61, 1892.

353. DEKABAN, A., AND DRAGER, G.: Metastases of the retinoblastoma to the central nervous system; advisability of a combined intraorbital and intracranial removal of the affected optic nerve. *Arch. Ophthal., 61*:239, 1959.

354. DEKKING, H. M.: Tropical nutritional amblyopia. *Ophthalmologica, 113*:5, 1947.

355. DELOGU, A.: Retinopatia in corso di dermatomiosite grave diffuse. *Arch. Ottal., 63*:143, 1959.

356. DENNY-BROWN, D.: Symposium on specific methods of treatment; treatment of recurrent cerebrovascular symptoms and question of "vasospasm." *Med. Clin. N. Amer., 35*:1457, 1951.

357. DENNY-BROWN, D.: Basilar artery syndromes. *Bull. Tufts New Engl. Med. Cent., 15*:53, 1953.

357a. DENNY-BROWN, D.: Hepatolenticular degeneration (Wilson's disease); two different components. *New Engl. J. Med., 270*:1149, 1964.

358. DENNY-BROWN, D., AND CHAMBERS, R. A.: Visuo-motor function in the cerebral cortex. *J. Nerv. Ment. Dis., 121*:288, 1955.

359. DENNY-BROWN, D.; MEYER, J. S., AND HORENSTEIN, S.: Significance of perceptual rivalry resulting from parietal lesion. *Brain, 75*:433, 1952.

360. DEUSCH, G.: Zur symptomatologie und ätiologie der Myelitis (Encephalomyelitis) disseminata acuta. *Deutsch. Z. Nervenheilk., 80*:211, 1923.

361. DEVINCENTIIS, M.: Considerazioni su una probabile etiologia virale in casi di neurite ottica retrobulbare. *Arch. Ottal., 61*:209, 1957.

362. DIACICOV, M.: [Purtscher's disease or traumatic angiopathy of the retina.] *Oftalmologia (Bucarest), 1*:67, 1956. (Abst. *Excerpta Med. XII, 12*: #145, 1958.)

363. DICKERSON, W. W.: Characteristic roentgenographic changes associated with tuberous sclerosis. *Arch. Neurol. Psychiat., 53*:199, 1945.

364. DICKMAN, G.; CRAMER, F., AND KAPLAN, A.: Opto-chiasmatic arachnoiditis; surgical treatment and results. *J. Neurosurg., 8*:355, 1951.

365. DIDE, M.: Diagnostic anatomo-clinique de desorientations temporospatiales. *Rev. Neurol. (Par.), 69*:720, 1938.

366. DIETER, W.: Untersuchungen zur Duplizitätstheorie; die angeborene familiäre-erbliche, stationäre (idiopathische) hemeralopie. *Pflueger Arch. Ges. Physiol. 222*:381, 1929.

367. DIEZEL, P. B., AND RICHARDSON, E. P.: Histochemical and neuropathological studies in leukodystrophy (degenerative diffuse cerebral sclerosis, Scholz, Bielschowsky and Henneberg type). Presented before the American Association of Neuropathologists, 1956. (Abst., *J. Neuropath. Exper. Neurol., 16*:130, 1957.)

368. DIFERDINANDO, R.: Eritema essudativo polimorfo e neurite ottica. *Arch. Ottal., 53*:385, 1959.

369. DIMSDALE, H.: Discussion on the neuro-ophthalmological aspects of the cerebral angiomas. *Proc. Roy. Soc. Med., 50*:85, 1957.

370. DOANE, B. K.: Changes in visual function with perceptual isolation. Doctoral Thesis, McGill University, 1955.

371. DODEN, W.: Zur semiologie der periphlebitis retinae. *Klin. Mbl. Augenheilk., 137*:328, 1960.

372. DODGE, H. W.; LOVE, J. G.; CRAIG, W. M.; DOCKERTY, M. B.; KEARNS, T. P.; HOLMAN, C. B., AND HAYLES, A. B.: Gliomas of the optic nerves. *Arch. Neurol. Psychiat., 79*:607, 1958.

373. DOEHRING, D. G., AND REITAN, R. M.: Language disorders in brain-damaged patients. The effects of homonymous visual field defects. *Arch. Neurol., 5*:294, 1961.

374. DOLMAN, C. L., AND CAIRNS, A. R.: Leukoencephalopathy associated with Hodgkin's disease. *Neurology, 11*:349, 1961.

375. DONDERS, P. C.: Eale's disease. *Docum. Ophthal., 12*:1, 1958.

376. DONDERS, P. C., IMHOF, J. W., AND BAARS, H.: Ophthalmological phenomena in Waldenström's disease with cryoglobulinemia. *Ophthalmologica, 135*:324, 1958.

377. DONNELLY, E. J.: Ocular complications of multiple myelomatosis. *Amer. J. Ophthal., 47*:211, 1959.

378. D'ORIO, R., AND SCARINCIA A.: L'emianopsia binasale. *Riv. Oto-Neuro-Oftal., 34*:617, 1959.

379. DOTT, N. M., AND BAILEY, P.: A consideration of the hypophysial adenomata. *Brit. J. Surg., 13*:314, 1925.

380. DOWLING, J. E., AND SIDMAN, R. L.: Inherited retinal dystrophy in the rat. *J. Cell Biol., 14*:73, 1962.

381. DOWLING, J. L., AND SMITH, T. R.: An ocular study of pulseless disease. *Arch. Ophthal., 64*:236, 1960.

382. DOWLING, J. E., AND WALD, G.: The biological function of vitamin A acid. *Proc. National Acad. Sci., 46*:587, 1960.

383. DOWLING, J. E., AND WALD, G.: On the mechanism of vitamin A deficiency and night blindness. In: *Vitamin Metabolism. Fourth International Congress of Biochemistry*, vol. XI, New York: Pergamon Press, 1960, p. 185.

384. DOWNER, J. L.: Changes in visual gnostic functions and emotional behaviour following unilateral temporal pole damage in the 'split-brain' monkey. *Nature, 191*:50, 1961.

385. DRANCE, S. M.: Quinine amaurosis. *Brit. J. Ophthal., 39*:178, 1955.

386. DREISLER, K. K.: Unilateral retinitis pigmentosa. *Acta Ophthal., 26*:385, 1948.

387. DREW, A. L., AND MAGEE, K. R.: Papilledema in Guillian-Barré syndrome. *Arch. Neurol. Psychiat., 66*:744, 1951.

388. DRUEZ, G.: Un nouveau cas d'acanthocytose: Dysmorphie érythrocytaire congénitale avec rétinite, troubles nerveux et stigmates dégéneratifs. *Rev. Hemat. (Par.), 14*:3, 1959.

389. DUANE, T. D.: Observations on the fundus oculi during black-out. *Arch. Ophthal., 51*:343, 1954.

390. DUBOIS-POULSEN, A.; GUILLAUME, AND MAGIS, C.: La ligature de l'artère choroïdienne antérieure. *Bull. Soc. Franc. Ophtal., 69*:451, 1956.

391. DUFOUR, R., AND WELTER, S.: Périartérite rétinienne et vasculite généralisée. *Ophthalmologica, 129*:316, 1955.

392. DUGUID, I. M.: Features of ocular infestation by toxocara. *Brit. J. Ophthal., 45*:789, 1961.

393. DUKE, J. R., AND NAQUIN, H. A.: Lethal midline granuloma. *Trans. Amer. Acad. Ophthal. Otolaryng., 61*:463, 1957.

394. DUKE, J. R., AND WALSH, F. B.: Metastic carcinoma to the retina. *Amer. J. Ophthal., 47*:44, 1959.

395. DUKE-ELDER, W. S.: The ocular circulation: Its normal pressure relationships on their physiological significance. *Brit. J. Ophthal., 10*:513, 1926.

396. DUKE-ELDER, W. S.: *Textbook of ophthalmology. II. Clinical methods of examination, congenital and developmental considerations, diseases of the outer eye*. St. Louis: Mosby, 1938, p. 1412.

397. DUKE-ELDER, W. S.: *Textbook of ophthalmology. IV. The neurology of vision, motor and optical anomalies.* St. Louis: Mosby, 1949, p. 3661.

398. DUNNING, H. S.: Intracranial and extracranial vascular accidents in migraine. *Arch. Neurol. Psychiat., 48*:397, 1942.

399. DUNPHY, E. B.: Ocular manifestations of Raynaud's disease. *Trans. Amer. Ophthal. Soc., 30*:420, 1932.

400. DYSON, C.: Chordomas of ocular interest. *Arch. Ophthal., 57*:19, 1957.

401. DZUGAIEVA, S. B.: [Direct connections of the optical tract with the cortex.] *Zh. Vyss. Nerv. Deiat. Pavlov, 8*:942, 1958. *(Excerpta Med. XII, 13:* #1658, 1951.)

402. Editorial: A new vascular syndrome-"The subclavian steal." *New Engl. J. Med., 265*:912, 1961.

403. EDMUND, J.: Visual disturbances associated with gliomas of the temporal and occipital lobe. *Acta Psychiat. Scand., 29*:291, 1954.

404. EDMUND, J.: Some clinical features of the symptomatology of gliomas of the temporal lobe. *Acta Psychiat. Scand., 29*:311, 1954.

405. EHLERS, H.: Ophthalmoscopical findings in proliferative diabetic retinopathy. *Acta Ophthal., 31*:289, 1953.

406. EISUM, E. F.: Crater-like hole in the optic disc. *Acta Ophthal., 35*:200, 1957.

407. ELKINGTON, J. C.: Arachnoiditis. In: *Modern Trends in Neurology.* Ed. A. Feiling, New York: Paul B. Hoeber, 1951, p. 149.

408. ELLIS, P. P., AND HAMILTON, H.: Retrobulbar neuritis in pernicious anemia. *Amer. J. Ophthal., 48*:95, 1959.

409. ELLIS, P. P., AND JACKSON, W. E.: Osteopetrosis. A clinical study of optic-nerve involvement. *Amer. J. Ophthal., 53*:943, 1962.

410. ELLIS, R. A.: Central retinal artery occlusion associated with cryoglobulinemia. *Arch.. Ophthal., 57*:327, 1957.

411. ELLIS, R. W. B., SHELDON, W., AND CAPON, N. B.: Gargoylism (chondro-osteo-dystrophy, corneal opacities, hepatosplenomegaly, and mental deficiency). *Quart. J. Med., 5*:119, 1936.

412. ELLSWORTH, R. J., AND ZELLER, R. W.: Chloroquine (Aralen)-induced retinal damage. *Arch. Ophthal., 66*:269, 1961.

413. ELSCHNIG, A.: Ueber den Einfluss des Verschlusses der Arteria ophthalmica und der Carotis auf das Sehorgan. *Graefe Arch. Ophthal., 39*:151, 1893.

414. EMERSON, E.: Retinitis: pigmentosa or rubella? *Amer. J. Ophthal., 45*:93, 1958.

415. ENGELHARDT, H.; REMKY, H., AND ROPER, K.: Beitrag zur Diagnose der Arachnopathia optico chiasmatica. *Nervenarzt, 24*:370, 1953.

416. ENNEMA, M. C., AND ZEEMAN, W. P. C.: Venous occlusions in the retina. *Ophthalmologica, 126*:329, 1953.

417. ENOKSSON, P., AND BYNKE, M.: Visual field defects in arteriovenous aneurysms of the brain. *Acta Ophthal., 36*:586, 1958.

418. ENOKSSON, P.; LUNDBERG, N.; SJOSTEDT, S., AND SKANSE, B.: Influence of pregnancy on visual fields in suprasellar tumours. *Acta Psychiat. Scand., 36*:524, 1961.

419. ERWIN, W.; WEBER, R. W., AND MANNING, R. T.: Complications of infectious mononucleosis. *Amer. J. Med. Sci., 238*:699, 1959.

420. ESBJERG, H. O.: Cerbral complications (papilledemas) in epidemic parotitis. *Acta Ophthal., 21*:119, 1943.
421. ETTLINGER, G.: Sensory deficits in visual agnosia. *J. Neurol. Neurosurg.
Psychiat., 19*:297, 1956.
422. ETTLINGER, G.; WARRINGTON, E., AND ZANGWILL, O. L.: A further study
of visual-spatial agnosia. *Brain, 80*:335, 1957.
423. EUSTIS, R. S:. Specific reading disability; familial syndrome associated with
ambidexterity and speech defects and frequent cause of problem behavior.
New Engl. J. Med., 237:243, 1947.
424. FALCONER, M. A., AND WILSON, J. L.: Visual field changes following anterior temporal lobectomy: Their significance in relation to Meyer's loop
of the optic radiation. *Brain, 81*:1, 1958.
425. FALLS, H. F., AND COTTERMAN, C. D.: Choroidoretinal degeneration: A
sex-linked form in which heterozygous women exhibit a tapetal-like retinal
reflex. *Arch. Ophthal., 40*:685, 1948.
426. FANTA, H.: Die Bedeutung des Augenbefundes bei Fällen mit suprasellarem
Tumor. *Wien. Klin. Wschr., 70*:916, 1958.
427. FANTA, H.: Das Gesichtefeld für Bewegung und Weiss bei intrakraniellen
Prozessen. *Graefe Arch. Ophthal., 161*:492, 1960.
428. FARMER, R. G.; COOPER, T., AND PASCUZZI, C. A.: Cryoglobulinemia. Report of twelve cases with bone marrow findings. *Arch. Intern. Med.,
106*:483, 1960.
429. FARNELL, F. J., AND GLOBUS, J. H.: Primary melanoblastosis of leptomeninges and brain. *Arch. Neurol. Psychiat., 25*:803, 1931.
430. FAUST, C.: Über Gestaltzerfall als Symptom des parieto-occipitalen
Übergangsgebietes bei doppelseitiger Verletzung nach Hirnschuss. *Nervenarzt, 18*:103, 1947.
431. FAUST, C.: Partielle Seelenblindheit nach Occipitalhirnverletzung mit
besonderer Beeinträchtigung des Physiognomieerkennens. *Nervenarzt,
18*:294, 1947.
432. FEDOTOVA, T. A.: [Visible vessels of the eye and retina in coarctation of
the aorta]. *Vestn. Oftal., 2*:3, 1958. (Abst., *Excerpta Med. XII, 13*:
#997, 1959.)
433. FEINDEL, W., AND PENFIELD, W.: Localization of discharge in temporal
lobe automatism. *Arch. Neurol. Psychiat., 72*:605, 1954.
434. FEINDEL, W.; PENFIELD, W., AND McNAUGHTON, F.: The tentorial nerves
and localization of intracranial pain in man. *Neurology 10*:555, 1960.
435. FELDMAN, S.; LANDAU, J., AND HALPERN, L.: Papilledema in Guillain-
Barré syndrome. *Arch. Neurol. Psychiat., 73*:678, 1955.
436. FERRIMAN, D. G., AND ANDERSON, A. B.: Macroglobulinæmia of Waldenström. *Brit. Med. J., 2*:402, 1956.
437. FIELD, E. J., AND BRIERLY, J. B.: The retro-orbital tissues as a site of outflow
of cerebrospinal fluid. *Proc. Roy. Soc. Med., 42*:447, 1949.
438. FIELD, E. J., and FOSTER, J. B.: Periphlebitis retinæ and multiple sclerosis.
J. Neurol. Neurosurg. Psychiat., 25:269, 1962.
439. FIELD, M., AND AUVERT: Conclusions à l'étude d'une statistique de 148
cas d'arachnoidite opto-chiasmatique opérés. *Rev. Otoneuroophtal., 19*:
315, 1947.
440. FILLENZ, M.: Binocular interaction in the lateral geniculate body of the cat.

In: *The visual system*. Ed. R. Jung and H. Kornhuber. Berlin: Springer-Verlag, 1961, pp. 110-116.

441. FINE, B. S.: Limiting membranes of the sensory retina and pigment. epithelium. An electron microscopic study. *Arch. Ophthal., 66*:847, 1961.

442. FINE, B. S.: Ganglion cells in the human retina, with particular reference to the macula lutea: An electron-microscopic study. *Arch. Ophthal., 69*: 83, 1963.

443. FINK, A. I.: Carbon-monoxide asphyxia with visual sequelæ. *Amer. J. Ophthal., 34*:1024, 1951.

444. FINKEMEYER, H.: Der Kollateralkreislauf zwischen A. carotis externa und interna im Arteriogramm. *Zbl. Neurochir., 16*:342, 1956.

445. FINLAY, C. E.: Bitemporal contraction of visual fields in pregnancy. *Int. Congress Ophthal., 1*:144, 1922.

446. FINNERTY, F. A., FOOTE, W. D., MASSARO, G. D., TUCKMAN, J., BUCHHOLZ, J. H., AND RYAN, M. J.: The significance of lateral and generalized retinal sheen. *Ann. Intern. Med., 52*:819, 1960.

447. FISCHER, F.: Retinitis diabetica proliferans. Bericht über 100 Fälle. *Graefe Arch. Ophthal., 161*:239, 1959.

448. FISHER, C. M.: Cranial bruit associated with occlusion of the internal carotid artery. *Neurology, 7*:299, 1957.

449. FISHER, C. M.: Ocular palsy in temporal arteritis. *Minnesota Med., 42*: 1258, 1959.

450. Not used.

451. Not used.

452. FISHER, C. M.: Concerning recurrent transient cerebral ischemic attacks. *Canad. Med. Ass. J., 86*:1091, 1962.

453. FISHER, C. M.; KARP, H. R. AND ADAMS, R. D.: Cerebrovascular diseases. In: *Principles of internal medicine*. Vol. 2 Ed., T. R. Harrison. 3rd ed. New York: McGraw-Hill, 1958, pp. 1560-1606.

454. FISHER, M.: Occlusion of the internal carotid artery. *Arch. Neurol. Psychiat., 65*:346, 1951.

455. FISHER, M.: Transient monocular blindness associated with hemiplegia. *Arch. Ophthal., 47*:167, 1952.

456. FISHER, R. G., AND FRIEDMAN, K. R.: Carotid artery thrombosis in persons fifteen years of age or younger. *J.A.M.A., 170*:1918, 1959.

457. FITZ-HUGH, G. S., AND WALLENBORN, W. M.: Tumors of the nasopharynx; A review of 52 cases. *Laryngoscope, 71*:457, 1961.

458. FLATLEY, F. J.; ATWELL, M. E., AND McEVOY, R. K.: Pseudoxanthoma elasticum with gastric hemorrhage. *Arch. Intern. Med., 112*:352, 1963.

459. FLEISHER, B.: Ueber myotonische Dystrophie mit Katarakt. *Graefe Arch. Ophthal., 96*:91, 1918.

460. FLYNN, J. A. F.: Eclipse blindness—Prevention is better than cure. *Trans. Ophthal. Soc. Aust., 12*:7, 1959.

461. FOIX, C. AND HILLEMAND, P.: Les artères de l'axe encephalique jusqu'au diencephali inclusivement. *Rev. Neurol. (Par.), 32*:705, 1925.

462. FORBES, A. P.; HENNEMAN, P. H.; GRISWOLD, G. C., AND ALBRIGHT, F.: Syndrome characterized by galactorrhea, amenorrhea and low urinary FSH: Comparison with acromegaly and normal lactation. *J. Clin. Endocr., 14*:265, 1954.

463. Forbes, W.; Carcinoma of the pituitary gland with metastases to the liver in a case of Cushing's syndrome. *J. Path. Bact.,59*:137, 1947.
464. Ford, F. R., and Walsh, F. B.: Guillain-Barré syndrome (Acute infective polyneuritis) with increased intracranial pressure and papilledema; Report of 2 cases. *Bull. Johns Hopkins Hosp., 73*:391, 1943.
465. Fornaro, L.: Azione dell'ACTH e del cortisone sulla neurite ottica allergica (Ricerche sperimentali). *Riv. Oto-Neuro-oftal., 28*:114, 1953.
466. Forster, H. W.: The clinical use of the Haidinger's brushes phenomenon. *Amer. J. Ophthal., 38*:661, 1954.
467. Foster, J. B., and Ingram, T. T. S.: Familial cerebro-macular degeneration and ataxia. *J. Neurol. Neurosurg. Psychiat., 25*:63, 1962.
468. Fountain, E. M., Baird, W. C., and Poppen, J. L.: Pituitary apoplexy: report of 3 cases with recovery. *Lahey Clin. Bull., 7*:117, 1951.
469. Frame, B., and Carter, S.: Pseudohypoparathyroidism; clinical picture and relation to convulsive seizures. *Neurology, 5*:297, 1955.
470. Franceschetti, A., and Babel, J.: La choriorétinite en "taches de bougie," manifestation de la maladie de Besnier-Boeck. *Ophthalmologica, 118*:701, 1949.
471. Franceschetti, A., and Bischler, V.: Les hémianopsies bilatérales inférieures d'origine hémorragique. *Bull. Soc. Franc. Ophtal., 62*:350, 1949.
472. Franceschetti, A.; Dieterle, P., and Schwartz, A.: Rétinite pigmentaire à virus: relation entre tableau clinique et électroétinogramme (ERG). *Ophthalmologica, 135*:545, 1958.
473. Franceschetti, A., and Rickli, J. H.: Névrite rétrobulbaire après intoxication aigüe aux hydrocarbures chlorés. *Ophthalmologica, 123*:255, 1952.
474. Francois, J.: L'Hémianopsie binasale. *Ophthalmologica, 113*:321, 1947.
475. Francois, J.: The differential diagnosis of tapetoretinal degenerations. *Arch. Ophthal., 59*:88, 1958.
476. Francois, J., and Deweer, J.-P.: Dissociation entre la fonction visuelle et la fonction pupillo-motrice du nerf optique. *Ann. Oculist. (Par.), 183*: 913, 1950.
477. Francois, J.; Hoffmann, G., and deBrabandere, J.: Le pronostic visuel des opérations pour tumeurs hypophysaires. *Ann. Oculist. (Par.), 193*: 993, 1960.
478. Francois, J., and Neetens, A.: Vascularization of the optic pathway. I. Lamina cribrosa and optic nerve. *Brit. J. Ophthal., 38*:472, 1954.
479. Francois, J., and Neetens, A.: Vascularization of the optic pathway. III. Study of intra-orbital and intra-cranial optic nerve by serial sections. *Brit. J. Ophthal., 40*:45, 1956.
480. Francois, J., and Neetens, A.: L'engainement des veines rétiniennes dans la sclérose in plaques. *Ophthalmologica, 138*:322, 1959.
481. Francois, J. and Neetens, A.: Central retinal artery and central optic nerve artery. *Brit. J. Ophthal., 47*:21, 1963.
482. Francois, J.; Neetens, A., and Collette, J. M.: Vascularization of the optic pathway: V. Chiasm. *Brit. J. Ophthal., 40*:730, 1956.
483. Francois, J.; Neetens, A., and Collette, J. M.: The vascularization of the primary optic pathways. Presented at Soc. Brit. Neurol. Surg., Dublin, May 1957. (Abstr., *J. Neurol. Neurosurg. Psychiat., 20*:230, 1957.)

484. FRANCOIS, J.; NEETENS, A., AND COLLETTE, J. M.: Vascularization of the primary optic pathways. *Brit. J. Ophthal., 42*:65, 1958.

485. FRANCOIS, J., NEETENS, A., AND COLLETTE, J. M.: Vascularization of the optic radiation and the visual cortex. *Brit. J. Ophthal., 43*:394, 1959.

486. FRANCOIS, J., AND RABAEY, M.: Tumeurs primitives du nerf optique (Meningoblastome et gliome). *Acta Ophthalmologica, 30*:203, 1952.

487. FRANCOIS, J.; RABAEY, M.; EVENS, L., AND DE VOS, E.: Étude histopathologique d'une rétinite de Coats probablement toxoplasmique. *Ophthalmologica, 132*:1, 1956.

488. FRANCOIS, J., AND VERRIEST, G.: Rétinopathie pigmentaire unilaterale. *Ophthalmologica, 124*:65, 1952.

489. FRANCOIS, J., AND VERRIEST, G.: Gomme syphilitique de l'hypophyse. *Ann. Oculist. (Par.), 189*:416, 1956.

490. FRANCOIS, J.; VERRIEST, G., AND DEROUCK, A.: La maladie d'Oguchi. *Ophthalmologica, 131*:1, 1956.

491. FRANCOIS, P.; WOILLEZ, M.; BISERTE, G., AND HAVEZ, R.: Rétinite dysorique, seule manifestation clinique d'un myélome. Importance de l'immunoélectrophorèse. *Bull. Soc. Ophthal. Franc.* p. 470, 1960.

492. FRANDSEN, S.: Visual manifestations of digitalis poisoning; Two cases of toxic amblyopia. *Acta. Med. Scand., 157*:51, 1957.

493. FRANKEL, K.: Relation of migraine to cerebral aneurysm. *Arch. Neurol. Psychiat., 63*:195, 1950.

494. FRASCA, G.: Sindrome emorragica oculocerebrale di terson. *Riv. Oto-Neuro-Oftal., 34*:544, 1959.

495. FREEDMAN, B. J.: Papilloedema, optic atrophy, and blindness due to emphysema and chronic bronchitis. *Brit. J. Ophthal., 47*:290, 1963.

496. FREEMAN, A. G., AND HEATON, J. M.: The aetiology of retrobulbar neuritis in Addisonian pernicious anaemia. *Lancet, 1*:908, 1961.

497. FRENCH, L. A.: Studies on the optic radiations. The significance of small field defects in the region of the vertical meridian. *J. Neurosurg., 19*:522, 1962.

498. FREY, E.: Zur pathologischen Anatomie der Neuromyelitis optica. *Ophthalmologica, 131*:294, 1956.

499. FRIEDENBERG, S.: Tryparsamide optic neuritis treated by 2,3 dimer-captopropanol (BAL) *J.A.M.A., 135*:1072, 1947.

500. FRIEDENWALD, J. S.: Ocular lesions in fetal syphilis. *Trans. Amer. Ophthal. Soc., 27*:203, 1929.

501. FRIEDENWALD, J. S.: A new approach to some problems of retinal vascular disease. *Amer. J. Ophthal., 32*:487, 1949.

502. FRIEDENWALD, J. S., AND RONES, B.: Ocular lesions in septicemia. *Arch. Ophthal., 5*:175, 1931.

503. FRIEDMAN, B.: The blue arcs of the retina. *Arch. Ophthal., 6*:663, 1931.

504. FRIEDMAN, M. W.: Bilateral papilledema in otherwise well patients. *Arch. Ophthal., 58*:59, 1957.

505. FRIEDMAN, M. W.: Occlusion of the cilioretinal artery. *Amer. J. Ophthal., 47*:684, 1959.

506. FRIEDMANN, W., AND MAGUN, R.: Ernährungsschäden des Nervensystems bei Kriegsgefangenen (unter besonderer Berücksichtigung der Sehstörungen). *Graefe Arch. Ophthal., 149*:437, 1949.

507. FROMM, G. H.: An unusual case of hemianopia from cerebral anoxia at high altitudes. *Amer. J. Ophthal., 50*:648, 1960.

508. FROVIG, A. G.: Bilateral obliteration of the common carotid artery. *Acta. Psychiat. Scand. supp., 39,* 1946.

509. FRUGH, A., AND RABINER, A. M.: Optic nerve changes in the Guillain-Barré syndrome. *New York J. Med., 57*:3861, 1957.

510. FUCHS, A.: *Die Erkrankungen des Augenhintergrundes.* Vienna: F. Deuticke, 1945, p. 27.

511. FUCHS, A.: White spots of the fundus combined with night blindness and xerosis (Uyemura's syndrome). *Amer. J. Ophthal., 48*:101, 1959.

512. FUCHS, E.: Senile changes of the optic nerve. *Amer. J. Ophthal., 5*:215, 1922.

513. FUJINO, T., AND GO, Y.: On the retinal representation in the lateral geniculate body. *Jap. J. Ophthal., 4*:1, 1960. (Abst., *Amer. J. Ophthal., 51*:206, 1961.)

514. GALDSTON, M.; GOVONS, S.; WORTIS, S. B.; STEELE, J. M., AND TAYLOR, H. K.: Thrombosis of the common internal and external carotid arteries: A report of two cases with a review of the literature. *Arch. Intern. Med., 67*:1162, 1941.

515. GALINDEZ IGLESIAS, F.: Patologia psico-visual. *Arch. Soc. Oftal. hisp.-amer., 11*:289, 1951. (Abst., *Excerpta Med. XII ,6*:#1439, 1952.)

516. GALLAGHER, P. G.; DORSEY, J. F.; STEFANINI, M., AND LOONEY, J. M.: Large intracranial aneurysm producing panhypopituitarism and frontal lobe syndrome. *Neurology, 6*:829, 1956.

517. GANGSTROM, K. O.: A family with glaucoma-like optic discs but no glaucoma. *Acta. Ophthal. (Kbh.), 36*:371, 1958.

518. GARCIN, G.; FERRAND, J., AND PERRIN, C.: Les dangers de l'acetylarsan pour le nerf optique. *Bull. méd. Afrique occident. Franc. (Dakar), 7*:67, 1950. (Abst., *Excerpta Med. XII, 6*:#574, 1952.)

519. GARDE, A., AND ETIENNE, R.: Névrite optique rétrobulbaire par chlorure de méthyle. *Rev. Otoneuroophtal., 23*:480, 1951.

520. GARDNER, W. J.: Otitic sinus thrombosis causing intracranial hypertension. *Arch. Otolaryng., 30*:253, 1939.

521. GARDNER, W. J., SPITLER, D. K., AND WHITTEN, C.: Increased intracranial pressure caused by increased protein content in the cerebrospinal fluid: An explanation of papilledema in certain cases of small intracranial and intraspinal tumors, and in the Guillain-Barré syndrome. *New Engl. J. Med., 250*:932, 1954.

522. GARTNER, S.: Optic neuropathy in multiple sclerosis. Optic neuritis. *Arch. Ophthal., 50*:718, 1953.

523. GASSEL, M. M.: False localizing signs. A review of the concept and analysis of the occurrence in 250 cases of intracranial meningioma. *Arch. Neurol., 4*:526, 1961.

524. GAYER, M. O.: Acquired hole in the disc. *Brit. J. Ophthal., 35*:437, 1951.

525. GEERAETS, W. J., AND GUERRY, D.: Angioid streaks and sickle-cell disease. *Amer. J. Ophthal., 49*:450, 1960.

526. GEERAETS, W. J., AND GUERRY, D.: Elastic tissue degeneration in sickle-cell disease. *Amer. J. Ophthal., 50*:213, 1960.

527. GEERAETS, W. J., McNEER, K. W., MAXEY, E. F., AND GUERRY, D.: Retinopathy in sarcoidosis. *Acta. Ophthal., 40*:492, 1962.

528. GERSTMANN, J.: Fingeragnosie. Eine umschriebene Störung der Orientierung am eigenen Körper. *Wien. Klin. Wschr., 37*:1010, 1924.
529. GERSTMANN, J.: Fingeragnosie und isolierte Agraphie, ein neues Syndrom. *Z. Ges. Neurol. Psychiat., 108*:152, 1927.
530. GERSTMANN, J.: Some notes on the Gerstmann syndrome. *Neurology, 7*:866, 1957.
531. GESCHWIND, N.: The anatomy of acquired disorders of reading disability. In: *Progress and Research Needs in Dyslexia.* Ed. J. Money. Baltimore: The Johns Hopkins Press, 1962, pp. 115-130.
532. GESCHWIND, N., AND KAPLAN, E.: A human cerebral deconnection syndrome: A preliminary report. *Neurology, 12*:675, 1962.
533. GEYER, K. H.: Zentrale Störungen des Formensehens: Zur Pathogenese der Metamorphopsie. *Deutsch. Z. Nervenheilk., 184*:378, 1963.
534. GILES, C. L.: Retinal hemorrhages in the newborn. *Amer. J. Ophthal.,49*: 1005, 1960.
535. GILES, C. L., AND ISAACSON, J. D.: The treatment of acute optic neuritis. Analysis of eighty cases. *Arch. Ophthal., 66*:176, 1961.
536. GILGER, A. P., FARKAS, I. S., AND POTTS, A. M.: Studies on the visual toxicity of methanol X. Further observations on the ethanol therapy of acute methanol poisoning in monkeys. *Amer. J. Ophthal., 48*:153, 1959.
537. GILLER, H., AND COGAN, D. C.: Papilledema as the outstanding sign in meningeal hydrops. *Arch. Ophthal., 48*:557, 1952.
538. GILLETTE, D. F.: Visual disturbances due to digitalis. *Trans. Amer. Ophthal. Soc., 44*:156, 1946.
539. GILLILAN, L. A.: The collateral circulation of the human orbit. *Arch. Ophthal., 65*:684, 1961.
540. GIOIRE, CHARBONNEL, COLAS, COLLET, VERCELLETTO, AND BESANCON: Un cas d'arachnoïdite opto-chiasmatique sévère, avec hydrocéphalie, consécutive à une myélographie lipsiodolée. *Rev. Otoneuroophtal., 34*:239, 1962.
541. GIVNER, I.: Bilateral uveitis, poliosis and retinal detachment with recovery: Report of a case. *Arch. Ophthal., 30*:331, 1943.
542. GIVNER, I.: Visual loss following cardiac arrest. *Arch. Ophthal., 51*:878, 1954.
543. GLEES, M., AND ZIELINSKI, H.: Über bitemporale zentrale und parazentrale Skotome bei verschiedenen krankhaften Prozessen im Sellabereich. *Klin. Mbl. Augenheilk., 129*:145, 1956.
544. GLEES, P.: Terminal degeneration and trans-synaptic atrophy in the lateral geniculate body of the monkey. In: *The Visual System.* Ed., R. Jung and H. Kornhuber. Berlin: Springer-Verlag, 1961, pp. 104-110.
545. GLEW, W. B., KEARNS, T. P., RUCKER, C. W., AND ESSEX, H. E.: The experimental production of papilledema. *Arch. Ophthal., 60*:1074, 1958.
546. GLOBUS, J. H., AND SILVERSTONE, S. M.: Diagnostic value of defects in the visual fields and other ocular disturbances. Associated with supratentorial tumors of the brain. *Arch. Ophthal., 14*:325, 1935.
547. GLONING, I.; GLONING, K., AND TSCHABITSCHER, H.: Die occipitale Blindheit auf vasculärer Basis; Untersuchungsergebnisse von 16 eiginen Fällen, *Graefe Arch. Ophthal., 165*:138, 1962.
548. GLUCKSMANN, A., AND TANSLEY, K.: Some effects of gamma radiation on the developing rat retina. *Brit. J. Ophthal., 20*:497, 1936.

549. GOAR, E. L., AND FLETCHER, M. C.: Toxic chorioretinopathy following the use of NP 207. *Amer. J. Ophthal., 44*:603, 1957.

550. GOLDBERG, F. R.: Impairment of the vestibular apparatus as a symptom in optic atrophy caused by Plasmocid. *Vestn. Oftal., 29*:42, 1950. (Abst., *Excerpta Med. XII, 5*:#2382, 1951.)

551. GOLDBERG, H. K.; MARSHALL, C., AND SIMS, E.: The role of brain damage in congenital dyslexia. *Amer. J. Ophthal., 50*:586, 1960.

552. GOLDBY, F.: A note on transneuronal atrophy in the human lateral geniculate body. *J. Neurol. Neurosurg. Psychiat., 20*:202, 1957.

553. GOLDING, A. M. B.: Retinitis punctata albescens with pigmentation. *Brit. J. Ophthal., 40*:242, 1956.

554. GOLDMAN, H.: Experimentelle Tetaniekatarakt. *Graefe Arch. Ophthal., 122*:146, 1929.

555. GOLDMAN, H.: Discussion of Huber, A.: Einseitige Stauungspapille Pseudoneuritis und Pseudopapillenödem. *Ophthalmologica, 123*:261, 1952.

556. GOLDSCHMIDT, M.: A new test for function of the macula lutea. *Arch. Ophthal., 44*:129, 1950.

557. GOLDSMITH, A. J. B.: Chiasmal arachnoiditis. *Proc. Roy. Soc. Med., 36*:163, 1943.

558. GOLDSMITH, J.: Neurofibromatosis associated with tumours of the optic papilla: Report of a case. *Arch. Ophthal., 41*:718, 1949.

559. GOLDSTEIN, I., AND WEXLER, D.: Bilateral atrophy of the optic nerve in periarteritis nodosa, a miscorcopic study. *Arch. Ophthal., 18*:767, 1937.

560. GOLDSTEIN, J. E. AND COGAN, D. G.: Exercise and the optic neuropathy of multiple sclerosis. *Arch. Ophthal., 72*:168, 1964.

561. GOOD, C. A.: The cortical localization of sight and hearing. Report of a case of blindness (slight perception remaining) and deafness due to cerebral lesions. *Amer. J. Med. Soc. Phila., 65*:648, 1900.

562. GOOD, P.: Choked discs in lead encephalopathy. *Amer. J. Ophthal., 24*:794, 1941.

563. GOODDY, W., AND REINHOLD, M.: Congenital dyslexia and asymmetry of cerebral function. *Brain, 84*:231, 1961.

564. GOODMAN, G.; VON SALLMANN, L., AND HOLLAND, M. G.: Ocular manifestations of sickle-cell disease. *Arch. Ophthal., 58*:655, 1957.

565. GOODSIDE, V.: The anterior limiting membrane and the retinal light reflexes. *Amer. J. Ophthal., 41*:288, 1956.

566. GORDON, N.: Ocular manifestations of internal carotid artery occlusion. *Brit. J. Ophthal., 43*:257, 1959.

567. GORODETSKAYA, A. M.: [Atrophy of the optic nerve in optochiasmatic arachnoiditis]. *Sborn. Trud. Azerbaüan. Oftal. Inst., 1*:146, 1956. (Abst., *Excerpta Med. XII, 12*:#901, 1958.)

568. GOULD, H., AND KAUFMAN, H. E.: Sarcoid of the fundus. *Arch. Ophthal., 65*:453, 1961.

569. GOVAN, C. D., AND WALSH, F. B.: Symptomatology of subdural hematoma in infants and in adults: Comparative study, with particular reference to the ocular signs; an observation concerning pathogenesis of subdural hematoma. *Arch. Ophthal., 37*:701, 1947.

570. GOWERS, W. R.: Simultaneous embolism of central retinal and middle cerebral arteries. *Lancet, 2*:794, 1875.

571. GRADEL, H. S.: The x-ray therapy of retinal-vein thrombosis. *Amer. J. Ophthal., 20*:1125, 1937.
572. VON GRAEFE, A.: Fälle von Cysticercus im Innern des Auges. *Graefe Arch. Ophthal., 1*:259, 1855.
573. GRAETHER, J. M.: Transient amaurosis in one eye with simultaneous dilatation of retinal veins in association with a congenital anomaly of the optic nerve head. *Arch. Ophthal., 70*:342, 1963.
574. GRAMBERG-DANIELSON, B.: Die Doppelversorgung der Macula. *Graefe Arch. Ophthal., 160*:543, 1959.
575. GRANIT, R.: *Sensory mechanisms of the retina, with an appendix on electroretinography.* Oxford: Oxford University Press, 1947.
576. GRANT, F. C., AND HEDGES, T. R.: Ocular findings in meningiomas of the tuberculum sellae. *Arch. Ophthal., 56*:163, 1956.
577. Not used.
578. GRANT, W. M.: *Toxicology of the eye.* Springfield, Ill. Charles C Thomas, Publisher, 1962.
579. GREENFIELD, J. G.: Retina in cerebrospinal lipidosis. *Proc. Roy. Soc. Med., 44*:686, 1951.
580. GREENFIELD, J. G.: *The spino-cerebellar degenerations.* Oxford: Blackwell Scientific Publications, 1954.
581. GREGERSEN, E.: Optic atrophy in a breast-fed infant and treatment of maternal cestode infection with filix. *Acta. Ophthal. (Kbh.), 36*:115, 1958.
582. GRIFFIN, A. O., AND BODIAN, M.: Segmental retinal periarteritis. A report of three cases. *Amer. J. Ophthal., 47*:544, 1959.
583. GRIFFITH, J. O., JEFFERS, W. A., FEWELL, A. G., AND FRY, W. E.: A study of the communication and direction of flow between cerebrospinal fluid and optic discs in the rat. *Amer. J. Ophthal., 20*:457, 1937.
584. GRIMM, R. J., AND TEDFORD, J.: Hereditary macular degeneration. Report of Best's disease in a family. *Amer. J. Ophthal., 55*:457, 1963.
585. GRINKER, R. R.: Tumors of the optic nerve. *Arch. Ophthal, 4*:497, 1930.
586. GRISCOM, J. M.: Hereditary optic atrophy. *Amer. J. Ophthal., 4*:347, 1921.
587. GRONBLAD, E.: Angioid streaks—pseudoxanthoma elasticum. *Acta. Ophthal., 7*:329, 1929.
588. GROSS, H.: Zur Pathogenese der Sehnerven-atrophie bei den turicephalen Schädel-dysostosin. *Graefe Arch. Ophthal., 157*:225, 1956.
589. GRUBER, E.: Complete avulsion of the optic nerve, associated with severe concussion injuries to the eyes. *Amer. J. Ophthal., 48*:528, 1959.
590. GRUBER, E.: Reading ability, binocular coordination and the ophthalmograph. *Arch. Ophthal., 67*:280, 1962.
591. GUNN, R. M.: Family optic atrophy in mother and two children. *Trans. Ophthal. Soc. U.K., 27*:221, 1907.
592. GUPTA, J. S.: Secondary glaucoma following occlusion of the central retinal artery. *Brit. J. Ophthal., 44*:52, 1960.
593. GURDJIAN, E. S., HARDY, W. G., LINDNER, D. W., AND THOMAS, L. M.: Diagnostic evaluation and treatment. In: Symposium: Occlusive cerebrovascular disease. *Trans. Amer. Acad. Ophthal. Otolaryng., 66*:149, 1962.
594. GUTHKELCH, A. N.: Subdural effusions in infancy: 24 cases. *Brit. Med. J., 1*:233, 1953.

595. GUYTON, T. B., EHRLICH, F., BLANC, W. A., AND BECKER, M. H.: New observations in generalized cytomegalic-inclusion disease of the newborn: report of a case with chorioretinitis. *N. Engl. J. Med., 257*:803, 1957.

596. HAARR, M.: Periphlebitis retinae in association with multiple sclerosis; contribution to discussion on pathogenesis of multiple sclerosis. *Acta Psychiat. Scand., 28*:175, 1953.

597. HAARR, M.: Uveitis with neurological symptoms. *Acta Ophthal., 39*:60, 1961.

598. HAEMIG, E.: Ueber die Möglichkeit traumatischer Genese des Verschlusses der Vena centralis retinae. *Schweiz. Med. Wschr., 71*:933, 1941.

599. HAGIWARA, H.: On Behçet's syndrome. *Acta. Soc. Ophthal. Jap., 63*:1504, 1959.

600. HAGUE, E. B.: Uveitis, dysacousia, alopecia, poliosis, and vitiligo.: A theory as to cause. *Arch. Ophthal. 31*:520, 1944.

601. HALLGREN, B.: Retinitis pigmentosa combined with congenital deafness; with vestibulo-cerebellar ataxia and mental abnormality in a proportion of cases. *Acta. Psychiat. Scand., 34*:1, 1959.

602. HALPERN, L.: Simultaneous visual and tactile illusions of size. *Confin. Neurol., 19*:301, 1959.

603. HALSTEAD, W. C.: Function of the frontal lobe in man: The dynamic visual field. Presented before Chicago Neurol. Soc. Oct. 15, 1942. (Abst., *Arch. Neurol. Psychiat., 49*:633, 1943.)

604. HAMILTON, H. E., ELLIS, P. P., AND SHEETS, R. F.: Visual impairment due to optic neuropathy in pernicious anemia: Report of a case and review of the literature. *Blood, 14*:378, 1959.

605. HAMLIN, H.: The case for transsphenoidal approach to hypophysial tumors. *J. Neurosurg., 19*:1000, 1962.

606. HANLON, D. G., BAYRD, E. D., AND KEARNS, T. P.: Macroglobulinemia—report of four cases. *J.A.M.A., 167*:1817, 1958.

607. HANNO, H. A., AND WEISS, D. I.: Pseudohypoparathyroidism, report of two new cases. *Arch. Ophthal., 65*:221, 1961.

608. HARDENBERGH, F. E.: Idiopathic central retinal artery occlusion, case report and presentation of a general guide to therapy. *Arch. Ophthal., 67*:556, 1962.

609. HARRINGTON, D. O.: Psychosomatic interrelationships in ophthalmology. *Amer. J. Ophthal., 31*:1241, 1948.

610. HARRINGTON, D. O.: Visual field character in temporal and occipital lobe lesions. *Arch. Ophthal., 66*:778, 1961.

611. HARRINGTON, D. O., AND FLOCKS, M.: Ophthalmoplegic migraine: Pathogenesis; report of pathological findings in a case of recurrent oculomotor paralysis. *Arch. Ophthal., 49*:643, 1953.

612. HARRIS, W.: Pseudo-glioma due to larval choroido-retinal granulomatosis. *Brit. J. Ophthal., 45*:144, 1961.

613. HARRISON, R., HOEFNAGEL, D., AND HAYWARD, J. N.: Congenital total color blindness: clinicopathological report. *Arch. Ophthal., 64*:685, 1960.

614. HARTMANN, E.: Optochiasmic arachnoiditis. *Arch. Ophthal., 33*:68, 1945.

615. HARTMANN, E., AND GILLES, E.: *Radiodiagnostic en ophthalmologie.* Paris: Masson et Cie, 1955.

616. HASCHKE, W., AND SICKEL, W.: Das Elektroretinogram des Menschen bei

Ausfall der Ganglienzellen und partieller Schädigung der Bipolaren. *Acta. Ophthal. Supp., 70*:164, 1962.

617. HATCH, H. A.: Bilateral optic neuritis following chicken pox. Report of a case with apparently complete recovery. *J. Pediat., 34*:758, 1949.

618. HAUGE, T.: Catheter vertebral angiography. *Acta. Radiol. Supp.,* 1954, p. 109.

619. HAUSMAN, L.: Syphilitic arachnoiditis of the optic chiasm. *Arch. Neurol. Psychiat., 37*:929, 1937.

620. HEAD, H.: *Aphasia and kindred disorders of speech.* Cambridge: University Press, 1926.

621. HEATH, P.: Measles encephalitis. A clinical report of some eye findings. *Trans. Amer. Ophthal. Soc., 29*:357, 1931.

622. HEATON, J. M.: Chronic cyanide poisoning and optic neuritis. *Trans. Ophthal. Soc. U.K., 82*:263, 1962.

623. HECAEN, H., AND AJURIAGUERRA, J.: L'apraxie de l'habillage; ses rapports avec la planototopoklinésie et les troubles de la somatognosie. *Encéphale, 35*:113, 1942-45.

624. HECAEN, H., AND ANGELERGUES, R.: Agnosia for faces (prosopagnosia). *Arch. Neurol., 7*:92, 1962.

625. HECAEN, H., PENFIELD, W., BERTRAND, C., AND MALMO, R.: Syndrome of apractognosia due to lesions of minor cerebral hemisphere. *Arch. Neurol. Psychiat., 75*:400, 1956.

626. HECHT, S., SHLAER, S., AND PIRENNE, M. H.: Energy, quanta and vision. *J. Gen. Physiol., 25*:819, 1942.

627. HEDGES, T. R., AND SCHEIE, H. G.: Visual field defects in exophthalmos associated with thyroid disease. *Arch. Ophthal., 54*:885, 1955.

628. HEDGES, T. R., AND WALSH, F. B.: Optic nerve sheath and subhyaloid haemorrhage as a complication of angiocardiography. *Arch. Ophthal., 54*:425, 1955.

629. HEILBRUN, A. B.: Lateralization of cerebral lesion and performance on spatial-temporal tasks. *Arch. Neurol., 1*:282, 1959.

630. HENDERSON, A. B.: Sickle cell anemia; clinical study of 54 cases. *Amer. J. Med., 9*:757, 1950.

631. HENDERSON, J. L., MACGREGOR, A. R., THANNHAUSER, S. J., AND HOLDEN, R.: Pathology and biochemistry of gargoylism; report of 3 cases with review of literature. *Arch. Dis. Child., 27*:230, 1952.

632. HENDERSON, J. W.: Optic neuropathy of exophthalmic goiter (Graves' disease). *Arch. Ophthal., 59*:471, 1958.

633. HENDERSON, R. H.: Retinitis punctata albescens and retinitis pigmentosa as affected by pregnancy. Report of a case. *Arch. Ophthal., 11*:763, 1934.

634. HENDERSON, W. R.: Pituitary adenomata; follow-up study of surgical results in 338 cases. *Brit. J. Surg., 26*:811, 1939.

635. HENRY, M. D., AND CHAPMAN, A. Z.: Vitreous hemorrhage and retinopathy associated with sickle-cell disease. *Amer. J. Ophthal., 38*:204, 1954.

636. HENSCHEN, S. E.: Ueber localization innerhalb des äusseren Knieganglions. *Neurol. Centralblatt, 17*:194, 1898.

637. HENSCHEN, S. E.: Vierzigjähriger Kampf um das Sehzentrum und seine Bedeutung für die Hirnforschung. *Z. Ges. Neurol. Psychiat., 87*:505, 1923.

638. HENTSCHEL, F.: Zu den arteriellen und venösen Zirkulationsstörungen der Netzhaut. *Klin. Mbl. Augenheilk., 125*:595, 1954.
639. HEPTINSTALL, R. H., PORTER, K. A., AND BARKLEY, H.: Giant-cell (temporal) arteritis. *J. Path. Bact., 67*:507, 1954.
640. HERRMAN, G., AND POTZL, O.: *Ueber die Agraphie.* Berlin: S. Karger, 1926.
641. HERVOUET, F., BARON, A., AND LENOIR, A.: Anatomie pathologique de la rétinose hespéranopique. *Arch. Ophtal., 15*:263, 1955.
642. HEUER, G. J., AND VAIL, D. T.: Chronic cisternal arachnoiditis producing symptoms of involvement of the optic nerves and chiasm, pathology and results of operative treatment in four cases. *Arch. Ophthal., 5*:334, 1931.
643. HEYDENREICH, A.: Zur Pathogenese des Pseudoglioms. *Klin. Mbl. Augenheilk., 134*:465, 1959.
644. HEYMAN, A., KARP, H. R., AND BLOOR, B. M.: Determination of retinal artery pressures in diagnosis of carotid artery occlusion. *Neurology, 7*:97, 1957.
645. HIERONS, R., AND LYLE, T. K.: Bilateral retrobulbar optic neuritis. *Brain, 82*:56, 1959.
646. HILL, K., COGAN, D. G., AND DODGE, P. R.: Ocular signs associated with hydranencephaly. *Amer. J. Ophthal., 51*:267, 1961.
647. VON HIPPEL, E.: Anatomischer Befund bei einem Fall von primärer syphilitischer Erkrankung der Retinalgefässe. *Graefe Arch. Ophthal., 117*:221, 1926.
648. VON HIPPEL, E.: Zur Frage der Perivasculitis retinae (recidivierende Glaskörper Blutungen bei Jugendlichen). *Graefe Arch. Ophthal., 134*:121, 1935.
649. VON HIPPEL, E.: Cited by Bürki, E. ref. 193.
650. HIRSCH, O.: Über Augensymptome bei Hypophysentumoren und ähnlichen Krankheitsbildern. *Z. Augenheilk., 45*:294, 1921.
651. HIRSCH, O.: Symptoms and treatment of pituitary tumors. *Arch. Otolaryng., 55*:268, 1952.
652. HIRSCH, O., AND HAMLIN, H.: Fate of visual fields and optic discs in pituitary tumors. *Amer. J. Ophthal., 37*:880, 1954.
653. HIRSCH, O., AND HAMLIN, H.: Symptomatology and treatment of the hypophyseal duct tumors (Craniopharyngiomas). *Confin. Neurol., 19*: 153, 1959.
654. HOBBS, H. E.: Fibrous dysplasia of the bony orbit. *XVII Concil. Ophthalmologicum, 3*:1756, 1955.
655. HOBBS, H. E., EADIE, S. P., AND SOMERVILLE, F.: Ocular lesions after treatment with chloroquine. *Brit. J. Ophthal., 45*:284, 1961.
656. HOBBS, H. E., SORSBY, A., AND FREEDMAN, A.: Retinopathy following chloroquine therapy. *Lancet, 2*:478, 1959.
657. HODGMAN, F. S. J., PARRY, H. B., RASKRIDGE, W. J., AND STEEL, J. D.: Progressive retinal atrophy in dogs. *Vet. Rec., 61*:185, 1949.
658. VAN DER HOEVE, J.: Augengeschwülste bei der tuberosen Hirnsklerose (Bourneville). *Graefe Arch. Ophthal., 105*:880, 1921.
659. VAN DER HOEVE, J.: Optic nerve and accessory sinuses. *Arch. Ophthal., 51*:210, 1922.
660. HOFF, H., GLONING, I., AND GLONING, K.: Die zentralen Störungen der optischen Wahrnemung. III. Die optischagnostischen Störungen. *Wien. Med. Wschr., 112*:450, 1962.

661. HOFF, H., AND POTZL, O.: Anisotropie des Sehraums bei occipitaler Herder-krankung. *Deutsch Z. Nervenheilk., 145*:179, 1938.

662. HOFFMAN, G. R., AND KLUYSKENS, J.: L'angiographie dans les tumeurs chiasmatiques et occipitales. *Bull. Soc. Belg. Ophtal., 102*:703, 1952.

663. HOFMAN, A.: Über das gleichzeitige Aufreten einer doppelseitigen retro-bulbären Neuritis bei zwei Brüdern und deren Vetter im annähernd gleichen Lebensalter. *Klin. Mbl. Augenheilk., 140*:192, 1962.

664. HOFMAN, H.: Tuberöse Hirnsklerose. *Graefe Arch. Ophthal., 161*:122, 1959.

665. HOGAN, M. J.: Symposium: toxoplasmosis. Ocular manifestations. *Trans. Amer. Acad. Ophthal. Otolaryng., 54*:183, 1950.

666. HOLLENHORST, R. W.: Ophthalmodynamometry and intracranial vascular disease. *Med. Clin. N. Amer., 42*:951, 1958.

667. HOLLENHORST, R. W.: Ocular manifestations of insufficiency or thrombosis of the internal carotid artery. *Amer. J. Ophthal., 47*:753, 1959.

668. HOLLENHORST, R. W.: Significance of bright plaques in the retinal arter-ioles. *J.A.M.A., 178*:23, 1961.

669. HOLLENHORST, R. W., BROWN, J. R., WAGENER, H. P., AND SHICK, R. M.: Neurologic aspects of temporal arteritis. *Neurology, 10*:490, 1960.

670. HOLLENHORST, R. W., AND HENDERSON, J. W.: The ocular manifestations of the diffuse collagen diseases. *Amer. J. Med. Sci., 221*:211, 1951.

671. HOLLENHORST, R. W., AND STEIN, H. A.: Ocular signs and prognosis in subdural and subarachnoid bleeding in young children. *Arch. Ophthal., 60*:187, 1958.

672. HOLLENHORST, R. W., AND WAGENER, H. P.: Loss of vision after distant hemorrhage. *Amer. J. Med. Sci., 219*:209, 1950.

673. HOLLENHORST, R. W., WILBUR, R. E., AND SVIEN, H. J.: Effect of occlu-sion of the common, external and internal carotid arteries upon the retinal arterial pressure. Presented before the Midwestern Section, Association for Research in Ophthalmology, 1957. (Abst., *Amer. J. Ophthal., 43*:778, 1957.)

674. HOLLOWAY, T. B.: Angioid streaks. A report concerning two cases. *Trans. Amer. Ophthal. Soc., 25*:173, 1927.

675. HOLM, A., SACHS, J., AND WILSON, A.: Glaucoma secondary to occlusion of central retinal artery. *Amer. J. Ophthal., 48*:530, 1959.

676. HOLMAN, C. B.: Roentgenologic manifestations of glioma of the optic nerve and chiasm. *Amer. J. Roentgenol., 82*:462, 1959.

677. HOLMBERG, C. G., AND LAURELL, C. B.: Investigations in serum copper. II. Isolation of the copper containing protein and a description of some of its properties. *Acta. Chem. Scand., 2*:550, 1948.

678. HOLMES, G.: Disturbances of visual orientation. *Brit. J. Ophthal., 2*:449 and 506, 1918.

679. HOLMES, G.: Cerebral integration of ocular movements. *Brit. Med. J., 2*:107, 1938.

680. HOLMES, G., AND HORRAX, G.: Disturbances of spatial orientation and visual attention, with loss of stereoscopic vision. *Arch. Neurol. Psychiat., 1*:385, 1919.

681. HOLMES, G., AND LISTER, W. T.: Disturbances of vision from cerebral lesions, with special reference to the cortical representation of the macula. *Brain, 39*:34, 1916.

682. HOLT, J. F., AND WRIGHT, E. M.: Radiologic features of neurofibromatosis. *Radiology, 51*:647, 1948.
683. HOPE-ROBERTSON, W. J.: Thrombosis of the central retinal vein following injury: report of 2 cases. *N. Z. Med. J.* (Supp.), 1952, p. 22.
684. HORRAX, G.: Visual hallucinations as a cerebral localizing phenomenon; with especial reference to their occurrence in tumors of the temporal lobes. *Arch. Neurol. Psychiat., 10*:532, 1923.
685. HORRAX, G.: Generalized cisternal arachnoiditis simulating cerebellar tumor: Its surgical treatment and end-results. *Arch. Surg., 9*:95, 1924.
686. HORRAX, G., AND PUTNAM, T. J.: Distortions of visual fields in cases of brain tumour; field defects and hallucinations produced by tumours of occipital lobe. *Brain, 55*:499, 1932.
687. HORRAX, G., AND WYATT, J. P.: Ectopic pinealomas in the chiasmal region report of three cases. *J. Neurosurg., 4*:309, 1947.
688. HOURLAY-STASSART, C., AND LAVERGNE, G.: Emboli of the central retinal artery after commissurotomy. *Amer. J. Ophthal., 47*:90, 1959.
689. HOWARD, G. M.: Angioid streaks in acromegaly. *Amer. J. Ophthal., 56*:137, 1963.
690. HOWARTH, C. H., AND HAVENER, W. H.: Differential diagnosis of an edematous optic disc. *Amer. J. Ophthal., 49*:150, 1959.
691. HOYT, W. F.: Vascular lesions of the visual cortex with brain herniation through the tentorial incisura. *Arch. Ophthal., 64*:44, 1960.
692. HOYT, W. F.: Charcot-Marie-Tooth disease with primary optic atrophy. Report of a case. *Arch. Ophthal., 64*:925, 1960.
693. HOYT, W. F.: Transient bilateral blurring of vision; considerations of an episodic ischemic symptom of vertebral-basilar insufficiency. *Arch. Ophthal., 70*:746, 1963.
694. HOYT, W. F., AND LUIS, O.: The primate chiasm, details of visual fiber organization studied by silver impregnation techniques. *Arch. Ophthal., 70*:69, 1963.
695. HOYT, W. F., AND PONT, M. E.: Pseudopapilledema: Anomalous elevation of optic disk. Pitfalls in diagnosis and management. *J.A.M.A., 181*:191, 1962.
696. HOYT, W. F., AND WALSH, F. B.: Cortical blindness with partial recovery following acute cerebral anoxia from cardiac arrest. *Arch. Ophthal., 60*:1061, 1958.
696a. HUBEL, D. H.: Personal communication.
697. HUBER, A.: *Eye symptoms in brain tumors.* Trans. S. van Wien. St. Louis: Mosby, 1961.
698. HUBER, A.: Papillenödem bei Leukamien. *Ophthalmologica, 141*:290, 1961.
699. HUBER, A., AND CAGIANUT, B.: Zur Differential-diagnose zwischen Papillenödem bei maligner Hypertonie und Stauungspapille. *Ophthalmologica, 135*:412, 1958.
700. HUDSON, A. C.: Primary tumors of the optic nerve. *Roy. Lond. Ophthal. Hosp. Rep., 18*:317, 1912.
701. HUGGERT, A., AND HULTQUIST, G. T.: True glioma of the retina. *Ophthalmologica, 113*:193, 1947.
702. HUGHES, B.: *The Visual Fields.* Oxford; Blackwell Scientific Publications, 1954.

703. HUGHES, B.: Blood supply of the optic nerves and chiasma and its clinical significance. *Brit. J. Ophthal., 42*:106, 1958.

704. HUGHES, B.: Indirect injury of the optic nerves and chiasma. *Bull. Johns Hopkins Hosp., 111*:98, 1962.

705. HUGHES, E. B. C.: Indirect injury of optic chiasma—case report. *Brit. J. Ophthal., 29*:629, 1945.

706. HUGHES, E. B. C.: Ocular sequelae of head injuries, general discussion: The visual fields in indirect injury of the optic nerves. *Trans. Ophthal. Soc. U.K., 65*:35, 1945.

707. HULLAY, J.: Results of 50 surgically treated temporal epileptic patients. *Acta. Neurochir. Wien, 6*:169, 1958.

708. HUMPHREY, J. G., AND NEWTON, T. H.: Internal carotid artery occlusion in young adults. *Brain, 83*:565, 1960.

709. HURLER, G.: Ueber einen Typ multipler Abartungen, vorwiegend am Skelettsystem. *Z. Kinderheilk., 24*:220, 1920.

710. HURXTHAL, L. M.: Increased intracranial pressure associated with chronic parathyroid tetany. *Lahey Clin. Bull., 2*:238, 1942.

711. HYALLESTED, K., AND MOLLER, P. M.: Follow-up on patients with a history of optic neuritis. *Acta. Ophthal., 39*:655, 1961.

712. IGERSHEIMER, J.: *Handbuch der Haut-und Geschlechtskrankheiten.* Vol. 17 no. 2 Syphilis und Auge. Berlin: Springer, 1928.

713. IGERSHEIMER, J.: Sehnervenerkrankung bei maligner Sklerose. *Z. Augenheilk., 69*:47, 1929.

714. IGERSHEIMER, J.: Ueber Anomalien und krankhafte Zustände der Kleinen Gefässe des Opticus. *Ophthalmologica, 103*:230, 1942.

715. IGERSHEIMER, J.: Atrophy of the optic nerve in tabes and dementia paralytica. *Arch. Ophthal., 42*:170, 1949.

716. IGERSHEIMER, J.: Visual changes in progressive exophthalmos. *Arch. Ophthal., 53*:94, 1955.

717. IMACHI, J., AND KAJIKAMA, I.: Pathohistological studies on arachnoiditis, with especial reference to circulation disturbances of the cerebrospinal fluid. Inquiry into etiology of neuritis retrobulbaris. *Jap. J. Ophthal., 4*:37, 1960.

718. IMACHI, J., YASO, I., AND MATSUMOTO, S.: On 32 craniotomized cases of Leber's disease with reference to its genetic problems. *Jap. J. Ophthal., 1*:236, 1957.

719. INGHAM, S. D.: The functional primary, secondary and tertiary visual cortical areas. *Bull. Los Angeles Neurol. Soc., 5*:12, 1940.

720. INGHIRAMI, L.: Frequenza e caratteristiche dei disturbivisivi nelle manifestazioni critiche della epilessia. *Sist. Ner., 10*:194, 1958. (Abst., *Excerpta Med. XII, 14*:#66, 1960.)

721. INGRAHAM, F. D., AND HEYL, H. L.: Subdural hematoma in infancy and childhood. *J.A.M.A., 112*:198, 1939.

722. INGRAHAM, F. D., MATSON, D. D., AND McLAURIN, R. L.: Cortisone and ACTH as an adjunct to the surgery of craniopharyngiomas. *New Engl. J. Med., 246*:568, 1952.

723. INGRAHAM, F. D., AND SCOTT, H. W.: Craniopharyngiomas in children. *J. Pediat., 29*:95, 1946.

724. IRVINE, S. R.: In discussion of Bedell, A. J.: Spots in the Ocular Fundus. *Trans. Amer. Ophthal. Soc., 57*:51, 1959.

725. IRVINE, W. C., AND IRVINE, A. R.: Nematode endophthalmitis: Toxocara canis. Report of one case. *Amer. J. Ophthal., 47*:185, 1959.

726. ISRAELS, M. G.: Neuromyelitis optica (Devic's disease). *Canad. Med. Ass. J., 65*:587, 1951.

727. ISSELBACHER, K. J., ANDERSON, E. P., KURAHASHI, K., AND KALCKAR, H. M.: Congenital galactosemia, single enzymatic block in galactose metabolism. *Science, 123*:635, 1956.

728. IVERSON, H. A., Hereditary optic atrophy. *Arch. Ophthal., 59*:850, 1958.

729. JACKSON, J. H.: Ophthalmoscopic examination during sleep. *Roy. Lond. Ophthal. Hosp. Rep., 4*:35, 1864.

730. JACOB, P., FAVORY, A., AND MALLARDS Un cas de névrite rétro-bulbaire au cours d'une méningite tuberculeuse traitée par la streptomycine. *Bull. Soc. Med. Hop. Paris, 65*:587, 1949.

731. JACOBS, L., FAIR, J. R., AND BICKERTON, J. H.: Adult ocular toxoplasmosis. Report of a parasitologically proved case. *Arch. Ophthal., 52*:63, 1954.

732. JACOBSON, J. H., AND STEPHENS, G.: Hereditary choroidoretinal degeneration: Study of a family including electroretinography and adaptometry. *Arch. Ophthal., 67*:321, 1962.

733. JAEGER, W.: Dominante vererbte opticusatrophie (Unter besonderer Berücksichtigung der dabei vorhandenen Farbensinnstörung). *Graefe Arch. Ophthal., 155*:457, 1954.

734. JAEGER, W.: Neuroretinitis nach Masern. Presented before the Vereinigung Bayerischer Augenärzte, May 23 and 24, 1959. (Abst., *Klin. Mbl. Augenheilk., 135*:438, 1959.)

735. JAEGER, W., AND NOVER, A.: Störungen des Lichtinsinns und Farbensinns bei chorioretinitis centralis serosa. *Graefe Arch. Ophthal., 152*:111, 1951.

736. JAGER, B. V., FRED, H. L., BUTLER, R. B., AND CARNES, W. H.: Occurrence of retinal pigmentation, ophthalmoplegia, ataxia, deafness and heart block.: Report of a case with findings at autopsy. *Amer. J. Med., 29*:888, 1960.

737. JAMPEL, R. S., AND FALLS, H. F.: Atypical retinitis pigmentosa, acanthrocytosis, and heredodegenerative neuromuscular disease. *Arch. Ophthal., 59*:818, 1958.

738. JAMPEL, R. S., OKAZAKI, H., AND BERNSTEIN, H.: Ophthalmoplegia and retinal degeneration associated with spinocerebellar ataxia. *Arch. Ophthal., 66*:247, 1961.

739. JANE, J. A., AND McKISSOCK, W.: Importance of failing vision in early diagnosis of suprasellar meningiomas. *Brit. Med. J., 2*:5, 1962.

740. JAYLE, G. E., BOYER, R., AND AUBERT, L.: L'Achromatopsie congenitale typique et son expression electro-retinographique. *Ann. Oculist., 195*:193, 1962.

741. JEBEJIAN, R., AND KALFAYAN, B.: Le syndrome Oculo-Bucco-Génital. *Ann. Oculist., 179*:841, 1946.

742. JEFFERSON, G.: Compression of chiasma, optic nerves, and optic tracts by intracranial aneurysms. *Brain, 60*:444, 1937.

743. JEFFERSON, G.: Extrasellar extensions of pituitary adenomas. *Proc. Roy. Soc. Med., 33*:433, 1940.

744. JEFFERSON, G.: On compression and invasion of the optic nerves and chiasma by neighboring gliomas. *Trans. Ophthal. Soc. U.K., 65*:262, 1945.

745. JEFFERSON, G.: Involvement of the optic chiasma and optic nerves in cerebral gliomas. *Trans. Ophthal. Soc. U.K., 79*:463, 1959.

746. JEFFERSON, G., POLLACK, E., AND YATES, P. O.: Invasion of the optic chiasma and optic nerves by neighboring gliomas. Presented at 55th Meeting: Society of British Neurological Surgeons. (Abst., *J. Neurol. Neurosurg. Psychiat., 20*:230, 1957.)

747. JOCHMUS, I., AND JOCHMUS, H.: Zum Krankheitsbild der tuberösen Sklerose. Psychopathologische und ophthalmologische Beobachtungen. *Z. Kinderheilk., 85*:543, 1961.

748. JOHNS, J. P.: The influence of pregnancy on the visual field. *Amer. J. Ophthal., 13*:956, 1930.

749. JOHNSON, H. C., AND WALKER, A. E.: The angiographic diagnosis of spontaneous thrombosis of the internal and common carotid arteries. *J. Neurosurg., 8*:631, 1951.

750. JOHNSON, L. C.: Flicker as a helicopter pilot problem. *Aerospace Med., 34*:306, 1963.

751. JOHNSON, M. L.: Degeneration and repair of the rat retina in avitaminosis A. *Arch. Ophthal., 29*:793, 1943.

752. JOHNSON, W. A., AND KEARNS, T. P.: Sludging of Blood in retinal veins. *Amer. J. Ophthal., 54*:201, 1962.

753. JOY, H. H.: Agnostic alexia without agraphia following trauma. *Amer. J. Ophthal., 31*:811, 1948.

754. JOY, H. H.: Suprasellar meningioma; report of an atypical case. *Trans. Amer. Ophthal. Soc., 49*:59, 1951.

755. JOY, H. H., ECKER, A., AND REIMENSCHNEIDER, P. A.: The role of cerebral angiography in ophthalmology. Normal anatomy: Presellar and suprasellar tumours: Ocular complications. *Amer. J. Ophthal., 37*:55, 1954.

756. JOY, R. J. T., SCALETTAR, R., AND SODEE, D. B.: Optic and peripheral neuritis; probable effect of prolonged chloramphenicol therapy. *J.A.M.A., 173*:1727, 1960.

757. JOYNT, R. J.: Mechanism of production of papilledema in the Guillain-Barré syndrome. *Neurology, 8*:8, 1958.

758. JUBB, K. V., SAUNDERS, L. Z., AND COATES, H. V.: The intraocular lesions of canine distemper. *J. Comp. Path. Ther., 67*:21, 1957.

759. KADLECOVA, V., AND MELICHAR, V.: [Retinal Folds in Children with Multiple Malformations]. *Cesk. Oftal., 13*:426, 1957. (Abst., *Excerpta Med. XII, 13*:#1855, 1959.)

760. KAGEYAMA, N., AND BELSKY, R.: Ectopic pinealoma in the chiasma region. *Neurology, 11*:318, 1961.

761. KAHN, A.: Some physiologic implications of craniopharyngiomas. *Neurology, 9*:82, 1959.

762. KANZER, M., AND BENDER, M. B.: Spatial disorientation with homonymous defects of the visual field. *Arch. Ophthal., 21*:439, 1939.

763. KARLIN, D. B., AND HIRSCHENFANG, S.: A comparison of visuosensory and visuomotor disturbances in right and left hemiplegics. *Amer. J. Ophthal., 50*:627, 1960.

764. KARPE, G.: The basis of clinical electroretinography. *Acta Ophthal. Supp.,* 24:1, 1945.
765. KARSTIEN, H.: Über die Sehschärfe bei Stauungspapille. *Fortschr. Neurol. Psychiat.,* 27:649, 1959.
766. KASS, J., MANDEL, W., COHEN, H., AND DRESSLER, S. H.: Isoniazid as a cause of optic neuritis and atrophy. *J.A.M.A., 164*:1740, 1957.
767. KATZ, J. L., VALSAMIS, M. P., AND JAMPEL, R. S.: Ocular signs in diffuse carcinomatous meningitis. *Amer. J. Ophthal., 52*:681, 1961.
768. KEARNS, T. P.: Fat embolism of the retina. *Amer. J. Ophthal., 41*:1, 1956.
769. KEARNS, T. P.: Ocular manifestations of vertebral-basilar arterial thrombosis. *Med. Clin. N. Amer., 44*:909, 1960.
770. KEARNS, T. P., SALASSA, R. M., KERNOHAN, J. W., AND MacCARTY, C. S.: Ocular manifestations of pituitary tumor in Cushing's syndrome. *Arch. Ophthal., 62*:242, 1959.
771. KEARNS, T. P., AND SAYRE, G. P.: Retinitis pigmentosa, external ophthalmoplegia, and complete heart block. Unusual syndrome with histologic study in one of two cases. *Arch. Ophthal., 60*:280, 1958.
772. KEARNS, T. P., AND WAGENER, H. P.: Ophthalmologic diagnosis of meningiomas of the sphenoidal ridge. *Amer. J. Med. Sci., 226*:221, 1953.
773. KEARNS, T. P., WAGENER, H. P., AND MILLIKAN, C. H.: Bilateral homonymous hemianopsia. *Arch. Ophthal., 53*:560, 1955.
774. KEEFE, R. J., AND TROWBRIDGE, D. H.: Neuromyelitis optica with increased intracranial pressure. *Arch. Ophthal., 57*:110, 1957.
775. KEEFE, W. P., YOSS, R. E., MARTENS, T. G., AND DALY, D. D.: Ocular manifestations of narcolepsy. *Amer. J. Ophthal., 49*:953, 1960.
776. KEELE, C. A.: Pathological changes in carotid sinus and their relation to hyptertension. *Quart. J. Med., 2*:213, 1933.
777. KEELER, C. E.: Rodless retina an ophthalmic mutation in house mouse, Mus musculus. *J. Exp. Zool., 46*:355, 1927.
778. KENEL, C.: Cinq cas d'Arachnoïdite optico-chiasmatique d'origine traumaitque, dont quatre confirmés operatoirement. *Ophthalmologica 96*:336, 1939.
779. KENNARD, M. A.: Alterations in response to visual stimuli following lesions of frontal lobe in monkeys. *Arch. Neurol. Psychiat., 41*:1153, 1939.
780. KENNEDY, C. AND CARROLL, F. D.: Optic neuritis in children. *Arch. Ophthal., 63*:747, 1960.
781. KENNEDY, C., AND CARTER, S.: Relation of optic neuritis to multiple sclerosis in children. *Pediatrics, 28*:377, 1961.
782. KENNEDY, F.: Retrobulbar neuritis as an exact diagnostic sign of certain tumors and abscesses in the frontal lobes. *Amer. J. Med. Sci., 142*:355, 1911.
783. KENNEDY, F.: A further note on the diagnostic value of retrobulbar neuritis in expanding lesions of the frontal lobes; with a report of this syndrome in a case of aneurysm of the right internal carotid artery. *J.A.M.A., 67*:1361, 1916.
784. KENNEDY, J. J., AND COPE, C. B.: Intraocular lesions associated with sickle-cell disease. *Arch. Ophthal, 58*:163, 1957.
785. KENNEDY, R. J., RUMMEL, W. D., McCARTHY, J. L., AND HAZARD, J. B.: Metastatic carcinoma of the retina. Report of a case and the pathologic findings. *Arch. Ophthal., 60*:12, 1958.

786. KERR, A. S.: Hormone replacement therapy in craniopharyngiomata. Presented at 55th Meeting: Society of British Neurological Surgeons. (Abst., *J. Neurol. Neurosurg. Psychiat., 20*:230, 1957.)

787. KERR, F. W. L.: The etiology of trigeminal neuralgia. *Arch. Neurol., 8*:15, 1963.

788. KERRINNES, F.: Das Fundusbild bei Herzoperationen mit Kreislaufunterbrechung in Hypothermie. *Graefe Arch. Ophthal., 161*:532, 1959.

789. KESCHNER, M., AND ROSEN, V. H.: Optic neuritis caused by a coal tar hair dye. *Arch. Ophthal., 25*:1020, 1941.

790. KEVORKIAN, J.: Rapid and accurate ophthalmoscopic determination of circulatory arrest. *J.A.M.A., 164*:1660, 1957.

791. KIEL, E.: Zur Histologie der Opticustumoren. *Graefe Arch. Ophthal., 112*: 64, 1923.

792. KING, L. S., AND BUTCHER, J.: Osteochondroma of base of skull. *Arch. Path., 37*:282, 1944.

793. KINOSHITA, J. H., MEROLA, L. O., AND DIKMAK, E.: Osmotic changes in experimental galactose cataracts. *Exp. Eye Res., 1*:405, 1962.

794. KINROSS-WRIGHT, V.: Newer phenothiazine drugs in treatment of nervous disorders. *J.A.M.A., 170*:1283, 1959.

795. KISSEL, P., ARNOLD, G., AND LEPOIRE, J.: Obésité et amaurose, séquelles de méningite tuberculeuse; découverte opératoire d'un tuberculome préchiasmatique et intrasellaire. *Rev. Neurol. (Par.), 90*:816, 1954.

796. KJER, P.: Hereditary infantile optic atrophy with dominant transmission, preliminary report. *Danish Med. Bull., 3*:135, 1956.

797. KJER, P.: Infantile optic atrophy with dominant mode of inheritance. *Acta Ophthal. (Kbh.) Supp.* 1959, p. 54.

798. KLAUDER, J. V. AND ELLIS, V. M.: Effective treatment of lupus erythematosus and exudative retinitis with a gold compound. *Arch. Ophthal., 21*:893, 1939.

799. KLAUDER, J. V., AND MEYER, G. P.: Chorio-Retinitis of congenital syphilis. *Arch. Ophthal., 49*:139, 1953.

800. KLEIST, K.: *Die Kriegsverletzungen des Gehirns.* Leipzig 1922.

801. KLEIST, K.: Die einzeläugigen Gesichtsfelder und ihre Vertretung in den beiden Lagen der verdoppelten inneren Körnerschicht der Sehrinde *Klin. Wschr., 5*:3, 1926.

802. KLENK, E.: La chimie des soi-disant thesaurismoses phosphatidiques du tissu nerveux. *Acta Neurol. Belg., 54*:586, 1954.

803. KLIEN, B. A.: Anticoagulant therapy of occlusion of central vein of retina. In relation to pathogenesis and differential diagnosis. *Arch. Ophthal., 29*: 699, 1943.

804. KLEIN, B. A.: Obstruction of the central retinal vein. A clinico-histopathologic analysis. *Amer. J. Ophthal., 27*:12, 1944.

805. KLEIN, B. A.: Prevention of retinal venous occlusion. *Amer. J. Ophthal., 33*: 175, 1950.

806. KLEIN, B. A.: The heredodegeneration of the macula lutea. Diagnostic and differential diagnostic considerations and a histopathologic report. *Amer. J. Ophthal., 33*:371, 1950.

807. KLEIN, B. A.: Retina and optic nerve. *Arch. Ophthal., 63*:862, 1960.

808. KLEIN, B. A.: Macular and extramacular serous chorioretinopathy, with

remarks upon the role of an extrabulbar mechanism in its pathogenesis. *Amer. J. Ophthal., 51*:231, 1961.

809. KLEIN, B. A.: Die Blutgefässe der retina und choroidea bei allgemeiner Sklerodermie. Presented before the Austrian Ophthalmological Society 1961. (Abst. *Z. Ges. Ophthal., 84*:71, 1962.)

810. KLEIN, B. A., AND OLWIN, J. H.: A survey of the pathogenesis of retinal venous occlusion; emphasis upon choice of therapy and an analysis of the therapeutic results in 53 patients. *Arch Ophthal., 56*:207, 1956.

811. KLINGER, M., AND CONDRAU, G.: Lokalisatorisch irreführende Gesichtsfeldsymptome bei Hirntumoren. *Ophthalmologica, 120*:270, 1950.

812. KLOPP, H. W.: Über Umgekehrt- und Verkehrtsehen. *Deutsch. Z. Nervenheilk., 165*:231, 1951.

813. KLÜVER, H.: Visual disturbances after cerebral lesions. *Psychol. Bull., 24*: 316, 1927.

814. KLÜVER, H.: AND BUCY, P. C.: Preliminary analysis of functions of temporal lobes in monkeys. *Arch. Neurol. Psychiat., 42*:979, 1939.

815: KLUYKENS, J., AND JANSSENS, J.: Obliteration des vaisseaux rétiniens et choroidiens dans un cas d'exsanguination. *Bull. Soc. Belg. Ophtal., 122*: 408, 1959.

816. KNAPP, A.: Course in certain cases of atrophy of the optic nerve with cupping and low tension. *Arch. Ophthal., 23*:41, 1940.

817. KNAPP, P.: Beitrag zur Symptomatologie und therapie der rezidivierenden hypopyoniritis und der begleitenden aphthösen Schleimhauterkrankungen. *Schweiz. Med. Wschr., 71*:1288, 1941.

818. KNOX, D. L., AND COGAN, D. G.: Eye pain and homonymous hemianopia. *Amer. J. Ophthal., 54*:1091, 1962.

819. KOCH, L. P., WOLF, A., COWEN, D., AND PAIGE, B. H.: Toxoplasmic encephalomyelitis. VII. Significance of ocular lesions in the diagnosis of infantile or congenital toxoplasmosis. *Arch. Ophthal., 29*:1, 1943.

820. KOK-VAN ALPHEN, C. C.: A family with the dominant infantile form of optical atrophy. *Acta Ophthal., 38*:675, 1960.

821. KOLAGNY, J., AND BYSTRICA, B.: Evulsio nervi optici. *Cesk. Oftal., 12*:389, 1956. (Abst., *Excerpta Med. XII 12*:#160, 1958.)

822. KONIG, A., AND KOTTGEN, E.: Sitzber. *Akad. Wiss.* Berlin 1894, p. 577.

823. KONSTAS, K., AND ARGLIAS, A.: [Angiospasm of the Retina]. *Arch. Soc. Ophtal. Grece N. 6*:320 and 164, 1957. (Abst., *Excerpta Med. XII, 13*: #145, 1959.)

824. KORFF, J.: Fibro-Kapillar-Angiom des Optikus. *Klin. Mbl. Augenheilk., 121*:68, 1952.

825. KORNZWEIG, A. L., AND BASSEN, F. A.: Retinitis pigmentosa, acanthrocytosis and heredodegenerative neuromuscular disease. *Arch. Ophthal., 58*:183, 1957.

826. KORNZWEIG, A. L., FELDSTEIN, M., AND SCHNEIDER, J.: The pathogenesis of senile macular degeneration. *Amer. J. Ophthal., 48*:22, 1959.

827. KOROVITSKI, L., AND SCHEIN, J.: [Affections of the visual organ in plasmocid intoxication and its treatment]. *Vestn. Oftal., 17*:747, 1940. (Abst., *Excerpta Med. XII, 2*:#786, 1948.)

828. KORSTEN, H. B., AND BERNEAUD-KOTZ, G.: Ein Frühes Stadium des Fundus paraproteinaemicus bei einem Fall von Makroglobulinämie. *Klin. Mbl. Augenheilk., 128*: 679, 1956.

829. KRABBE, K.: A new infantile form of diffuse brain-sclerosis. *Brain, 39*:74, 1916.

830. KRANENBURG, E. W.: Crater-like holes in the optic disc and central serous retinopathy. *Arch. Ophthal., 64*:912, 1960.

831. KRAUS, A. M., AND O'ROURKE, J.: Lymphomatous optic neuritis. *Arch. Ophthal., 70*:173, 1963.

832. KRAVITZ, D.: The value of quadrant field defects in the localization of temporal lobe tumors. *Amer. J. Ophthal., 14*:781, 1931.

833. KRAVITZ, D: Arachnoiditis. *Arch. Ophthal., 37*:199, 1947.

834. KRAYENBUHL, H.: Die Bedeutung der Gesichtsfeldbestimmung in der Diagnostik von Tumoren des Schläfen und Hinterhauptlappens. *Schweiz. Med. Wschr., 69*:1028, 1939.

835. KREIBIG, W.: Das epipapillare Melanom. *Klin. Mbl. Augenheilk., 115*: 354, 1949.

836. KREIBIG, W.: Optikomalazie, die Folge eines Gefässverschlusses im retrobulbären Abschnitt des Schnerven. *Klin. Mbl. Augenheilk., 122*: 719, 1953.

837. KREIBIG, W.: Zoster lesions of the eye. *Wien. Med. Wschr., 109*:636, 1959.

838. KRILL, A. E., AND FOLK, M. R.: Retinitis punctata albescens. A functional evaluation of an unusual case. *Amer. J. Ophthal., 53*:450, 1962.

839. KRILL, A. E., WIELAND, A. M., AND OSTFELD, A. M.: The effect of two hallucinogenic agents on human retinal function. *Arch. Ophthal., 64*:724, 1960.

840. KUBIK, C. S., AND ADAMS, R. D.: Occlusion of the basilar artery—a clinical and pathological study. *Brain, 69*:73, 1946.

841. KUPER, J.: Familiäre sektorenförmige Retinitis pigmentosa. *Klin. Mbl. Augenheilk., 136*:97, 1960.

842. KUNKLE, E. E.: Diseases of nerve roots, plexuses and nerves. In *A Textbook of Medicine*. Ed. R. L. Cecil and R. F. Loeb. 9th ed. Philadelphia: W. B. Saunders, 1955, pp. 1616-1627.

843. KUNKEL, E. C., AND ANDERSON, W. B.: Significance of minor eye signs in headache of migraine type. *Arch. Ophthal., 65*:504, 1961.

844. KUPFER, C.: The projection of the macula in the lateral geniculate nucleus of man. *Amer. J. Ophthal., 54*:597, 1962.

845. KURZ, J.: [Remarks on some ophthalmological signs of intracranial lesions]. *Cesk. Oftal., 13*:241, 1957. (Abst., *Ophthal. Lit., 11*:#372, 1958.)

846. KURZ, O.: Über Papillitis arteriosclerotica. *Ophthalmologica, 116*:281, 1948.

847. KUWABARA, T.: Unpublished.

848. KUWABARA, T., AND COGAN, D. G.: Studies of retinal vascular patterns. I. Normal architecture. *Arch. Ophthal., 64*:904, 1960.

849. KUWABARA, T., AND COGAN, D. G.: Tetrazolium studies on the retina. III. Activity of metabolic intermediates and miscellaneous substrates. *J. Histochem. Cytochem., 8*:214, 1960.

850. KUWABARA, T., AND COGAN, D. G.: Retinal glycogen. *Arch. Ophthal., 66*: 680, 1961.

851. KUWABARA, T., AND COGAN, D. G.: Retinal vascular patterns. VI. Mural cells of the retinal capillaries. *Arch. Ophthal., 69*:492, 1963.

852. KWITTKEN, J., AND BAREST, H. D.: The neuropathology of hereditary

optic atrophy (Leber's disease); the first complete anatomic study. *Amer. J. Path., 34*:185, 1958.

853. KYRIELEIS, W.: Über atypische Gefässtuberkulose der Netzhaut. *Arch. f. Augenheilk., 107*:182, 1933.

854. KYTILA, J., AND MIETTINEN, P.: On bilateral aplasia of the optic nerve. *Acta Ophthal., 39*:416, 1961.

855. LADWIG, H. A., MURPHY, J. H., MURPHY, R. E., AND BURGERT, E. O.: Papilledema in poliomyelitis. *Guildcraft, 32*:21, 1958.

856. LAKATOS, I.: Arachnoiditis opticochiasmatica. *Ophthalmologica, 123*:46, 1962.

857. LANDERS, P. H.: Vitreous lesions observed in Boeck's sarcoid. *Amer. J. Ophthal., 32*:1740, 1949.

858. LANDOLT, E.: Zur Opticusschädigung bei Schädeltrauma. *Acta Neurochir., 4*:128, 1955.

859. LANDOLT, E.: Ein Fall von Fettembolie der Augen. *Klin. Mbl. Augenheilk., 131*:538, 1957.

860. LANDOLT, E.: Zur einseitigen Retinitis pigmentosa. *Ophthalmologica, 137*: 155, 1959.

861. LANGE, F.: Doppelseitige Optikusatrophie nach akuter Thalliumvergiftung. *Klin. Mbl. Augenheilk., 121*:221, 1952.

862. LANSCHE, R. K., AND RUCKER, C. W.: Progression of defects in visual fields produced by hyaline bodies in optic discs. *Arch. Ophthal., 58*:115, 1957.

863. LARSEN, H.: Demonstration mikroskopischer Präparate von einem monochromatischen Auge. *Z. Augenheilk., 46*:228, 1921.

864. LARSSON, S., AND NORD, B.: Klinisk bild av retrobulbärneurit vid intrakraniella tumörer. *Nord. Med., 34*:1059, 1947 (Abst., *Excerpta Med. XII, 2*:#609, 1948.)

865. LARSSON, S., AND NORD, B.: Some remarks on retinal vein thrombosis and its treatment with anticoagulants. *Acta Ophthal., 28*:187, 1950.

866. LARUELLE, AND REUMONT: Lésions anatomopathologiques du chiasma optique au cours de la poliomyélite antérieure aigüe. *Bull. Soc. Belg. Ophthal., 102*:659, 1952.

867. LASATER, G. M.: Reading epilepsy. *Arch. Neurol., 6*:492, 1962.

868. LASCO, F., MINCULESCO, C., AND SIMONESCO, M.: L'aspect ophthalmoscopique des métastases cérébrales. La stase papillaire hémorragique. *Arch. Ophtal., 19*:165, 1959.

869. LASCO, F., AND NICOLESCO, M.: Le syndrome de l'excavation de la lame criblée - le pseudoglaucome. *Ophthalmologica 136*:90, 1958.

870. LASCO, F., NICOLESCO, M., AND NICULIU, I.: Pseudonévrite rétrobulbarie par métastase endocranienne. *Arch. Ophtal., 19*:19, 1959.

871. LASCU, F., NICULESCU, M., AND NICULIU, I.: Pseudonévrita retrobulbara în metastazele endocraniene. *Oftalmologia, 1*:84, 1956.

872. LASHLEY, K. S.: The mechanism of vision. XVIII. Effects of destroying the visual "associative areas" of the monkey. *Genet. Psychol. Monogr., 37*:107, 1948.

873. LASSMAN, L. P., CULLEN, J. F., LOND, D. O., AND HOWAT, J. M. L.: Stenosis of the aqueduct of Sylvius. *Amer. J. Ophthal., 49*:261, 1960.

874. LATERZA, A.: La Papilla da stasi nelle compressioni del cono e della cauda equina. *Riv. Oto-Neuro-Oftal., 34*:336, 1959.

875. Lauber, H. L., and Lewin, B.: Über optische Halluzinationen bei Ausschaltung des Visus, Klinisch und Tiefenpsychologisch betrachtet. *Arch. Psychiat. Nervenkr., 197*:15, 1958.
876. Laval, J.: Ocular sarcoidosis. *Amer. J. Ophthal., 35*:551, 1952.
877. Lavy, S., and Neuman, E.: Changes of the optic nerve after cataract extraction simulating the Foster Kennedy syndrome. *Confin. Neurol., 19*: 383, 1959.
878. Lazarus, J. D., and Levine, G.: Blindness in whooping cough. *Amer. J. Dis. Child., 47*:1310, 1934.
879. Lazorthes, G., and Anduze, H.: L'ouverture du canal optique dans les lésions traumatiques récentes du nerf optique. (A propos de 10 cas opérés.) *Rev. Neurol., 7*:540, 1952.
880. Leber, T.: Ueber Retinitis Pigmentosa und angeborene Amaurose. *Graef. Arch. Ophthal., 15*:1, 1869.
881. Leber, T.: Ueber hereditäre und congenital-angelegte Sehnervenleiden. *Graefe Arch. Ophthal., 17*:249, 1871.
882. Leber, T.: Die Cirkulations- und Ernährungsverhältnisse des Auges. In: *Graefe-Saemisch Hb. Gesamten Augenheilkunde,* Vol. 2, Part 2, Ch. 11 Leipzig: Wilhelm Engelmann, 1903.
883. Lees, F.: The migrainous symptoms of cerebral angiomata. *J. Neurol. Neurosurg. Psychiat., 25*:45, 1962.
884. LeGrand, M., Dehage, and Lecomte: Quinine amaurosis. *Bull. Soc. Belg. Ophtal., 125*:965, 1960.
885. LeGros-Clark, W. E.: The laminar pattern of the lateral geniculate nucleus in relation to colour vision. *Docum. Ophthal., 3*:327, 1949.
886. Lehrer, G. M.: Arteriographic demonstration of collateral circulation in cerebrovascular disease. *Neurology, 8*:27, 1958.
887. Leiderman, H., Mendelson, J. H., Wexler, D., and Solomon, P.: Sensory deprivation: Clinical aspects. *Arch. Intern. Med., 101*:389, 1958.
888. Leinfelder, P. S.: Pathogenesis of papilledema. *Amer. J. Ophthal., 48*:107, 1959.
889. Leishman, R.: Gastric function in tobacco amblyopia. *Trans. Ophthal. Soc. U.K., 71*:319, 1951.
890. Leishman, R.: The eye in general vascular disease: Hypertension and arteriosclerosis. *Brit. J. Ophthal., 41*:641, 1957.
891. Leitholf, O.: Traumatische Optikusschädigungen. *Zbl. Neurochir., 20*:19, 1959. (Abst., *Excerpta Med. XII, 14*:#1177, 1960.
892. Lelong, M., Habib, E.-C., Kreisler, L., Bader, J.-C., and Delaru, R.: L'épilepsie photogénique avec autostimulation intermittente. *Arch. Franc. Pediat., 18*:163, 1961.
893. Lenz, H.: Raumsinnstörungen bei Hirnverletzungen. *Deutsch. Nervenheilk., 157*:22, 1944.
894. Lepoire, J., and Pertuiset, B.: Les kystes epidermoïdes cranio-encéphaliques. *Neurochirurgica, 1*:1, 1958.
895. Lerman, S., and Feldman, A. L.: Centrocecal scotomata as the presenting sign in pernicious anemia. *Arch. Ophthal., 65*:381, 1961.
896. Lesenne, E.: Névrite optique au cours d'une intoxication botulinique. *Bull. Soc. Ophtal. Franc., 3*:345, 1947.
897. Levatin, P.: Atrophy of the optic nerve following hemorrhage. *Arch. Ophthal., 37*:18, 1947.

898. LEVATIN, P.: Increased intracranial pressure without papilledema. *Arch. Ophthal., 58*:683, 1957.

899. LEVITT, J. M.: Unilateral ophthalmoplegia totalis; parasellar osteochondroma: Report of a case. *Arch. Ophthal., 12*:877, 1934.

900. LEVITT, J. M.: Boeck's sarcoid with ocular localization. Survey of the literature and report of a case. *Arch. Ophthal., 25*:358, 1941.

901. LEVY, E. Z., RUFF, G. E., AND THALER, V. H.: Studies in human isolation. *J.A.M.A., 169*:236, 1959.

902. LEY, A.: Compression of the optic nerve by a fusiform aneurism of the carotid artery. *J. Neurol. Neurosurg. Psychiat., 13*:75, 1950.

903. LHERMITTE, F.: Les leuco-encéphalites; étude anatomoclinique, nosologique et expérimentale. Paris, University Faculty of Medicine, Thesis 1950.

904. LHERMITTE, J.: Syndrome de la calotte du pédoncule cérébral. Les troubles psycho-sensoriels dans lésions du mésocéphale. *Rev. Neurol. (Par.), 29*: 1359, 1922.

905. LHERMITTE, J.: Les fondements anatomophysiologiques de certaines hallucinations visuelles. *Confin. Neurol., 9*:43, 1949.

906. LHERMITTE, J. J., AND AJURIAGUERRA, J.: *Psychopathologie de la Vision.* Paris: Masson, 1942.

907. LHEMITTE, J., AND TRELLES, J. O.: L'artério-sclerose du tronc basilaire et ses consequences anatomo-cliniques. *Jahrb. Psychiat. Neurol., 51*:91, 1934.

908. LIEB, W. A., GEERAETS, W. J., AND GUERRY, D.: Sickle-cell retinopathy. Ocular and systemic manifestations of sickle-cell disease. *Acta Ophthal. (Kbh.) supp., 58*:7, 1959.

909. LIEB, W. A., GEERAETS, W. J., AND GUERRY, D.: Retinopathie bei der Sichelzellenerkrankung. *Klin. Mbl. Augenheilk., 137*:60, 1960.

910. LILLIE, W. I.: Ocular phenomena produced by temporal lobe tumors. *J.A.M.A., 85*:1465, 1925.

911. LILLIE, W. I.: Prechiasmal syndrome produced by chronic local arachnoiditis. *Arch. Ophthal., 24*:940, 1940.

912. LINCOFF, H. A., WISE, G. N., AND ROMAINE, H. H.: Total detachment and reattachment of the retina (in herpes zoster ophthalmicus). *Amer. J. Ophthal., 41*:253, 1956.

913. LINCOFF, M. H.: Quinine amblyopia. Report of a case. *Arch. Ophthal., 53*: 382, 1955.

914. LINDGREN, E.: Percutaneous angiography of vertebral artery. *Acta Radiol. (Stockh.), 33*:389, 1950.

915. LINHART, R. W.: Lethal granuloma of the orbit. *Trans. Penn. Acad. Ophthal., 9*:121, 1956.

916. LISS, L., AND JAMPEL, R. S.: Chromophobe adenoma of the pituitary; clinicopathologic report of a case. *Neurology, 9*:501, 1959.

917. LISS, L., AND WOLTER, J. R.: The histology of the glioma of the optic nerve. *Arch. Ophthal., 58*:689, 1957.

918. LIST, C. F.: Osteochondromas arising from base of skull. *Surg. Gynec. Obstet., 76*:480, 1943.

919. LIST, C. F., WILLIAMS, J. R., AND BALYEAT, G. W.: Vascular lesions in pituitary adenomas. *J. Neurosurg., 9*:177, 1952.

920. LIVERSEDGE, L. A., AND SMITH, V. H.: Neuro-medical and ophthalmic

aspects of central retinal artery occlusion. *Trans. Ophthal. Soc. U.K., 82*:571, 1962.

921. LLOYD, L. A.: Optic neuritis in children. *Trans. Canad. Ophthal. Soc., 22*: 108, 1959.

922. LOCKE, S., AND TYLER, H. R.: Pituitary apoplexy. Report of two cases with pathological verification. *Amer. J. Med., 30*:643, 1961.

923. LODBERG, C. V., AND LUND, A.: Hereditary optic atrophy with dominant transmission; three Danish families. *Acta Ophthal. (Kbh.), 28*:437, 1950.

924. LOHLEIN, W., AND TONNIS, W.: Die operative Behandlung der das Foramen opticum überschreitenden Sehnerven-geschwülste. *Graefe Arch. Ophthal., 149*:318, 1949.

925. LOEWE, I.: Gefässveränderungen in der Netzhaut bei Sclerosis multiplex. *Z. Aertzl. Fortbild., 52*:976, 1958.

926. LOEWENSTEIN, A.: Cavernous degeneration, necrosis and other regressive processes in optic nerve with vascular disease of eye. *Arch. Ophthal., 34*: 220, 1945.

927. LOGOTHETIS, J., SILVERSTEIN, P., AND COE, J.: Neurologic aspects of Waldenström's macroglobulinemia: Report of a case. *Arch. Neurol., 3*: 564, 1960.

928. LONGFELLOW, D. W., DAVIS, F. S., AND WALSH, F. B.: Unilateral intermittent blindness with dilation of retinal veins. Undetermined etiology. *Arch. Ophthal., 67*:554, 1962.

929. LOPES D'ANDRADE: Uma hemianopsia inferior consecutiva a hemorragia uterina. *Arg. Port. Oftal. (Lisbon), 1*:23, 1949. (Abst., *Excerpta Med. XII, 4*:#2298, 1950.)

930. LORENTZEN, S. E.: Microaneurysms of unknown nature observed ophthalmoscopically. *Acta Ophthal. (Kbh.),37*:279, 1959.

931. LORENTZEN, S. E.: Drusen of the optic disk, an irregularly dominant hereditary affection. *Acta Ophthal. (Kbh.), 39*:626, 1961.

932. LOSSIUS, H. M.: Transitory visual disturbances after ventriculography. *Acta Psychiat. Scand., 31*:81, 1956.

933. LOVE, J. G., DODGE, H. W., AND BAIR, H. L.: Complete removal of glioma affecting the optic nerve. *Arch. Ophthal., 54*:386, 1955.

934. LOVE, J. G., WAGENER, H. P., AND WOLTMAN, H. W.: Tumors of spinal cord associated with choking of optic disks. *Arch. Neurol. Psychiat., 66*: 171, 1951.

935. LOW, N. L., AND CARTER, S.: Multiple sclerosis in children. *Pediatrics, 18*:24, 1956.

936. LOWE, R. F.: Harada's disease. *Trans. Ophthal. Soc. Aust., 10*:11, 1950.

937. LUBECK, M. J.: Papilledema caused by iron deficiency anemia. *Trans. Amer. Acad. Ophthal. Otolaryng., 63*:306, 1959.

938. LUBOW, M.: Carotid-cavernous fistula. Comments on ocular complications. *Amer. J. Ophthal., 53*:121, 1962.

939. LUCAS, D. R., AND NEWHOUSE, J. P.: The toxic effect of sodium 1-glutamate on the inner layers of the retina. *Arch. Ophthal., 58*:193, 1957.

940. LUFT, R. et al.: Hypophysectomy in diabetes mellitus with vascular complications. *Nord. Med., 55*:715, 1956.

941. LUNDBERG, A.: Über Oligodendrozytome des Sehnervs. *Acta Ophthal. (Kbh.), 14*:271, 1936.

942. LYLE, D. J.: Arteriosclerotic optic atrophy. *Proc. Roy. Soc. Med., 50*:937, 1957.
943. LYLE, D. J.: Compression atrophy of the optic nerve. *Amer. J. Ophthal., 45*:133, 1958.
944. LYLE, D. J.: Ophthalmological involvement in the primary demyelinating disease. *Arch. Ophthal., 62*:255, 1959.
945. LYLE, T. K.: Some pitfalls in the diagnosis of plerocephalic oedema. *Trans. Ophthal. Soc. U.K., 73*:87, 1953.
946. LYLE, T. K., AND CLOVER, P.: Ocular symptoms and signs in pituitary tumours. *Proc. Roy. Soc. Med., 54*:611, 1961.
947. LYLE, T. K., AND WYBAR, K.: Retinal vasculitis. *Brit. J. Ophthal., 45*:778, 1961.
948. McCREA, W. B. E.: Glioma of the retina. A review of twelve cases. *Brit. J. Ophthal., 27*:259, 1943.
949. McCULLOCH, C., AND McCULLOCH, R. J. R.: A hereditary and clinical study of choroideremia. *Trans. Amer. Acad. Ophthal. Otolaryng., 53*:160, 1948.
950. MacDONALD, A. E.: Ocular lesions caused by intracranial hemorrhage. *Trans. Amer. Ophthal. Soc., 29*:418, 1931.
951. McFIE, J., PIERCY, M. F., AND ZANGWILL, O. L.: Visual-spatial agnosia associated with lesions of the right cerebral hemisphere. *Brain, 73*:167, 1950.
952. McFIE, J., AND ZANGWILL, O. L.: Visual-constructive disabilities associated with lesions of the left cerebral hemisphere. *Brain, 83*:243, 1960.
953. McKAY, R. A., AND SPIVEY, B. E.: Generalized choroidal angiosclerosis. *Arch. Ophthal., 67*:727, 1962.
954. MacKENZIE, I.: Clinical presentation of cerebral angioma; review of 50 cases. *Brain, 76*:184, 1953.
955. MacKENZIE, I., MEIGHAN, S., AND POLLACK, E. N.: On the projection of the retinal quadrants on the lateral geniculate bodies, and the relationship of the quadrants to the optic radiations. *Trans. Ophthal. Soc. U.K., 53*:142, 1933.
956. McKISSOCK, W., RICHARDSON, A., AND BLOOM, W. H.: Subdural haematoma; a review of 389 cases. *Lancet, 1*:1365, 1960.
957. McLEAN, J. M.: Astrocytoma (true glioma) of the retina, report of a case. *Arch. Ophthal., 18*:255, 1937.
958. McLEAN, J. M.: Glial tumours of the retina in relation to tuberous sclerosis. *Amer. J. Ophthal., 41*:428, 1956.
959. McLEAN, J. M., AND RAY, B. S.: Soft glaucoma and calcification of the internal carotid arteries. *Arch. Ophthal., 38*:154, 1947.
960. McPHAUL, J. J., AND ENGEL, F. L.: Heterotopic calcification, hyperphosphatemia and angioid streaks of the retina. *Amer. J. Med., 31*:488, 1961.
961. McPHERSON, S. D.: Primary drusen (hyaline bodies) of the optic nerve. *Amer. J. Ophthal., 39*:294, 1955.
962. MACRAE, D., AND TROLLE, E.: Defect of function in visual agnosia. *Brain, 79*:94, 1956.
963. McREYNOLDS, W. V., HAVENER, W. H., AND PETROHELOS, M. A.: Bilateral optic neuritis following smallpox vaccination and diphtheria—tetanus toxoid. *Amer. J. Dis. Child., 86*:601, 1953.

964. MADDOX, E. E.: See-saw nystagmus with bitemporal hemianopia. *Proc. Roy Soc. Med.,* 7:12, 1914.

965. MAEDA, J.: Electron microscopy of the retinal vessels. I. *Jap. J. Ophthal.,* 3:37, 1959.

966. MAGDER, H.: Test for central serous retinopathy based on clinical observations and trial. *Amer. J. Ophthal.,* 49:147, 1960.

967. MAIONE, M.: Atrofia ottica da piccoli traumi della regione orbito-fronto-parietale. (Contribute clinico e considerazioni generali.) *Ann. Ottal.,* 78:33, 1952. (Abst., *Excerpta Med. XII.,* 8:#801, 1954.)

968. MAISON, G. L., SETTLAGE, P., AND GRETHER, W. F.: Experimental study of macular representation in the monkey. *Arch. Neurol. Psychiat.,* 40:981, 1938.

969. MAJKOWSKI, J.: [Case of a complication infantile atrophy of optic nerves (Behr's disease)]. *Klin. Oczna,* 29:403, 1959. (Abst., *Zbl. Ophthal.,* 79:326, 1960.)

970. MAKLEY, T. A.: Retinoblastoma in a 52-year-old man. *Arch. Ophthal.,* 69:325, 1963.

971. MALTBY, G. L.: Visual field changes and subdural hematomas. *Surg. Gynec. Obstet.,* 74:496, 1942.

972. MANCELL, I. T.: Opticociliary neuritis. *Arch. Ophthal.,* 54:436, 1955.

973. MANDELL, M. M., AND STEINMETZ, C. G.: Subdural membrane with arachnoiditis of the optic chiasm. *Arch. Ophthal.,* 62:419, 1959.

974. MANFREDI, F., MERWARTH, C. R., BUCKLEY, C. E., AND SIEKER, H. O.: Papilledema in chronic respiratory acidosis. Report of a case, with studies on the blood-cerebrospinal fluid barrier for carbon dioxide. *Amer. J. Med.,* 30:175, 1961.

975. MANN, I.: Congenital retinal fold. *Brit. J. Ophthal.,* 19:641, 1935.

976. MANN, I.: *Developmental abnormalities of the eye.* 2nd. ed. Philadelphia: Lippencott, 1957, p. 151.

977. MANN, W. A.: Hysterical amblyopia. *Quart. Bull. Northw. Univ. Med. Sch.,* 34:215, 1960.

978. MANNICK, J. A., SUTER, C. G., AND HUME, D. M.: The "subclavian steal" syndrome. A further documentation. *J.A.M.A.,* 182:254, 1962.

979. MANSCHOT, W. A.: The fundus oculi in subarachnoid haemorrhage. *Acta. Ophthal.,* 22:281, 1944.

980. MANSCHOT, W. A.: Subarachnoid hemorrhage: intraocular symptoms and their pathogenesis. *Amer. J. Ophthal.,* 38:501, 1954.

981. MANSCHOT, W. A.: Embolism of the central retinal artery, originating from an endocardial myxoma. *Amer. J. Ophthal.,* 48:381, 1959.

982. MANSCHOT, W. A., AND DAEMEN, C. B.: A case of cytomegalic inclusion disease with ocular involvement. *Ophthalmologica,* 143:137, 1962.

983. MANSCHOT, W. A., AND HAMPE, J. F.: The origin of ocular symptoms in spontaneous subarachnoid haemorrhage. *Int. Congress Ophthal.,* 1:356, 1950.

984. MARCHESANI, O.: Die Morphologie der Glia in Nervus Opticus und in der Retina, dargestellt nach den neuesten Untersuchungesmethoden und Untersuchungsergebnissen. *Graefe Arch. Ophthal.,* 117:575, 1926.

985. MARGAILLAN, A., GAUE, H., AND GOURE, P.: À propos d'un cranio-pharyngiome: valeur localisatrice de la chronologie des symptômes ocu-

laires, récupération total de la vision centrale d'un oeil aveugle. *Rev. Otoneuroophtal., 33*:175, 1961.

986. MARIE, P., AND CHATELIN, C.: Les troubles visuels dûs aux lésions des voies optiques intra-cérébrales et de la sphéré visuelle dans les blessures du crâne per coup de feu. *Rev. Neurol. (Par.), 28*:882, 1915.

987. MARIN-AMAT, M.: Atrofia total de ambas papilas ópticas consecutiva a grandes hemorragias. *Arch. Soc. Oftal. hisp-amer., 10*:1227, 1950. (Abst., *Excerpta Med. XII, 5*:#1990, 1951.)

988. MARINHO DE QUEIROZ, J.: Seráa retinite de Coats uma xantomatose? *Rev. Bras. Oftal., 15*:136, 1956.

989. MARK, V. H., SMITH, J. L., AND KJELLBERG, R. D.: Suprasellar epidermoid tumor; a case report with the presenting complaint of see-saw nystagmus. *Neurology, 10*:81, 1960.

990. MARKS, E. O., WILLIS, R. A., AND ANDERSON, J. R.: Glioma of the optic disc. *Trans. Ophthal. Soc. Aust., 1*:46, 1939.

991. MARKS, V.: Cushing's syndrome occurring with pituitary chromophobe tumors. *Acta. Endocr. (Kbh.), 32*:527, 1959.

992. MARQUART, G.: Pseudostauungspapille. *Klin. Mbl. Augenheilk., 127*:546, 1955.

993. MARR, W. G., AND CHAMBERS, R. G.: Pseudotumor cerebri syndrome, following unilateral radical neck dissection. *Amer. J. Ophthal., 51*:605, 1961.

994. MARSHALL, D.: Glioma of the optic nerve, as a manifestation of von-Recklinghausen's disease. *Amer. J. Ophthal., 37*:15, 1954.

995. MARTELLI, A., AND STRAZZI, A.: Resultati dell'intervento chirurgico precoce nelle amaurosi secondarie a trauma cranico. *Riv. Oto-Neuro-Oftal., 31*:9, 1956.

996. MARTHINSEN, R.: Supraclinoid carotid aneurysm. *Acta. Ophthal. (Kbh.), 19*:141, 1941.

997. MARTIN, P., AND CUSHING, H.: Primary gliomas of the chiasm and optic nerves in their intracranial portion. *Arch. Ophthal., 52*:209, 1923.

998. MASPES, P. E.: Le syndrome expérimental chez l'homme de la section du splénium du corps calleux; alexie visuelle pure hémianopsique. *Rev. Neurol. (Par.), 80*:100, 1948.

999. MASSON, C. B.: Disturbances in vision and in visual fields after ventriculography. *Bull. Neurol. Inst. N.Y., 3*:190, 1933.

1000. MATHUR, S. P., AND MATHUR, B. P.: Optic atrophy after small-pox. *Brit. J. Ophthal., 43*:378, 1959.

1001. MATSON, D. D., AND CRIGLER, J. F.: Radical treatment of craniopharyngioma. *Ann. Surg., 152*:699, 1960.

1002. MAUMENEE, A. E.: Retinal lesions in lupus erythematosus. *Amer. J. Ophthal., 23*:971, 1940.

1003. MAWDSLEY, C.: Epilepsy and television. *Lancet, 1*:190, 1961.

1004. MAYER-GROSS, W.: Some observations on apraxia. *Proc. Roy. Soc. Med., 28*:1203, 1935.

1005. MAYER-GROSS, W.: Question of visual impairment in constructional apraxia. *Proc. Roy. Soc. Med., 29*:1396, 1936.

1006. MAYNARD, R. B.: Blindness among prisoners of war. *Trans. Ophthal. Soc. Aust., 6*:92, 1946.

1007. MEADOWS, S. P.: Optic nerve compression and its differential diagnosis. *Proc. Roy. Soc. Med., 42*:1017, 1949.

1008. MEADOWS, S. P.: Intracranial aneurysms. In *Modern Trends in Neurology.* Ed. A. Feiling. N.Y.: Paul B. Hoeber, 1951. p. 391.

1009. MEADOWS, S. P.: Intracavernous aneurysms of the internal carotid artery, their clinical features and natural history. *Arch. Ophthal., 62*:566, 1959.

1010. MERKULOV, I. I., AND KHALFINA, F. A.: [The dynamics of papilloedema in intracerebral tumours]. *Zh. Oftalm., 4*:195, 1956. (Abst., *Excerpta Med. XII, 12*:#802, 1958.)

1011. MERLE, C., CANTAT, M. A., AND ROUHER, F.: Benign melanotic tumours of the optic disc. *Bull. Soc. Ophtal. Franc.,* p. 447, 1959.

1012. MESSINGER, H. C., AND CLARKE, B. E.: Retinal tumors in tuberous sclerosis, review of the literature and report of a case, with special attention to microscopic structure. *Arch. Ophthal., 18*:1, 1937.

1013. MEURER, T. C.: Optic neuritis following measles. *Trans. Ophthal. Soc. Aust., 7*:106, 1947.

1014. MEVES, H.: Zur Differentialdiagnose des Foster Kennedyschen Syndroms. *Z. Augenheilk., 78*:242, 1932.

1015. MEYER, A.: The connections of the occipital lobes and the present status of the cerebral visual affections. *Trans. Ass. Amer. Physicians 22*:7, 1907.

1016. MEYER, J. E.: Über eine "Ödemkrankheit" des Zentralnervensystems im frühen Kindesalter. *Arch. Psychiat., 185*:35, 1950.

1017. MEYER, J. S., AND DENNY-BROWN, D.: The cerebral collateral circulation I. Factors influencing collateral blood flow. *Neurology, 7*:477, 1957.

1018. MEYERRATKEN, E.: Über Häufigkeit und Besonderheiten der sogenannten Arteritis temporalis. *Klin. Mbl. Augenheilk., 141*:641, 1962.

1019. MEYERSON, L., AND PIENAAR, B. T.: Intra-ocular cysticercus. *Brit. J. Ophthal., 45*:148, 1961.

1020. MIER, M., SCHWARTZ, S. O., AND BOSHES, B.: Acanthrocytosis, pigmentary degeneration of the retina and ataxic neuropathy: A genetically determined syndrome and associated metabolic disorder. *Blood, 16*:1586, 1960.

1021. MILLER, R. D., BASTRON, J. A., AND KEARNS, T. P.: Papilledema in patients with severe pulmonary emphysema. *Dis. Chest, 37*:350, 1960.

1022. MILLER, W. A., AND VAN HERICK, W.: Primary optic atrophy in von Recklinghausen's disease. *Amer. J. Ophthal., 37*:36, 1954.

1023. MILLICHAP, J. G.: Benign intracranial hypertension and otitic hydrocephalus. *Pediatrics, 23*:257, 1959.

1024. MILLIKAN, C. H., AND SIEKERT, R. G.: Studies in cerebrovascular disease; syndrome of intermittent insufficiency of basilar arterial system. *Proc. Mayo Clin., 30*:61, 1955.

1025. MILLIKAN, C. H., SIEKERT, R. G., AND SHICK, R. M.: Studies in cerebrovascular disease; use of anticoagulant drugs in treatment of intermittent insufficiency of internal carotid arterial system. *Proc. Mayo Clin., 30*:578, 1955.

1026. MILLIKAN, C. H., SIEKERT, R. G., AND WHISNAUT, J. P.: The syndrome of occlusion of the labyrinthine division of the internal auditory artery. *Trans. Amer. Neurol. Ass., 84*:11, 1959.

1027. MILLMAN, G. G., AND WHITTICK, J. W.: Sex-linked variant of gargoylism. *J. Neurol. Neurosurg. Psychiat., 15*:253, 1952.

1028. MILNER, B.: Psychological defects produced by temporal lobe excision. *Res. Publ. Ass. Res. Nerv. Ment. Dis., 36*:244, 1958.

1029. MINKOWSKI, M.: Zur Kenntnis der cerebral Sehbanen. *Schweiz. Med. Wschr., 69*:990, 1939.

1030. MINOR, R. H., KEARNS, T. P., MILLIKAN, C. H., SIEKERT, R. G., AND SAYRE, G. P.: Ocular manifestations of occlusive disease of the vertebral-basilar arterial system. *Arch. Ophthal., 62*:84, 1959.

1031. MISHKIN, M.: Visual discrimination performance following partial ablations of temporal lobe: ventral surface vs. hippocampus. *J. Comp. Physiol. Psychol., 47*:187, 1954.

1032. MISHKIN, M., AND PRIBRAM, K. H.: Visual discrimination performance following partial ablations of temporal lobe. ventral vs. lateral. *J. Comp. Physiol. Psychol., 47*:14, 1954.

1033. MISRA, S. M., AND MISRA, N. P.: Optic atrophy in tuberculous meningitis. (A preliminary report) *Indian J. Child. Health, 7*:721, 1957. (Abst., *Excerpta Med. XII, 12*:#1097, 1958.

1034. MIURA, K., AND ORSUKA, K.: [Two cases of embolism on the branch of the retinal artery caused by angiography]. *J. Clin. Ophthal. (Jap.), 13*:972, 1959. (Abst., *Excerpta Med. XII, 14*:#964, 1960.)

1035. MONES, R. J., CHRISTOFF, N., AND BENDER, M. B.: Posterior cerebral artery occlusion; a clinical and angiographic study. *Arch. Neurol., 5*:68, 1961.

1036. MONEY, J., Ed.: *Reading Disability: Progress and Research Needs in Dyslexia.* Baltimore: Johns Hopkins Press, 1962.

1037. MONTANA, J. A., AND HEDGES, T. R.: Carcinoma of the maxillary sinus with ocular involvement; report of four cases. *Amer. J. Ophthal., 49*:1337, 1960.

1038. MOOLTEN, S. E.: Hamartial nature of tuberous sclerosis complex and its bearing on tumor problem; report of case with tumor anomaly of kidney and adenoma sebaceum. *Arch. Intern. Med., 69*:589, 1942.

1039. MOONEY, A. J.: Some ocular sequelae of tuberculous meningitis. A preliminary survey, 1953-1954, *Amer. J. Ophthal., 41*:753, 1956.

1040. MOONEY, A. J.: Further observations on the ocular complications of tuberculous meningitis and their implications. *Amer. J. Ophthal., 48*:297, 1959.

1041. MOONEY, A. J., AND McCONNELL, A. A.: Visual scotomata with intracranial lesions affecting the optic nerve. *J. Neurol. Neurosurg. Psychiat., 12*:205, 1949.

1042. MOORE, R. F.: Subjective lightning streaks. *Brit. J. Ophthal., 19*:545, 1935.

1043. MOORE, T.: In *Symposium on Nutrition.* Ed., R. M. Herriott. Baltimore: Johns Hopkins Press, 1958.

1044. MOORREES, H. G.: Bijdrage tot de Kennis van de deficientieamblyopie ('kampogen') Thesis 1947. Rejksuniversiteit, Utrecht. (Abst., *Excerpta Med. XII, 2*:#2369, 1948.)

1045. MORALES, M.: [Optic neuritis during lactation]. *Arch. Chil. Oftal., 16*:143, 1959. (Abst., *Amer. J. Ophthal., 50*:1279, 1960.)

1046. MORELLO, A., AND COOPER, I. S.: Visual field studies following occlusion of the anterior choroidal artery. *Amer. J. Ophthal., 40*:786, 1955.

1047. MORELLO, A., AND PONTE, F.: A case of intrasellar aneurysm simulating a pituitary adenoma. The role of cerebral arteriography in the diagnosis of chiasmatic lesions. *Acta. Neurochir. (Wein.), 7*:391, 1959.

1048. MORENO CADIERNO, M., AND CRESPE CARCAR, F.: Sobre la significación del pulso venoso en el síndrome hipertensivo intracraneal. *Arch. Soc. Oftal hisp-amer., 19*:499, 1959. (Abst., *Excerpta Med. XII, 14*:#1437, 1960.)

1049. MORRICE, G., HAVENER, W. H., AND KAPETANSKY, F.: Vitamin A intoxication as a cause of pseudotumor cerebri. *J.A.M.A., 173*:1802, 1960.

1050. MOSHER, H. A.: The prognosis in temporal arteritis. *Arch. Ophthal., 62*:641, 1959.

1051. MOUNT, L. A., AND TAVERAS, J. M.: Arteriographic demonstration of the collateral circulation of the cerebral hemispheres. *Arch. Neurol. Psychiat., 78*:235, 1957.

1052. MÜLLER, H.: Zur Klinik und Histologie der Angiitis retinae bei einer 31 jährigen Patienten mit tödlichem arteriellem Gefässleiden. *Klin. Mbl. Augenheilk., 126*:150, 1955.

1053. MÜLLER, H., AND PRESBERGEN, H. J.: Zur Pathogenese und Morphologie der endogenen Uveitis, insbesondere zur segmentalen Vasculitis. *Graefe Arch. Ophthal., 153*:333, 1952.

1054. MULOCK-HOUWER, A. W.: Amblyopia cum polyneuropathia caused by starvation. *Ophthalmologica, 112*:177, 1946.

1055. MULOCK-HOUWER, A. W.: Kampoogen. *Medisch. Maandblad., 1*:4, 1946. (Abst., *Excerpta Med. XII, 1*:#692, 1947.)

1056. MUNCASTER, S. B., AND ALLEN, H. E.: Bilateral uveitis and retinal periarteritis as a focal reaction to the tuberculin test. *Arch. Ophthal., 21*:509, 1939.

1057. MUNK, O., AND ANDERSEN, S. R.: Accessory outer segment, a re-discovered cilium-like structure in the layer of rods and cones of the human retina: Preliminary report. *Acta. Ophthal. (Kbh.), 40*:526, 1962.

1058. MUNRO, S., AND WALKER, C.: Ocular complications in sickle-cell haemoglobin disease. *Brit. J. Ophthal., 44*:1, 1960.

1059. MURPHY, S. B.: Visual field defects following temporal lobe surgery. *Trans. Canad. Ophthal. Soc., 8*:104, 1956.

1060. MYERS, R. E.: Inter-ocular transfer of pattern discrimination in cats following section of crossed optic fibres. *J. Comp. Physiol. Psychol., 48*:470, 1955.

1061. MYERS, R. E.: Function of corpus callosum in interocular transfer. *Brain, 79*:358, 1956.

1062. MYERS, R. E.: Commissural connections between occipital lobes of the monkey. *J. Comp. Neurol., 118*:1, 1962.

1063. MYERSON, R. M., AND HINGSTON, W. L.: Cushing's syndrome associated with chromophobe adenoma of pituitary. *Arch. Intern. Med., 109*:609, 1962.

1064. NAFFZIGER, H. C.: Progressive exophthalmos. *Bull. Amer. Coll. Surg., 40*:33, 1955.

1065. NAGY, F.: Über die einseitige Hypoplasie der Sehnerven. *Klin. Mbl. Augenheilk., 141*:924, 1962.

1066. NEBEL, B. R.: The phosphene of quick eye motion. *Arch. Ophthal., 58*:235, 1957.

1067. NECTOUX, R., AND GALLOIS, R. A.: Quatre cas de névrite rétro-bulbaire par le sulfure de carbone. *Bull. Soc. Ophtal. Franc.,* p. 750, 1931.

1068. NELSON, D. H., MEAKIN, J. W., DEALY, J. B., MATSON, D. D., EMERSON,

K., AND THORN, G. W.: ACTH-producing tumor of the pituitary gland. *New Engl. J. Med., 259*:161, 1958.

1069. NELSON, M. G., AND WEAVER, J. A.: Case of Addisonian pernicious anaemia presenting with optic atrophy, iron-deficiency anaemia and pigmentation of skin. *Irish J. Med. Sci.,* p. 229, 1956.

1070. NETTLESHIP, E.: Central amblyopia as an early symptom in tumour at the chiasma. *Trans. Ophthal. Soc. U.K., 17*:277, 1897.

1071. NETTLESHIP, E.: A history of congenital stationary night-blindness in nine consecutive generations. *Trans. Ophthal. Soc. U.K., 27*:269, 1907.

1072. NETTLESHIP, E.: On retinitis pigmentosa and allied diseases. *Roy. Lond. Ophthal. Hosp. Rep. 17*:1, 151, 1908.

1073. NEWTON, T. H., BURHENNE, H. J., AND PALUBINSKAS, A. J.: Primary carcinoma of the pituitary. *Amer. J. Roentgenol., 87*:110, 1962.

1074. NICHOLLS, J. V. V.: Congenital dyslexia: a problem in aetiology. *Trans. Canad. Ophthal. Soc., 22*:45, 1959.

1075. NICHOLLS, J. V. V.: Metastatic carcinoma of the optic nerve: Report of two cases. *Trans. Canad. Ophthal. Soc., 24*:18, 1961.

1076. NIEBELING, H.-G.: Ophthalmologische Befunde bei Arachnoiditis optico-chiasmatica. *Klin. Mbl. Augenheilk., 129*:161, 1956.

1077. NIELSON, J. M.: Unilateral cerebral dominance as related to mind blindness; minimal lesion capable of causing visual agnosia for objects. *Arch. Neurol. Psychiat., 38*:108, 1937.

1078. NIELSON, J. M., AND FRIEDMAN, A. P.: The temporal isthmus and its clinical syndromes. *Bull. Los Angeles Neurol. Soc., 7*:1, 1942.

1079. NJA, A.: A sex-linked type of gargoylism. *Acta Paediat. (Upps.), 33*:267, 1945-46.

1080. NOELL, W. K.: Effect of iodoacetate on vertebrate retina. *J. Cell. Comp. Physiol., 37*:283, 1951.

1081. NOELL, W. K.: Experimentally induced toxic effects on structure and function of visual cells and pigment epithelium. *Amer. J. Ophthal., 36*:103, 1953.

1082. NOELL, W. K.: Metabolic injuries of the visual cell. *Amer. J. Ophthal., 40*:60, 1955.

1083. NOELL, W. K.: Differentiation, metabolic organization, and viability of the visual cell. *Arch. Ophthal., 60*:702, 1958.

1084. NONNENMACHER, H.: Neuritis bei Laktation. *Klin. Mbl. Augenheilk., 127*:228, 1955.

1085. NORBURY, F. B., AND LOEFFLER, J. D.: Primary reading epilepsy. *J.A.M.A., 184*:661, 1963.

1086. NORMAN, R. M., AND WOOD, N.: Congenital form of amaurotic family idiocy. *J. Neurol. Psychiat., 4*:175, 1941.

1087. NORRIE, G.: Causes of blindness in children. *Acta Ophthal. (Kbh.), 5*:357, 1927.

1088. NORTH, R. R., FIELDS, W. S., DEBAKEY, M. E., AND CRAWFORD, E. S.: Brachial-basilar insufficiency syndrome, *12*:810, 1962.

1089. NORTON, E. W. D.: Supratentorial mass lesions presenting brain stem signs. *Arch. Ophthal., 62*:284, 1959.

1090. NOVER, A.: Über das Verhalten des Optikus nach längerdeuernder Kompression. *Fortschr. Neurol. Psychiat., 30*:228, 1962.

1091. Nover, A., and Zielinski, H. W.: Zur Differentialdiagnose der Orbita und Optikustumoren. *Klin. Mbl. Augenheilk., 131*:577, 1957.

1092. O'Connell, J. E. A.: Some observations on cerebral veins. *Brain, 57*:484, 1934.

1093. O'Donnell, J. M.: Behçet's triple syndrome. *Med. J. Aust., 1*:730, 1947.

1094. Offret, B., and Godde-Jolly, D.: Les anévrismes de l'artère ophthalmique. *Arch. Ophtal. (Par.), 16*:388, 1956.

1095. Ogucchi, C.: Über die eigenartige Hemeralopie mit diffuser weiss-graulicher Verfärbung des Augenhintergrundes. *Graefe Arch. Ophthal., 81*:109, 1912.

1096. Okun, E.: Gross and microscopic pathology in autopsy eyes. I. Introduction and long posterior ciliary nerves. *Amer. J. Ophthal., 50*:424, 1960.

1097. Okun, E.: Gross and microscopic pathology in autopsy eyes. II. Peripheral chorioretinal atrophy. *Amer. J. Ophthal., 50*:547, 1960.

1098. Okun, E.: Chronic papilledema simulating hyaline bodies of the optic disc; a case report. *Amer. J. Ophthal., 53*:922, 1962.

1099. Olivarius, B. F., and Jensen, L.: Retrobulbar neuritis and optic atrophy in pernicious anemia. *Acta Ophthal. (Kbh.), 39*:190, 1961.

1100. Olivecrona, H.: On suprasellar cholesteatomas. *Brain, 55*:122, 1932.

1101. Orteza, J.: A case of ependymoma simulating Devic's syndrome. *Arch. Ophthal., 64*:940, 1960.

1102. Orton, R. H., and Willis, R. A.: Rare retinal tumour probably derived from Müller's fibres. *J. Path. Bact., 56*:255, 1944.

1103. Orton, S. T.: cited by Critchley, M. ref. 312.

1104. Østerberg, G.: Traumatic bitemporal hemianopia (sagittal tearing of the optic chiasma). *Acta Ophthal. (Kbh.), 16*:466, 1938.

1105. Otradovec, J.: [Prosopagnosia, a contribution to disorders of the higher visual functions]. *Sborn. Lek., 64*:240, 1962. (Abst., *Ophthal. Lit., 16*: #2534, 1963.)

1106. Paillas, J. E., Bremond, J., Sedan, R., and Winninger, J.: Syndromes chiasmatiques d'origine traumatique. *Rev. Otoneuroophtal., 31*:390, 1959.

1107. Paillas, J. E., Darcourt, G., and Righini, C.: Essai de distinction des agnosies visuelles pour les formes selon l'hemisphere cerebrallèse. *Sem. Hop. Paris, 38*:1210, 1962. (Abst., *Excerpta Med. XII, 17*:#539, 1963.)

1108. Pallares, J.: Sugerencias sobre la etiologia, patogenia y tratamiento de ciertas neuritis ópticas de origen desconocids. *Arch. Soc. Oftal. hisp. -amer., 16*:1123, 1956.

1109. Palmer, R. F., Searles, H. H., and Boldrey, E. A.: Papilledema in hypoparathyroidism simulating brain tumor. *J. Neurosurg., 16*:378, 1959.

1110. Pantelakis, S. N., Bower, B. D., and Jones, H. D.: Convulsions and television viewing. *Brit. Med. J., 2*:663, 1962.

1111. Parin, P.: Opticusatrophie durch Arteriosklerose der Carotis interna. *Schweiz. Arch. Neurol. Psychiat., 67*:139, 1951.

1112. Parker, W. R.: Uveitis associated with alopecia, poliosis, vitiligo and deafness. *Amer. J. Ophthal., 14*:577, 1931.

1113. Parkinson, C. D.: Tumours of the brain, occipital lobe; their signs and symptoms. *Canad. Med. Ass. J., 64*:111, 1951.

1114. Parks, M. M., and Zimmerman, L. E.: Retinoblastoma. *Clin. Proc. Child. Hosp. (Wash.), 16*:77, 1960.

1115. PARRY, H. B.: Degeneration of the dog retina. II. Generalized progressive atrophy of hereditary origin. *Brit. J. Ophthal., 37*:487, 1953.

1116. PARSONS-SMITH, G.: Sudden blindness in cranial arteritis. *Brit. J. Ophthal., 43*:204, 1959.

1117. PATERSON, A., AND ZANGWILL, O. L.: Disorders of visual space perception associated with lesions of the right cerebral hemisphere. *Brain, 76*:331, 1944.

1118. PATERSON, A., AND ZANGWILL, O. L.: Case of topographical disorientation associated with unilateral cerebral lesion. *Brain, 68*:188, 1945.

1119. PATERSON, M. W.: Melanoma of the optic disc. *Brit. J. Ophthal., 36*:447, 1952.

1120. PATON, D.: Angioid streaks and sickle cell anemia; a report of two cases. *Arch. Ophthal., 62*:852, 1959.

1121. PATON, D.: Angioid streaks and acromegaly; Letter-to-the-Editor. *Amer. J. Ophthal., 56*:841, 1963.

1122. PATON, L.: A clinical study of optic neuritis in its relationship to intracranial tumours. *Brain, 32*:65, 1909.

1123. PATZ, A.: Oxygen inhalation in retinal arterial occlusion, a preliminary report. *Amer. J. Ophthal., 40*:789, 1955.

1124. PAUFIQUE, L., AND ETIENNE, R.: Le tuberculome du chiasma. *Bull. Soc. Franc. Ophthal., 65*:97, 1952.

1125. PEARS, M. A., AND PICKERING, G. W.: Changes in the fundus oculi after haemorrhage. *Quart. J. Med., 29*:153, 1960.

1126. PEDLER, C.: The inner limiting membrane of the retina. *Brit. J. Ophthal., 45*:423, 1961.

1127. PEIFFER, J., AND VON HIRSCH, T.: Histochemical studies on leucodystrophy. Presented at the Second International Congress of Neurology. (Abst., *Excerpta Med. VIII, 8*:#3687, 1955.)

1128. PEMBERTON, J. W.: Optic atrophy in herpes zoster ophthalmicus. *Amer. J. Ophthal., 58*:852, 1964.

1129. PEMBERTON, J. W., AND FREEMAN, J. M.: Craniosynostosis; a review of experience with forty patients with particular reference to ocular aspects and comments on operative indications. *Amer. J. Ophthal., 54*:641, 1962.

1130. PENDERGRASS, E. P., AND PERRYMAN, C. R.: Optochiasmatic arachnoiditis. *Amer. J. Roentgenol., 56*:279, 1946.

1131. PENFIELD, W.: The interpretive cortex. *Science, 129*:1719, 1959.

1132. PENFIELD, W., AND JASPER, H. H.: *Epilepsy and the functional anatomy of the human brain.* London: Churchill, 1934.

1133. PENFIELD, M., AND MILNER, B.: Memory deficit produced by bilateral lesions in the hippocampal zone. *Arch. Neurol. Psychiat., 79*:475, 1958.

1134. PENFIELD, W., AND RASMUSSEN, T.: *The Cerebral Cortex of Man; A Clinical Study of Localization of Function.* N.Y.: Macmillan, 1950.

1135. PENNYBACKER, J.: Intracranial tumours in aged (Honyman Gillespie Lecture). *Edinburgh Med. J., 56*:590, 1949.

1136. PENTA, P.: Due casi di visione capovolta. *Cervello, 25*:377, 1949. (Abst., *Excerpta Med. XII, 4*:#2027, 1950.)

1137. PERERA, C. A., AND STOUT, A. P.: Intraorbital melanosis and intracranial neuroepithelioma of the optic nerve. *Arch. Ophthal., 35*:678, 1946.

1138. PERRAULT, L. E., AND ZIMMERMAN, L. E.: The occurrence of glaucoma following occlusion of the central retinal artery. *Arch. Ophthal., 61*:845, 1959.

1139. PERRETT, L. V., AND BULL, J. W.: Some aspects of subarachnoid haemorrhage: a symposium. III. The accuracy of radiology in demonstrating ruptured intracranial aneurysms. *Brit. J. Radiol., 32*:85, 1959.

1140. PESTALOZZI, D., AND MARTENET, A. C.: The case history of arteritis temporalis with affection of the eye (report on 11 cases). *Ophthalmologica, 141*:155, 1961.

1141. PETERS, W.: Über die Neuritis optici arteriosklerotischer Genese. *Klin. Mbl. Augenheilk., 132*:363, 1958.

1142. PETIT-DULAILLIS, D., GUILLAUMAT, L., AND ROUGERIE, J.: Syndrome de compression du nerf optique droit. Découverte opératoire d'un anévrisme de l'artère ophtalmique. Traitement par la méthode du 'trapping.' *Neurochurugie, 3*:22, 1957.

1143. PEVEHOUSE, B. C., BLOOM, W. H., AND McKISSOCK, W.: Ophthalmologic aspects of diagnosis and localization of subdural hematoma. An analysis of 389 cases and review of the literature. *Neurology, 10*:1037, 1960.

1144. PEVZNER, S., BORNSTEIN, B., AND LOEWENTHAL, M.: Prosopagnosia. *J. Neurol. Neurosurg. Psychiat., 25*:336, 1962.

1145. PEYTON, W. T., AND SIMMONS, D. R.: Neurofibromatosis with defect in wall of orbit; report of 5 cases. *Arch. Neurol. Psychiat., 55*:248, 1946.

1146. PHILLIPS, D. L., AND SCOTT, J. S.: Recurrent genital and oral ulceration with associated eye lesions; Behçet's syndrome. *Lancet, 1*:366, 1955.

1147. PICKLES, W.: Acute focal edema of the brain in children with head injuries. *New Engl. J. Med., 240*:92, 1949.

1148. PIETRUSCHKA, G.: Weitere Mitteilungen über die Marmorknochenkrankheit (Albers-Schönbergsche Krankheit) nebst Bemerkungen zur Differentialdiagnose. *Klin. Mbl. Augenheilk., 132*:509, 1958.

1149. PIETRUSCHKA, G.: Zur Symptomatik der Neurofibromatosis multiplex nach von Recklinghausen im Bereich des Sehorgans. *Med. Bilddienst., 4*:8, 1961.

1150. PILLAT, A.: Beitrag zur Morphologie des Alterns der Netzhaut. *Wien Klin. Wschr., 64*:927, 1952.

1151. PINKHAM, R. A.: The ocular manifestations of the pulseless syndrome. *Acta 17 Conc. Ophthal.* (1954), *1*:348, 1955.

1152. PIPER, H. F.: Über cavernose Angiome in der Netzhaut. *Ophthalmologica, 128*:99, 1954.

1153. PIPER, H. F., AND UNGER, L.: Hemianopsia horizontalis inferior bei akuten Durchblutungsstörungen des Sehnerven. *Ophthalmologica, 134*:169, 1957.

1154. PIERENNE, M. H.: Absolute sensitivity of eye and variation of visual acuity with intensity. *Brit. Med. Bull., 9*:61, 1953.

1155. PITTER, J.: [A rare case of atrophy of the optic nerves]. *Cesk. Oftal, 4*:151, 1948. (Abst., *Excerpta Med. XII, 3*:#1279, 1949.)

1156. PITTER, J., AND VRAHEC, F.: [Interesting case of tumor of the optic discs and the optic nerve]. *Cesk. Oftal., 7*:187, 1951. (Abst., *Excerpta Med. XII, 6*:#204, 1952.)

1157. PITTS, F. W.: Variations of collateral circulation in internal carotid occlusion: comparison of clinical and x-ray findings. *Neurology, 12*:467, 1962.

1158. PLAIR, C. M., AND PERRY, S.: Hypothalamic-pituitary sarcoidosis, a clinical and pathological entity: report of a case. *Arch. Pathol., 74*:527, 1962.
1159. POTZL, O.: *Aphasielehre vom Standpunkte der Klinischen Psychiatrie. I. Die optisch-agnostischen Störungen (die Verschiedenen Formen der Seelenblindheit).* Wein: Franz Deuticke, 1928.
1160. POLLACK, I. P., AND BECKER, B.: Cytoid bodies of the retina, in a patient with scleroderma. *Amer. J. Ophthal., 54*:655, 1962.
1161. POLYAK, S.: A contribution to the cerebral representation of the retina. *J. Comp. Neurol., 57*:541, 1933.
1162. POLYAK, S.: *The Retina: The Anatomy and the Histology of the Retina in Man, Ape, and Monkey, Including the Consideration of Visual Functions, The History of Physiological Optics, and the Histological Laboratory Technique.* Chicago: University of Chicago Press, 1941.
1163. POLYAK, S.: *The Vertebrate Visual System.* Chicago: University of Chicago Press, 1957.
1164. POPEK, K.: [Recurrent Guillain-Barré syndrome with recurrent papilledema.] *Cesk. Neurol., 20*:380, 1957. (Abst., *Excerpta Med. XII, 13*: #242, 1959).
1165. POPPELREUTER, W.: *Die psychischen Schädigungen durch Kopfschuss im Kriege 1914-1916.* Leipzig: L. Voss, 1917.
1166. POPPEN, J. L.: Tumors of the sella turcica in the presence of a prefixed chiasma, temporal approach. In *The Surgical Clinics of North America* Vol. 39 Phila: W. B. Saunders, 1959, p. 841.
1167. POSER, C. M., AND VAN BOGAERT, L.: Natural history and evolution of the concept of Schilder's diffuse sclerosis. *Acta Psychiat. Scand., 31*:285, 1956.
1168. POTTS, A. M.: The concentration of phenothiazines in the eye of experimental animals. *Invest. Ophthal., 1*:522, 1962.
1169. POTTS, A. M., AND JOHNSON, L. V.: Studies on the visual toxicity of methanol. I. The effect of methanol and its degradation products on retinal metabolism. *Amer. J. Ophthal., 35*:107, 1952.
1170. POTTS, A. M., MODRELL, R. W., AND KINGSBURY, C.: Permanent fractionation of the electroretinogram by sodium glutamate. *Amer. J. Ophthal., 50*:900, 1960.
1171. PRAGLIN, J., SPURNEY, R., AND POTTS, A. M.: An experimental study of electroretinography. I. The electroretinogram in experimental animals under the influence of methanol and its oxidation products. *Amer. J. Ophthal., 39*:52, 1955.
1172. PRIBRAM, H. B., AND BARRY, J.: Further behavioral analysis of parieto-temporo-preoccipital cortex. *J. Neurophysiol., 19*:99, 1956.
1173. PUISCARIU, H., LASCO, F., AND ARSENI, M. C.: L'influence de l'ophtalmotonus sur l'apparition et l'évolution de la stase papillaire. *Rev. Otoneuroophtal., 31*:471, 1959.
1174. PUTNAM, T. J., AND LIEBMAN, S.: Cortical representation of the macula lutea, with special reference to the theory of bilateral representation. *Arch. Ophthal., 28*:415, 1942.
1175. PYGOTT, F., AND HUTTON, C. F.: Vertebral arteriography by percutaneous brachial artery catheterisation. *Brit. J. Radiol., 32*:114, 1959.
1176. QUARANTA, C. A., AND VOZZA, R.: Studio istologico comparativo delle alterazioni corioretiche da ditezone, iodato e iodacetato di sodio. *Boll. Oculist., 38*:665, 1959. (Abst., *Zbl. Ges. Ophthal., 80*:161, 1960.)

1177. QUINTIERI, C.: [Pseudo-glaucomatous syndrome caused by intracranial arterial aneurysm]. *Boll. Oculist., 35*:293, 1956.

1178. RADOS, A.: Bilateral uveitis associated with detachment of the retina (Harada's disease). *Arch. Ophthal., 23*:534, 1940.

1179. RAE, A. S.: Bilateral infarction of calcarine cortex with lateral geniculate degeneration. *Confin. Neurol., 21*:225, 1961.

1180. RAND, C. W.: Alterations in visual fields following craniocerebral injuries. *Arch. Surg., 32*:945, 1936.

1181. RANEY, R. B., AND NEILSEN, J. M.: Spatial disorientation. Diagnostic differentiation between frontal and occipital lesions. *Bull. Los Angeles Neurol. Soc., 5*:73, 1940.

1182. REDLICH, F. C., AND DORSEY, J. F.: Denial of blindness by patients with cerebral disease. *Arch. Neurol. Psychiat., 53*:407, 1945.

1183. REDSLOB, E.: Problèmes concernant la circulation rétinienne. *Ann. Oculist., 186*:585, 1953.

1184. REESE, A. B.: Massive retinal fibrosis in children. *Amer. J. Opthal., 19*:576, 1936.

1185. REESE, A. B.: Relation of drusen of the optic nerve to tuberous sclerosis. *Arch. Opthal., 24*:187, 1940.

1186. REESE, A. B.: Telangiectasis of the retina and Coats' disease. *Amer. J. Ophthal., 42*:1, 1956.

1187. REESE, A. B.: Medullo-epithelioma (dictyoma) of the optic nerve. *Amer. J. Ophthal., 44*:4, 1957.

1188. REESE, A. B., AND CARROLL, F. D.: Optic neuritis following cataract extraction. *Amer. J. Ophthal., 45*:659, 1958.

1189. REESE, F. M.: Bilateral homonymous hemianopia. *Amer. J. Ophthal., 38*:44, 1954.

1190. REFSUM, S.: Heredo-ataxia hemeralopica polyneuritiformis, familial syndrome not previously described; preliminary report. *Nord. Med., 28*:2682, 1945.

1191. REFSUM, S.: Heredopathia atactica polyneuritiformis; a familial syndrome not hitherto described. *Acta Psychiat. Scand.* supp. 38, p. 1, 1946.

1192. REID, W. L., AND CONE, W. V.: The mechanism of fixed dilatation of the pupil. *J.A.M.A., 112*:2030, 1939.

1193. REIN, G.: Über melanoblastome der Papille und Tumoren des retinalen Pigmentepithels. *Graefe Arch. Ophthal., 161*:519, 1960.

1194. REINECKE, R. D.: Migrainoid symptoms associated with intracranial vascular anomalies, a case report. *Arch. Ophthal., 65*:808, 1961.

1195. REIVICH, M., HOLLING, H. E., ROBERTS, B., AND TOOLE, J. F.: Reversal of blood flow through the vertebral artery and its effect on cerebral circulation. *New Engl. J. Med., 265*:878, 1961.

1196. RENARD, G., DAVID, M., AND BREGEAT, P.: La névrite optique intra-canaliculaire oedémateuse aiguë. *Arch. Ophtal. (Par.), 9*:584, 1949.

1197. RENARD, G., DHERMY, P., AND AMAR, L.: Consideration sur les degenerescences vitelliformes de la macula. *Arch. Ophtal. (Par.), 20*:797, 1960.

1198. RENPENNING, H. J., AND WACASER, L. E.: Ipsilateral blindness after common carotid ligation for carotid-cavernous fistula. *Arch. Ophthal., 69*:186, 1963.

1199. RICCI, A., AND WERNER, A.: Vérification neurochirurgical du rôle des carotides internes dans certains symptoms chiasmatiques. *Schweiz. Med. Wschr., 87*:1190, 1957.

1200. RICH, W. M.: Permanent homonymous quadrantanopia after migraine. *Brit. Med. J., 1*:592, 1948.

1201. RICHARDS, W. W., AND THOMPSON, M. C.: Suprasellar osteochondroma with chiasmal syndrome. *Arch. Ophthal., 65*:437, 1961.

1202. RICHARDSON, E. P., ASTROM, K., AND MANCALL, E. L.: Progressive multifocal leuko-encephalopathy. *Brain, 81*:93, 1958.

1203: RICKFORD, R. G.: Ocular movement related to normal and pathological electrocortical discharge. Symposium on neurological aspects of oculomotor system, N. Y., April 14-15, 1961. (Abst., *Arch. Ophthal., 66*:300, 1961.)

1204. RICKLEFS, G.: Über das Uhthoffsche Symptom bei multipler Sklerose. *Klin. Mbl. Augenheilk., 139*:385, 1961.

1205. RIDDOCH, G.: Dissociation of visual perceptions due to occipital injuries, with especial reference to appreciation of movement. *Brain, 40*:15, 1917.

1206. RIDDOCH, G.: Visual disorientation in homonymous half-fields. *Brain, 58*:376, 1935.

1207. RIEGER, H.: Zur Pathologie des Ganglion ciliare. *Klin. Mbl. Augenheilk., 120*:337, 1952.

1208. RIEHM, W.: Akute Pigmentdegeneration der Netzhaut nach Intoxikation mit Septojod. *Arch. Augenheilk., 100-101*:872, 1929.

1209. RIESE, W.: Hughlings Jackson's doctrine of aphasia and its significance today. *J. Nerv. Ment. Dis., 122*:1, 1955.

1210. RIFFENBURGH, R. S.: Metastatic malignant melanoma to the retina. *Arch. Ophthal., 66*:487, 1961.

1211. RIFFENBURGH, R. S.: Ocular manifestations of mumps. *Arch. Ophthal., 66*:739, 1961.

1212. RIGGS, H. E., AND GRIFFITHS, J. O.: Anomalies of the circle of Willis in persons with nervous and mental disorders. *Arch. Neurol. Psychiat., 39*:1353, 1938.

1213. RIGGS, L. A.: Continuous and reproducible records of electrical activity of human retina. *Proc. Soc. Exp. Biol. Med., 48*:204, 1941.

1214. RINALDI, I., BOLTON, J. E., AND TROLAND, C. E.: Cortical visual disturbances following ventriculography and/or ventricular decompression. *J. Neurosurg., 19*:568, 1962.

1215. RINTELEN, F.: Fundusveränderungen bei tuberöser Hirnsklerose. *Z. Augenheilk., 88*:15, 1935.

1216. RINTELEN, F.: Über arteriosklerotische Opticusatrophie. *Ophthalmologica, 111*:285, 1946.

1217. RINTELEN, F.: Zur Kenntnis der Leitungsstorungen des Fasciculus opticus, insbesondere der "Apoplexia papillae". *Ophthalmologica, 141*:283, 1961.

1218. RINTELEN, F., HOTZ, G., AND WAGNER, P.: Zur klinik und experimentellen pathologie der pigmentepithelerkrankung nach medikation mit einem Piperidinphenothiazin. *Ophthalmologica, 133*:277, 1957.

1219. DEL RIO-HORTEGA, P.: Discussion of Tumours of the Optic Nerve. Presented before the Section of Ophthalmology and Section of Neurology, Royal Society of Medicine, Feb. 22, 1940. (Abst., *Proc. Roy. Soc. Med., 33*:686, 1940.)

1220. DEL RIO HORTEGA, P.: Contribucion al conocimiento citologico de los tumores du nervio y guiasma opticos. *Arch. Histol. (B. Air.)*, *2*:307, 1943.
1221. RISER, R. O.: Marble bones and optic atrophy. *Amer. J. Ophthal.*, *24*:874, 1941.
1222. ROBERT, F.: Sarcoidosis of the central nervous system, report of a case and review of the literature. *Arch. Neurol.*, *7*:442, 1962.
1223. ROBINSON, B. E.: Permanent homonymous migraine scotomata. *Arch. Ophthal.*, *53*:566, 1955.
1224. ROCHE, M., AND MARTIN, J. F.: L'aspect ophtalmologique d'un cas de chordome. *Bull. Soc. Franc. Ophtal.*, *50*:70, 1937.
1225. RODA, J. RAMON: Tratamiento quirugico de los tumores del nervio optico que traspasan el agujere optico. *Estud. Inform. Oftalmol. Barcelona*, *3*:1, 1951. (Abst., *Excerpta Med. XII*, *7*:#542, 1953.)
1226. RODGER, P. C.: Nutritional amblyopia. A statistical report of the course and progress in two hundred and thirty-eight cases. *Arch. Ophthal.*, *47*:570, 1952.
1227. ROE, O.: The ganglion cells of the retina in cases of methanol poisoning in humans and experimental animals. *Acta. Ophthal.*, *26*:169, 1948.
1228. RONNE, G.: The physiological basis of sensory fusion. *Acta. Ophthal. (Kbh.)*, *34*:1, 1956.
1229. RONNE, H.: Pathologisch-anatomische Untersuchungen über alkoholische Intoxikationsamblyopie. *Graefe Arch. Ophthal.*, *77*:1, 1910.
1230. RONNE, H.: Zur pathologischen Anatomie der diabetischen Intoxikationsamblyopie. *Graefe Arch. Ophthal.*, *84*:489, 1913.
1231. RONNE, H.: Ueber akute Retrobulbärneuritis, im Chiasma lokalisiert (Klinische und pathologisch-anatomische Untersuchungen). *Klin. Mbl. Augenheilk.*, *55*:68, 1915.
1232. RONNE, H.: On non-hypophyseal affections of the chiasma. *Acta. Ophthal. (Kbh.)*, *6*:332, 1928.
1233. RONNE, H.: *Den menneskelige Synsbanes Arkitektur.* Copenhagen: Munksgaard, 1943. Cited by Edmund, J. ref. 404.
1234. ROOT, H. F., MIRSKY, S., AND DITZEL, J.: Proliferative retinopathy in diabetes mellitus: review of 847 cases. *J.A.M.A.*, *169*:903, 1959.
1235. ROPER-HALL, M. J.: Optic disc oedema in the absence of raised intracranial pressure. *Brit. J. Ophthal.*, *42*:91, 1958.
1236. ROSEN, E.: Immunological significance of demyelination of medullated nerve fibres in the eye. *Brit. J. Ophthal.*, *34*:242, 1950.
1237. ROSS, E. J.: The endocrinology of pituitary tumours. *Proc. Roy. Soc. Med.*, *54*:621, 1961.
1238. ROSS, R. S., AND McKUSICK, V. A.: Aortic arch syndromes; diminished or absent pulses in arteries arising from arch of aorta. *Arch. Intern. Med.*, *92*:701, 1953.
1239. ROSSELET, E., ZANDER, E., AND SECRETAN, P.: Symptomatic hemianopic migraine in occipital aneurysm. *Confin. Neurol.*, *21*:197, 1961.
1240. ROSSI, G., CANOSSI, G. C., AND PASQUINELLI, C.: Impiego Diagnostico e possibili effetti terapeutici della pneumografia cerebrale nella aracnite ottico chiasmatica. *Riv. Oto-Neuro-Oftal.*, *33*:611, 1958. (Abst., *Excerpta Med. XII*, *14*:#1252, 1958.)

1241. ROTH, J. H.: Ocular syphilis: Early changes in retinal vessels. *Amer. J. Syph., 12*:216, 1928.

1242. ROTH, M.: Disorders of body image caused by lesions of right parietal lobe. *Brain, 72*:89, 1949.

1243. ROVITA, D. A., AND MANDEL, M. M.: Hemangioma of the brain simulating the migraine syndrome. *Delaware Med. J., 32*:118, 1960.

1244. ROWLAND, W. D.: Cited by Regan, J. J. in Angioid streaks. *Amer. J. Ophthal., 16*:61, 1933.

1245. ROZANSKI, J.: Peduncular hallucinosis following vertebral angiography. *Neurology, 2*:341, 1932.

1246. RUCKER, C. W.: Defects in visual fields produced by hyaline bodies in the optic disks. *Arch. Ophthal., 32*:56, 1944.

1247. RUCKER, C. W.: Sheathing of the retinal veins in multiple sclerosis. *J.A.M.A., 127*:970, 1945.

1248. RUCKER, C. W.: The concept of a semidecussation of the optic nerves. *Arch. Ophthal., 59*:159, 1958.

1249. RUCKER, C. W., AND KEARNS, T. P.: Mistaken diagnoses in some cases of meningioma. Clinics in Perimetry No. 5. *Amer. J. Ophthal., 51*:15, 1961.

1250. RUCKER, C. W., AND KEARNS, T. P.: Tobacco amblyopia. Clinics in Perimetry No. 4. *Amer. J. Ophthal., 51*:509, 1961.

1251. RUCKER, C. W., AND KERNOHAN, J. W.: Notching of the optic chiama by overlying arteries in pituitary tumors. *Arch. Ophthal., 51*:161, 1954.

1252. RUSHTON, W. A. H.: *Visual pigments in man.* Springfield, Ill. Charles C Thomas, Publisher, 1962.

1253. RUSSELL, R. W., AND PENNYBACKER, J. B.: Craniopharyngioma in the elderly. *J. Neurol. Neurosurg. Psychiat., 24*:1, 1961.

1254. RYAN, E. R.: Optochiasmic arachnoiditis, report of three cases. *Arch. Ophthal., 29*:818, 1943.

1255. RYAN, H.: Intra-orbital meningioma of the optic nerve. *Brit. J. Ophthal., 37*:506, 1953.

1256. RYAN, H.: Massive retinal gliosis. *Trans. Ophthal. Soc. Aust., 14*:77, 1954.

1257. RYAN, H.: Total blindness from temporal arteritis. *Med. J. Aust., 47*:978, 1960.

1258. RYCHENER, R. M., AND MURPHEY, F.: Periorbital fibrous dysplasia. *Trans. Amer. Ophthal. Soc., 53*:155, 1955.

1259. SABRA, F.: Observations on one hundred cases of cerebral angioma. *J.A.M.A., 170*:1522, 1959.

1260. SACHS, E.: Arteriographic demonstration of collateral circulation through ophthalmic artery in internal carotid artery thrombosis; report of two cases. *J. Neurosurg., 11*:405, 1954.

1261. SAFAR, K.: Über Drucksteigerung im Gefolge der juvenilen Netzhaut-Glaskörperblutungen und Verschluss der Zentralvene infolge tuberkulöser Phlebitis, nebst Bemerkungen über die Entstehungsweise der Netzhautge-fässtuberkulose. *Graefe Arch. Ophthal., 119*:624, 1928.

1262. SALASSA, R. M., KEARNS, T. P., KERNOHAN, J. W., SPRAGUE, R. G., AND MACCARTY, C. S.: Pituitary tumors in patients with Cushing's syndrome. *J. Clin. Endocr., 19*:1523, 1959.

1263. DE SALES, J. M.: Neurits ótica de lactaçao. *Rev. Ginec. Obstet. (Rio), 47*:384, 1953. (Abst., *Excerpta Med. XII, 8*:#665, 1954.)

1264. SALZMANN, M.: *The Anatomy and Histology of the Human Eyeball in the Normal State; Its Development and Senescence.* Trans. E. V. L. Brown. Chicago: University of Chicago Press, 1912.

1265. SALZMANN, M.: *Glaukom und Netzhautzirkulation.* Berlin: S. Karger, 1933.

1266. SALZMANN, M.: Einige Worte zur Oguchischen Krankheit. *Ophthalmologica, 118*:145, 1949.

1267. SANFORD, H. S., AND BAIR, H. L.: Visual disturbances associated with tumors of the temporal lobe. *Arch. Neurol. Psychiat., 42*:21, 1939.

1268. SANNA, M.: Le druse della papilla del nervo ottico nella malattia di Bourneville. *Riv. Oto-Neuro-Oftal., 34*:272, 1959.

1269. SARAUX, H., ESTEVE, P., GRAVELEAU, O., AND GOUPIL, H.: Syndrome de Balint et Apraxie Oculo-Motrice. *Ann. Oculist. (Par.), 195*:456, 1962.

1270. SAUNDERS, L. Z., JUBB, K. V., AND JONES, L. D.: The intraocular lesions of hog cholera. *J. Comp. Path. Ther., 68*:375, 1958.

1271. SCHAEFFER, J. P.: Some points in the regional anatomy of the optic pathway, with especial reference to tumors of the hypophysis cerebri and resulting ocular changes. *Anat. Rec., 28*:243, 1924.

1272. SCHAPPERT-KIMMIJSER, J., HENKES, H. E., AND VAN DEN BOSCH, J.: Amaurosis congenita (Leber). *Arch. Ophthal., 61*:211, 1959.

1273. SCHEERER, R.: Zur pathologischen Anatomie der Netzhautzentralgefässe beider sog. Thrombose der Zentralvene und Embolie der Zentralarterie mit besonderer Berücksichtigung ihrer Beziehungen zu anderweitigen Veränderungen an Sehnervenkopf bei Glaukom und verwandten Zuständen II. Die Entwicklung des Verschlusses der Zentralvene. *Graefe Arch. Ophthal., 112*:206, 1923.

1274. SCHEERER, R.: Akuter Zerfall des retinalen Pigmentepithels nach intravenöser Injektion von Septojod in Wochenbett. *Klin. Mbl. Augenheilk., 76*:524, 1926.

1275. SCHEERER, R.: Netzhaut und Sehnerv. Bericht über die Jahre 1906-1925. *Ergebn. Allg. Path., 21*:71, 1928.

1276. SCHEIE, H. G., AND HOGAN, T. F.: Angioid streaks and generalized arterial disease. *Arch. Ophthal., 57*:855, 1957.

1277. SCHEINBERG, I. H., AND GITLIN, D.: Deficiency of ceruloplasmin in patients with hepatolenticular degeneration (Wilson's disease). *Science, 116*:484, 1952.

1278. SCHELLER, H., AND SEIDEMANN, H.: Zur Frage der optischräumlichen Agnosie (Zugleich ein Beitrag zur Dyslexie). *Mschr. Psychiat. Neurol., 81*:97, 1931.

1279. SCHENK, H.: Über das Auftreten einer Retinopathia traumatica Purtscher nach Unterbindung der Arteria carotis communis. *Klin. Mbl. Augenheilk., 127*:669, 1955.

1280. SCHILDER, P.: Zur Kenntnis der sogenannten diffusen Sklerose (Ueber Encephalitis periaxialis diffusa). *Z. Ges. Neurol. Psychiat., 10*:1, 1912.

1281. SCHIRMER, R.: Herpes zoster gangraenosus trigemini I mit Sehnervenbeteilligung. *Klin. Mbl. Augenheilk., 130*:262, 1956.

1282. SCHLEZINGER, N. S., ALPERS, B. J., AND WEISS, B. P.: Suprasellar meningiomas associated with scotomatous field defects. *Arch. Ophthal., 35*:624, 1946.

1283. SCHLEZINGER, N. S., WALDMAN, J., AND ALPERS, B. J.: Drusen of the optic nerve simulating cerebral tumor. *Arch. Ophthal., 31*:509, 1944.

1285. SCHMIDT, I.: Diagnostic value of foveal entoptic phenomena in glaucoma. *Arch. Ophthal., 52*:583, 1954.

1286. SCHMIDT, R.: Über zwei seltene Druckschädigungen des Sehnerven. *Klin. Mbl. Augenheilk., 123*:546, 1953.

1287. SCHNECK, J. M.: Micropsia. *Amer. J. Psychiat., 118*:232, 1961-62.

1288. SCHNELLE, G. B.: Progressive retinal atrophy in a dog. *J. Amer. Vet. Med. Ass., 121*:177, 1952.

1289. SCHNITKER, M. T., AND AYER, D.: Primary melanomas of leptomeninges; clinico-pathologic study with review of literature and report of additional case. *J. Nerv. Ment. Dis., 87*:45, 1938.

1290. SCHOLZ, R. O.: Angioid streaks. *Arch. Ophthal., 26*:677, 1941.

1291. SCHROTT, E.: Worm seen wiggling, dissolving in case of ascaris retinopathy. *Med. Tribune 2* (30)2; 1961.

1292. SCHULZE, A.: Zur Differentialdiagnose der suprasellären Tumoren. *Klin. Mbl. Augenheilk., 136*:166, 1960.

1293. SCHUR, P. H., AND APPEL, L.: Waldenstrom's macroglobulinemia with pleural effusion. *New York J. Med., 61*:2431, 1961.

1294. SCHURR, P. H., McLAURIN, R. L., AND INGRAHAM, F. D.: Experimental studies on circulation of cerebrospinal fluid and methods of producing communicating hydrocephalus in dog. *J. Neurosurg., 10*:515, 1953.

1095. SCHWAB, F. I.: Einiges zur Histologie der tuberösen Hirnsklerose. *Wien. Med. Wschr., 110*:228, 1960.

1296. SCHWABER, J. R., AND BLUMBERG, A. G.: Papilledema associated with blood loss anemia. *Ann. Intern. Med., 55*:1004, 1961.

1297. SCHWARTZ, J. F., ROWLAND, L. P., EDER, H., MARKS, P. A., OSSERMAN, E. F., HIRSCHBERG, E., AND ANDERSON, H.: Bassen-Kornzweig syndrome: deficiency of serum beta-lipoprotein; a neuromuscular disorder resembling Friedreich's ataxia, associated with steatorrhea, acanthocytosis, retinitis pigmentosa, and a disorder of lipid metabolism. *Arch. Neurol., 8*:438, 1963.

1298. SCOTT, G. I.: Neuromyelitis optica. *Amer. J. Ophthal., 35*:755, 1952.

1299. SCOTT, G. I., Ed.: *Traquair's clinical perimetry.* 7th ed. St. Louis: Mosby, 1957, p. 94.

1300. SCOTT, J. G.: Hereditary optic atrophy with dominant transmission and early onset. *Brit. J. Ophthal., 25*:461, 1941.

1301. SCOVILLE, W. B., AND MILNER, B.: Loss of recent memory after bilateral hippocampal lesions. *J. Neurol. Neurosurg. Psychiat., 20*:11, 1957.

1302. SEEGAR, W., AND SCHRADER, K. E.: [Intrasellar epidermoid with unusual visual field findings]. *Acta. Neurochir. (Wien), 8*:81, 1960.

1303. SEITZ, R.: Beitrag zur Chorioretinitis centralis serosa. *Klin. Mbl. Augenheilk., 127*:676, 1955.

1304. SEITZ, R., AND KERSTING, G.: Die Drusen der Sehnervenpapille und des Pigmentepithels. *Klin. Mbl. Augenheilk., 140*:75, 1962.

1305. SELBY, G., AND LANCE, J. W.: Observations on 500 cases of migraine and allied vascular headache. *J. Neurol. Neurosurg. Psychiat., 23*:23, 1960.

1306. SELENKOW, H. A., TYLER, H. R., MATSON, D. D., AND NELSON, D. H.:

Hypopituitarism due to hypothalamic sarcoidosis. *Amer. J. Med. Sci.,* 238:456, 1959.

1307. SEZER, F. N.: The isolation of a virus as the cause of Behçet's disease. *Amer. J. Ophthal., 36:*301, 1953.

1308. SHAPIRO, M. F., AND BENDER, M.: Diagnosis and treatment in vascular diseases of the nervous system. *New York J. Med., 59:*2727, 1959.

1309. SHAW, D. A., AND DUNCAN, L. J.: Optic atrophy and nerve deafness in diabetes mellitus. *J. Neurol. Neurosurg. Psychiat., 21:*47, 1958.

1310. SHECHTER, F. R., LIPSIUS, E. I., AND RASANSKY, H. N.: Retrobulbar neuritis. A complication of infectious mononucleosis. *Amer. J. Dis. Child., 89:*58, 1955.

1311. SHEEHAN, B.: Optic atrophy with altitudinal hemianopia in neurofibromatosis. *Brit. J. Ophthal., 36:*506, 1952.

1312. SHELDON, W. H., GOLDEN, A., AND BONDY, P. K.: Cushing's syndrome produced by a pituitary basophil carcinoma with hepatic metastases. *Amer. J. Med., 17:*134, 1954.

1313. SHENKIN, H. A.: Relief of amblyopia in pituitary apoplexy by prompt surgical intervention. *J.A.M.A., 59:*1622, 1955.

1314. SHERMAN, N. S.: Significance of phthisis bulbi in retinoblastoma. *Amer. J. Ophthal., 47:*403, 1959.

1315. SHERMAN, N. S., AND POLLACK, S.: Retinal vascular occlusion, associated with gastro-intestinal hemorrhage. *Amer. J. Ophthal., 54:*851, 1962.

1316. SHERWOOD, D.: Chronic subdural hematomas in infants. *Amer. J. Dis. Child., 39:*980, 1930.

1317. SHIMIZU, K., AND SANO, K.: Pulseless disease. *J. Neuropath. Clin. Neurol., 1:*37, 1951.

1318. SHINKLE, C. E.: A case of Raynaud's disease involving the feet, the left retina and the heart wall. *J.A.M.A., 83:*355, 1924.

1319. SHLOSSBERG, F. R., AND PRIZER, M.: Retinal changes with marked impairment of vision in measles.: report of a case. *Amer. J. Ophthal., 23:*998, 1940.

1320. SIBLEY, W. A., AND WEISBERGER, A. S.: Demyelinating disease of the brain in chronic lymphatic leukemia. Occurrence of a case in the husband of a patient with multiple sclerosis. *Arch. Neurol., 5:*300, 1961.

1321. SIDLER-HUGUENIN: Über die hereditär-syphilitischen Augenhintergrundsveränderungen, nebst einigen allgemeinen Bemerkungen über Augenerkrankungen bei angeborener Lues. *Beitr. Augenheilk., 51:*1, 1904.

1322. SIE BOEN LIAN: Camp amblyopia. *Ophthalmologica, 113:*38, 1947.

1323. SIEKERT, R. G., AND MILLIKAN, C. H.: Studies in cerebrovascular disease; some clinical aspects of thrombosis of basilar artery. *Proc. Mayo Clin., 30:*93, 1955.

1324. SIEKERT, R. G., AND MILLIKAN, C. H.: Syndrome of intermittent insufficiency of the basilar arterial system. *Neurology, 5:*625, 1955.

1325. SILBERPFENNIG, J.: Contributions to the problem of eye movements. III. Disturbances of ocular movements with pseudohemianopsia in frontal lobe tumors. *Confin. Neurol., 4:*1, 1941.

1326. SILFVERSKIOLD, B. P.: Retinal periphlebitis and chronic disseminated encephalomyelitis. *Acta. Psychiat. Scand.* supp. 74. pp. 55-57, 1951.

1327. SILVERMAN, S. M., BERGMAN, P. S., AND BENDER, M. B.: The dynamics of transient cerebral blindness. Report of nine episodes following vertebral angiography. *Arch. Neurol., 4*:333, 1961.

1328. SILVERSTEIN, A., GILBERT, H., AND WASSERMAN, L. R.: Neurologic complications of polycythemia. *Ann. Intern. Med., 57*:909, 1962.

1329. SIMMONS, R. J., AND COGAN, D. G.: Occult temporal arteritis., *Arch. Ophthal., 68*:8, 1962.

1330. SINCLAIR, A. H.: Developmental aphasia. *Brit. J. Ophthal., 32*:522, 1948.

1331. SINGLETON, A. O.: Intracranial arteriovenous aneurysms. *Ann. Surg., 110*:525, 1939.

1332. SJOSTRAND, F. S.: Ultrastructure of outer segments of rods and cones of eye as revealed by electron microscope. *J. Cell. Comp. Physiol., 42*:15, 1953.

1333. SKANSE, B., AND AREN, O.: Disappearance of bitemporal hemianopsia following correction of myxedema in a case of chromophobe pituitary tumour. *Acta. Endocr. (Kbh.), 23*:289, 1956.

1334. SKILLERN, P. G., AND LOCKHART, G.: Optic neuritis and uncontrolled diabetes mellitus in 14 patients. *Ann. Intern. Med., 51*:468, 1959.

1335. SKIPPER, E., AND FLINT, F. J.: Symmetrical arterial occlusion of upper extremities, head and neck: rare syndrome. *Brit. Med. J., 2*:9, 1952.

1336. SLADE, H. W., AND WEEKLEY, R. D.: Glioma of the optic tract: report of a case. *Amer. J. Ophthal., 42*:585, 1956.

1337. SLOAN, L. L., AND BROWN, D. J.: Progressive retinal degeneration with selective involvement of the cone mechanism. *Amer. J. Ophthal., 54*:629, 1962.

1338. SLOAN, L. L., AND NAQUIN, H. A.: A quantitative test for determining the visibility of the Haidinger brushes: Clinical applications. *Amer. J. Ophthal., 40*:393, 1955.

1339. SMALL, R. G.: Optic neuroencephalomyelopathy (Devic's diseases). *Arch. Ophthal., 50*:368, 1953.

1340. SMITH, A. R.: Optic atrophy following inhalation of carbon tetrachloride. *Arch. Indust. Hygiene Occupational Med., 1*:348, 1950.

1341. SMITH, B. F., RIPPS, H., AND GOODMAN, G.: Retinitis punctata albescens. *Arch. Ophthal., 61*:93, 1959.

1342. SMITH, D. C., KEARNS, T. P., AND SAYRE, C. P.: Pre-retinal and optic nerve-sheath haemorrhage: pathologic and experimental aspect in subarachnoid haemorrhage. *Trans. Amer. Acad. Ophthal. Otolaryng., 61*:201, 1957.

1343. SMITH, H. E.: Aplasia of the optic nerve: report of three cases. *Amer. J. Ophthal., 37*:498, 1954.

1344. SMITH, J. L.: Progressive multifocal leukoencephalopathy. *Arch. Ophthal., 62*:828, 1959.

1345. SMITH, J. L.: Central retinal and internal carotid arterial occlusions: ophthalmodynamometric differentiation. *Arch. Ophthal., 65*:550, 1961.

1346. SMITH, J. L.: Chloroquine macular degeneration. *Arch. Ophthal., 68*:186, 1962.

1347. SMITH, J. L.: The ophthalmodynamometric carotid compression test. *Amer. J. Ophthal., 56*:369, 1963.

1348. SMITH, J. L., AND COGAN, D. G.: Optokinetic nystagmus: a test for parietal lobe lesions. A study of 31 anatomically verified cases. *Amer. J. Ophthal.,* 48:187, 1959.

1349. SMITH, J. L., AND COGAN, D. G.: Ophthalmodynamometric diagnosis of acute renal hypertension in pulseless syndrome. *Amer. J. Ophthal.,* 48:326, 1959.

1350. SMITH, J. L., AND COGAN, D. G.: The ophthalmodynamometric posture test. *Amer. J. Ophthal., 48*:735, 1959.

1351. SMITH, J. L., NASHOLD, B. S., AND KRESHON, M. J.: Ocular signs after stereotactic lesions in the pallidum and thalamus. *Arch. Ophthal.,* 65:532, 1961.

1352. SMITH, K. V.: Learning and the associative pathways of the human cerebral cortex. *Science, 114*:117, 1951.

1353. SNELL, P. A.: The entoptic phenomenon of the blue arcs. A study of the secondary excitation in the retina. *Arch. Ophthal., 1*:475, 1929.

1354. SNELLMAN, A., MAKELA, T., AND NYSTROM, S.: Considérations sur les anévrysmes de la région située entre les artères cérébrales antérieures (A propos d'une série de cinquante-deux cas opérés). *Neurochururgie,* 5:143, 1959.

1355. SODERBERG, V., AND ARDEN, G. B.: Single unit activity in the rabbit lateral geniculate body during experimental epilepsy. In *The Visual System: Neurophysiology* and *Psychophysics.* Ed. R. Jung and H. Kornhuber. Berlin: Springer-Verlag, 1961, p. 133.

1356. SOKOLOWSKI, S., AND SEGAL, P.: [Symmetric hemianopsia following a direct mechanical trauma to the optic tract]. *Neurol. Neurochir. Psychiat. (Pol.), 6*:343, 1956. (Abst., *Excerpta Med. XII, 11*:#1514, 1957.)

1357. SOMERVILLE, F.: Uniocular aplasia of the optic nerve. *Brit. J. Ophthal.,* 46:51, 1962.

1358. SORSBY, A.: *Genetics in ophthalmology.* London: Butterworth, 1951, p. 165.

1359. SORSBY, A., NEWHOUSE, J. P., AND LUCAS, D. R.: Experimental degeneration of the retina I. Thiol reactors as inducing agents. *Brit. J. Ophthal.,* 41:309, 1957.

1360. SOSMAN, M. C.: Roentgen therapy of pituitary adenomas. *J.A.M.A.,* 113:1282, 1939.

1361. SPAETH, E. B.: Swelling of the nerve heads with arachnoiditis and unusual changes in the visual fields. *Arch. Ophthal., 12*:167, 1934.

1362. SPALDING, J. M. K.: Wounds of the visual pathway. I. The visual radiation. *J. Neurol. Neurosurg. Psychiat., 15*:99, 1952.

1363. SPALTER, H. F.: Abnormal serum proteins and retinal vein thrombosis. *Arch. Ophthal., 62*:868, 1959.

1364. SPALTER, H. F.: Ophthalmodynamometry and carotid artery thrombosis. *Amer. J. Ophthal., 47*:453, 1959.

1365. SPALTER, H. F., AND BRUCE, G. M.: Ocular changes in pulmonary insufficiency. *Trans. Amer. Acad. Ophthal. Otolaryng., 68*:661, 1964.

1366. SPAULDING, W. L.: Glioma of the optic nerve and its management. *Amer. J. Ophthal., 46*:654, 1958.

1367. SPENCER, W. H., AND HOYT, W. F.: A fatal case of giant-cell arteritis (temporal or cranial arteritis) with ocular involvement. *Arch. Ophthal.,* 64:862, 1960.

1368. STALLARD, H. B.: The conservative treatment of retinoblastoma. *Trans. Ophthal. Soc. U.K., 82*:473, 1962.

1369. STANKOVIC, M. I.: L'Angiosclérose Choroidïenne familiale liée au sexe. *Bull. Soc. Franc. Ophtal., 71*:411, 1958.

1370. STANSBURY, F. C.: Neuromyelitis optica (Devic's disease): Presentation of five cases, with pathologic study and review of literature. *Arch. Ophthal., 42*:292, 1949.

1371. STANSBURY, F. C.: Neuromyelitis optica (Devic's disease): Presentation of five cases, with pathologic study, and review of literature. (Concluded.) *Arch. Ophthal., 42*:465, 1949.

1372. STANSBURY, J. R.: Optic atrophy in diabetes mellitus: a report of three cases in one family. *Amer. J. Ophthal., 31*:1153, 1948.

1373. STANWORTH, A., AND NAYLOR, E. J.: Haidinger's brushes and the retinal receptors: with a note on the Stiles-Crawford effect. *Brit. J. Ophthal., 34*:282, 1950.

1374. STARGARDT, K.: Ueber familiäre progressive degeneration in der Maculagegend des Auges. *Graefe Arch. Ophthal., 71*:534, 1909.

1375. STATTEN, T.: Subdural haematoma in infancy. *Canad. Med. Ass. J., 58*:63, 1948.

1376. STATTON, R., BLODI, F. C., AND HANIGAN, J.: Sarcoidosis of the optic nerve. *Arch. Ophthal., 71*:834, 1964.

1377. STEELE, E. J., AND BLUNT, M. J.: The blood supply of the optic nerve and chiasma in man. *J. Anat., 90*:486, 1956.

1378. STEELMAN, H. F., HAYES, G. J., AND RIZZOLI, H. V.: Surgical treatment of saccular intracranial aneurysms; report of 56 consecutively treated patients. *J. Neurosurg., 10*:564, 1953.

1379. STEGER, J., AND STEGER, R.: Die Störungen des Kupfer- und Aminosäuren-Stoffwechsels bei der hepatocerebralen Degeneration und deren Behandlung mit BAL. *Deutsch. Z. Nervenheilk., 172*:321, 1954.

1380. STENGEL, E.: The syndrome of visual alexia with colour agnosia. *J. Ment. Sci., 94*:46, 1948.

1381. STEVENS, H.: Carotid artery occlusion in childhood. *Pediatrics, 23*:699, 1959.

1382. STEVENS, P. M., AUSTEN, F., AND KNOWLES, J. H.: Prognostic significance of papilledema in course of respiratory insufficiency. *J.A.M.A., 183*:161, 1963.

1383. STEWARD, J. K., SMITH, J. L. S., AND ARNOLD, E. L.: Spontaneous regression of retinoblastoma. *Brit. J. Ophthal., 40*:449, 1956.

1384. STIEFEL, J. W., AND SMITH, J. L.: Hyaline bodies (drusen) of the optic nerve and intracranial tumor. *Arch. Ophthal., 65*:814, 1961.

1385. STREIFF, E. B.: Artérite rétinienne et polyarthrite chronique évolutive grave. *Bull. Soc. Franc. Ophtal., 70*:405, 1957.

1386. STREIFF, M. E. B.: Traumatismes des voies optiques. *Riv. Oto-Neuro-Oftal., 26*:356, 1951. (Abst., *Excerpta Med. XII, 7*:#130, 1953.)

1387. STROM, T.: [Acute blindness as post-measles complication]. *Acta. Paediat. (Upps.), 42*:60, 1953. (Abst., *Excerpta Med. XII, 7*:#1871, 1953.)

1388. STRONG, J. B., DEMPSEY, H., AND HILL, S. R.: The successful management of hepatolenticular degeneration with penicillamine: studies on three generations of a family. *Ann. Intern. Med., 54*:198, 1961.

1389. SUGAR, H. S.: Place of hemorrhagic glaucoma in etiologic classification of glaucoma. *Arch. Ophthal., 28*:587, 1942.

1390. SUGAR, H. S., WEBSTER, J. E., AND GURDJIAN, E. S.: Ophthalmologic findings in spontaneous thrombosis of the carotid artery. *Arch. Ophthal., 44*:823, 1950.

1391. SULLIVAN, P. R., KUTEN, J., ATKINSON, M. S., ANGEVINE, J. B., AND YAKOVLEV, P. I.: Cell count in the lateral geniculate nucleus of man. *Neurology, 8*:566, 1958.

1392. SUTTON, P. H., AND BEATTIE, P. H.: Optic atrophy after administration of isoniazid with P.A.S. *Lancet, 1*:650, 1955.

1393. SUZUKI, H., AND TAIRA, N.: Effect of reticular stimulation upon synaptic transmission in cat's lateral geniculate body. *Jap. J. Physiol., 11*:641, 1961.

1394. SVAETICHIN, G., LAUFER, M., MITARAI, G., FATEHCHAND, R., VALLECALLE, E., AND VILLEGAS, J.: Glial control of neuronal networks and receptors. In *The Visual System: Neurophysiology and Psychophysics.* Ed. R. Jung and H. Kornhuber. Berlin: Springer-Verlag, 1961, pp. 445-456.

1395. SVANE-KNUDSEN, P.: Bilateral ophthalmic arteritis as part of the temporal arteritis syndrome. *Acta. Ophthal. (Kbh.), 38*:708, 1960.

1396. SVIEN, H. J., AND HOLLENHORST, R. W.: Pressure in retinal arteries after ligation or occlusion of the carotid artery. *Proc. Mayo Clin., 31*:684, 1956.

1397. SWIETLICZKO, I.: [The aspect of the optic disc at a low intra-ocular pressure]. *Klin. Oczna, 29*:37, 1959. (Abst., *Ophthal. Lit., 13*:#335, 1959.)

1398. SWIETLICZKO, I., SZAPIRO, J., AND POLIS, Z.: Value of retinal artery pressure determination, in the diagnosis of internal carotid artery thrombosis: the role of the carotid compression test. *Amer. J. Ophthal., 52*:862, 1961.

1399. SYKOWSKI, P.: Digitoxin intoxication. Resulting in retrobulbar optic neuritis. *Amer. J. Ophthal., 32*:572, 1949.

1400. SYKOWSKI, P.: Diabetic retrobulbar neuritis. *Amer. J. Ophthal., 32*:1589, 1949.

1401. SYMONDS, C. P.: Contribution to clinical study of Schilder's encephalitis. *Brain, 51*:24, 1928.

1402. SYMONDS, C. P.: Otitic hydrocephalus. *Neurology, 6*:681, 1956.

1403. SYMONDS, C., AND MACKENZIE, I.: Bilateral loss of vision from cerebral infarction. *Brain, 80*:415, 1957.

1404. Symposium: Influence of hypophysectomy and of adrenalectomy on diabetic retinopathy. *Diabetes, 11*:461, 1962.

1405. SZOBOR, A., AND SZEGEDY, L.: Beiträge zur Frage der Neuromyelitis optica. Klinisch-pathologische Studie. *Psychiat. Neurol (Basel), 143*:100, 1962.

1406. TAKAGI, R., AND KAWAKAMI, R.: Ueber das Wesen der Oguchischen Krankheit. *Klin. Mbl. Augenheilk., 72*:349, 1924.

1407. TAKAYASU, S.: A case with unusual changes of the central vessels in the retina. *Acta. Soc. Ophthal. Jap., 12*:554, 1908.

1408. TALBOT, A. N.: A review of some cases of pituitary tumours. *N.Z. Med. J., 9*:46, 1957.

1409. TAMLER, E., AND EISSLER, R.: The intraocular pathology in Schilder's disease. *Arch. Ophthal., 65*:514, 1961.

1410. TAMLER, E., AND TAKAHASHI, E.: Collateral circulation to the eye. *Amer. J. Ophthal., 52*:381, 1961.

1411. TANSLEY, K.: Regeneration of visual purple; its relation to dark adaptation and night blindness. *J. Physiol. (Lond.), 71*:442, 1931.

1412. TANSLEY, K.: The formation of rosettes in the rat retina. *Brit. J. Ophthal., 17*:321, 1933.

1413. TARLAU, M., AND McGRATH, H.: Pathological changes in the fundus oculi in tuberous sclerosis. Clinical and pathological report of a case of a tumor arising from the optic nerve head with a review of the literature. *J. Nerv. Ment. Dis., 92*:22, 1940.

1414. TASSMAN, I. S.: Foster Kennedy syndrome with fusiform aneurysm of internal carotid arteries. *Arch. Ophthal., 32*:125, 1944.

1415. TAUB, R. G., AND HOLLENHORST, R. W.: Sulfonamides as a cause of toxic amblyopia. *Amer. J. Ophthal., 40*:486, 1955.

1416. TAUB, R. G., AND RUCKER, C. W.: The relationship of retrobulbar neuritis to multiple sclerosis. *Amer. J. Ophthal., 37*:494, 1954.

1417. TENG, P.: Suprachiasmal meningioma in a 2-year-old child. *J. Neurol. Neurosurg. Psychiat., 24*:379, 1961.

1418. TERRAGNA, A., AND STRADOLINI, L.: Comportamento del fundus oculi nella malattia di Heine-Medin. *G. Mal. Infett., 11*:288, 1959. (Abst., *Excerpta Med. XII, 14*:#548, 1960.)

1419. TERRY, T. L.: Angioid streaks and osteitis deformans. *Trans. Amer. Ophthal. Soc., 32*:555, 1934.

1420. TERRY, T. L.: Fibroblastic overgrowth of persistent tunica vasculosa lentis in premature infants. II. Report of cases—clinical aspects. *Arch. Ophthal., 29*:36, 1943.

1421. TERRY, T. L., AND DUNPHY, E. B.: Metastatic carcinoma in both optic nerve simulating retrobulbar neuritis. *Arch. Ophthal., 10*:611, 1933.

1422. TEUBER, H.-L.: Neuere Beobachtungen über Sehstrahlung und Sehrinde. In *The Visual System*. Ed. R. Jung and H. Kornhuber. Berlin: Springer-Verlag, 1961, p. 256-274.

1423. TEUBER, H.-L., BATTERSBY, W. S., AND BENDER, M. B.: *Visual Field Defects after Penetrating Missile Wounds of the Brain*. Cambridge, Mass.: Harvard Univ. Press, 1960.

1424. TEUNS, J.: Neuritis optica door het virus van parotitis epidemica. *Ned. T. Geneesk., 98*:2137, 1954. (Abst., *Excerpta Med. XII, 9*:#697, 1955.)

1425. THEOBOLD, G. D.: Cytomegalic inclusion disease. *Amer. J. Ophthal., 47*:52, 1959.

1426. THIEBAUT, F., AND GUILLAUMAT, L.: Hémianopsie relative. Presented before the Société de Neurologie de Paris, 1945. (Abst., *Rev. Neurol. (Par.), 77*:129, 1945.)

1427. THEIL, H.-L.: Zur Diagnostik und Therapie der Arachnoiditis opti-cochiasmatica. *Graefe Arch. Ophthal., 162*:227, 1960.

1428. THIEL, R.: Sonnenblumenstar bei hepato-lentikularer Degeneration (Pseudosklerose). *Klin. Mbl. Augenheilk., 93*:12, 1934.

1429. THOMAS, C., CORDIER, J., LARCAN, A., AND STREIFF, F.: Manifestations ophthalmologiques au cours de la macroglobulinémie de Waldenstrom: Le fond d'oeil dysprotéinemique. *Arch. Ophtal. (Par.), 19*:609, 1959.

1430. THOMAS, J. E., SCHIRGER, A., LOVE, J. G., AND HOFFMAN, D. L.: Orthostatic hypotension as the presenting sign in craniopharyngioma; case report. *Neurology, 11*:418, 1961.

1431. THOMPSON, A. H., AND CASHELL, G. T. W.: Pedigree of congenital optic atrophy embracing 16 affected cases in 6 generations. *Proc. Roy. Soc. Med., 28*:1415, 1935.

1432. THOMPSON, A. M. W.: Peri-arteritis retinae. *Brit. J. Ophthal., 36*:268, 1952.

1433. THURLBECK, W. M., AND CURRENS, J. H.: The aortic arch syndrome. *Circulation, 19*:499, 1959.

1434. THYGESON, P.: Prognosis in disseminated sclerosis and disseminated encephalomyelitis evaluated in relation to initial stage of disorders; differential diagnosis during this stage. *Nord. Med., 35*:1779, 1947.

1435. TIBERIN, P., GOLDBERG, G. M., AND SCHWARTZ, A.: Craniopharyngiomas in the aged. *Neurology, 8*:51, 1958.

1436. TIMBERLAKE, W. H., AND KUBIK, C. S.: Follow-up report with clinical and anatomical notes on 280 patients with subarachnoid hemorrhage. *Trans. Amer. Neurol. Ass., 77*:26, 1952.

1437. TIMM, G.: Zur pathologischen Anatomie des Auges bei der Makroglobulinämie Waldenstrom. *Klin. Mbl. Augenheilk., 137*:772, 1960.

1438. TISSINGTON TATLOW, W. F.: The prognosis of retrobulbar neuritis. *Brit J. Ophthal., 32*:488, 1948.

1439. TORMA, T., AND KOSKINEN, K.: A case of unilateral optic foramen meningioma. *Acta Ophthal., 39*:460, 1961.

1440. TOPILOW, A., AND BISLAND, T.: Diabetes mellitus as a cause of papillitis *Amer. J. Ophthal., 35*:855, 1952.

1441. TOULANT, P., LARMANDE, A., AND TOULANT, M.: Les lésions du nerf optique au cours de la trypanosomiose africaine. *Bull. Acad. Nat. Med. (Par.), 133*:23, 1949.

1442. TOUR, R. L.: Military retinal aneurysms. *Trans. Pacif. Coast. Otoophthal. Soc., 37*:121, 1956.

1443. TOUR, R. L., AND HOYT, W. F.: The syndrome of the aortic arch. Ocular manifestations of "pulseless disease" and a report of a surgically treated case. *Amer. J. Ophthal., 47*:35, 1959.

1444. TRAQUAIR, H. M.: Bitemporal hemiopia: the later stages and the special features of the scotoma. *Brit. J. Ophthal., 1*:216, 281, 337, 1917.

1445. TRAQUAIR, H. M.: *Introduction to Clinical Perimetry.* 6th ed. St. Louis: Mosby, 1949.

1446. TRAQUAIR, H. M., DOTT, N. M., AND RUSSELL, W. R.: Traumatic lesions of the optic chiasma. *Brain, 58*:398, 1935.

1447. TRESCHER, J. H., AND FORD, F. R.: Colloid cyst of third ventricle; report of case; operative removal with section of posterior half of corpus callosum. *Arch. Neurol. Psychiat., 37*:959, 1937.

1448. TURCK, L.: Über Compression und Ursprung des Sehnerven, *Z. Gesch. Artze Wien, 8*:299, 1852.

1449. TUREEN, L. L.: Lesions of fundus associated with brain hemorrhage. *Arch. Neurol. Psychiat., 42*:664, 1939.

1450. TURNBULL, D. C.: Optic neuritis associated with Bornholm disease. *Amer. J. Ophthal., 46*:81, 1958.

1451. TURPIN, R., JEROME, H., AND SCHMITT, H.: Study of variations of ceruloplasmin by easy technique. *Proc. Roy. Soc. Med., 46*:1061, 1953.

1452. TURTZ, C. A.: Visual toxic symptoms from digitalis. *Amer. J. Ophthal., 38*: 400, 1954.

1453. TURTZ, C. A.: Transient loss of vision following use of quinine. *Amer. J. Ophthal., 44*:110, 1957.

1454. TURTZ, C. A., AND TURTZ, A. I.: Vitamin-A intoxication. *Amer. J. Ophthal., 50*:165, 1960.

1455. TYTUS, J. S., SELTZER, H. S., AND KAHN, E. A.: Cortisone as an aid in the surgical treatment of craniopharyngiomas. *J. Neurosurg., 12*:555, 1955.

1456. UDVARHELYI, G. B., AND WALSH, F. B.: Complications involving the optic nerves and chiasm during the early period after neurosurgical operations. *J. Neurosurg., 19*:51, 1962.

1357. UNGER, L.: Das Verhalten des optokinetischen Nystagmus bei psychogenen Sehstörungen. *Klin. Mbl. Augenheilk., 127*:411, 1955.

1458. UNGER, L.: Chromatopie nach Digitalis. *Ophthalmologica, 136*:326, 1958.

1459. UTERMANN, D.: Beitrag zur Behandlung der Arachnoiditis opticochiasmatica. *Klin. Mbl. Augenheilk., 139*:640, 1961.

1460. UZMAN, L. L.: Chemical nature of storage substance in gargoylism; Hurler-Pfaundler's disease. *Arch. Path., 60*:308, 1955.

1461. UZMAN, L. L., IBER, F. L., CHALMERS, T. C., AND KNOWLTON, M.: The mechanism of copper deposition in the liver in hepatolenticular degeneration (Wilson's disease). *Amer. J. Med. Sci., 231*:511, 1956.

1462. UZMAN, L. L., AND JAKUS, M. A.: The Kayser-Fleischer ring; a histochemical and electron microscope study. *Neurology, 7*:341, 1957.

1463. VAERNET, K.: Collateral ophthalmic artery circulation in thrombotic carotid occlusion. *Neurology, 4*:605, 1954.

1464. VAIL, D. T.: Optochiasmic arachnoiditis, importance of a mixed type of atrophy of the optic nerve as a diagnostic sign. *Arch. Ophthal., 20*:384, 1938.

1465. VALIERE-VIALIEIX, CHASSAING, CELLIER, AND ROBIN, A.: Cas trés rare de gliome rétinien au sens histologique du mot. *Bull. Soc. Franc. Ophtal., 68*:263, 1955.

1466. VANCEA, P., AND TUDOR, E.: Dégénerescence maculaire familiale progressive (maladie de Stargardt). *Ann. Oculist. (Par.), 193*:914, 1960.

1467. VANNAS, S., HERNBERG, C. A., AND BJORKESTEN, G.: Hypophysectomy as a therapeutical method for proliferative diabetic retinopathy. *Arch. Ophthal., 62*:370, 1959.

1468. VANNINI, A.: Neurite ottica retrobulbare bilaterale da herpes zoster oftalmico monolaterale. *Rass. Ital. Ottal., 22*:401, 1953. (Abst., *Excerpta Med. XII, 8*:#1366, 1954.)

1469. VASTOLA, E. F.: A direct pathway from lateral geniculate body to association cortex. *J. Neurophysiol., 24*:469, 1961.

1470. VAUTHIER, D., AND ZANEN, J.: Fossettes Papillaires. *Bull. Soc. Belg. Ophtal., 110*:162, 1955.

1471. VEDEL-JENSEN, N.: Optic tract neuritis in multiple sclerosis. *Acta Ophthal. (Kbh.), 37*:573, 1959.

1472. DE VEER, J. A.: Melanotic tumors of the optic nerve head: a pathologic study. *Arch. Ophthal., 65*:536, 1961.

1473. DE VEER, J. A., AND CRAPOTTA, J. A.: Malignant melanoma or retinoblastoma in an adult: a differential diagnostic problem. *Arch. Ophthal., 63:* 70, 1960.

1474. VENTURI, G., AND VOLPI, U.: Rilievi adattometrici in soggeti con retinite sierosa centrale. *Ann. Ottal., 86:*65, 1960.

1475. VERHOEFF, F. H.: A rare tumor arising from the pars ciliaris retinae (terato-neuroma), of a nature hitherto unrecgonized, and its relation to the so-called glioma retinae. *Trans. Amer. Ophthal. Soc., 10:*351, 1904.

1476. VERHOEFF, F. H.: Obstruction of the central retinal vein. *Arch. Ophthal., 36:*1, 1907.

1477. VERHOEFF, F. H.: The effect of chronic glaucoma on the central retinal vessels. *Arch. Ophthal., 42:*145, 1913.

1478. VERHOEFF, F. H.: Primary intraneural tumors (gliomas) of the optic nerve, a histologic study of eleven cases, including a case showing cystic involvement of the optic disk, with demonstration of the origin of cytoid bodies of the retina and cavernous atrophy of the optic nerve. *Arch. Ophthal., 51:*120, 239, 1922.

1479. VERHOEFF, F. H.: The nature and pathogenesis of angioid streaks in the ocular fundus. *Trans. Amer. Med. Ass. Section Ophthal.,* p. 243, 1928.

1480. VERHOEFF, F. H.: Retinoblastoma: report of a case in a man aged forty-eight. *Arch. Ophthal., 2:*643, 1929.

1481. VERHOEFF, F. H.: A new theory of binocular vision. *Arch. Ophthal., 13:* 151, 1935.

1482. VERHOEFF, F. H.: A new answer to the question of macular sparing. *Arch. . Ophthal., 30:*421, 1943.

1483. VERHOEFF, F. H.: Are Moore's lightning streaks of serious portent. *Amer. J. Ophthal., 14:*837, 1956.

1484. VERHOEFF, F. H., AND GROSSMAN, H. P.: Pathogenesis of disciform degeneration of the macula. *Arch. Ophthal., 18:*561, 1937.

1485. VERHOEFF, F. H., AND SIMPSON, G. V.: Tubercle within central retinal vein; hemorrhagic glaucoma; periphlebitis retinalis in other eye. *Arch. Ophthal., 24:*645, 1940.

1486. VERREY, F.: Dégénérescence pigmentaire de la rétine d'origine médicamenteuse. *Ophthalmologica, 131:*296, 1956.

1487. VICTOR, M.: Tobacco-alcohol amblyopia: critique of current concepts of this disorder, with special reference to the role of nutritional deficiency in its causation. *Arch. Ophthal., 70:*313, 1963.

1488. VICTOR, M., MANCALL, E. L., AND DREYFUS, P. M.: Deficiency amblyopia in the alcoholic patient. *Arch. Ophthal., 64:*1, 1960.

1489. VOGELSANG, H.: Über eine angiographisch selten nachzuweisende Anastomose zwischen den A. carotis interna- und den A. carotis externa-Kreislauf (Variante des Blutzuflusses zur A. meningea media über Anastomosen von der A. ophthalmica) *Nervenarzt, 32:*518, 1961.

1490. VOGELSANG, K.: Optikusatrophie und Ophthalmoplegie und Ophthalmoplegie bei Zoster ophthalmicus. *Klin. Mbl. Augenheilk., 141:*116, 1962.

1491. VOISIN, J., AND CORNU, P.: L'atrophie optique primitive des méningites tuberculeuses traitée par la streptomycine. *Rev. Neurol. (Par.), 90:*823, 1954.

1492. VULPE, M., MEYER, J. S., AND GOODMAN, M.: Optic neuritis and encephalomyelitis in monkey produced with human optic nerve. *Nature,* *196*:901, 1962.

1493. WAARDENBURG, P. J.: Angio-sclérose familiale de la choroïde. *J. Genet. Hum., 1*:83, 1952.

1494. WAARDENBURG, P. J.: Does agenesis or dysgenesis neuroepithelialis retinae, whether or not related to keratoglobus, exist? *Ophthalmologica, 133*:454, 1957.

1495. WAGENER, H. P.: Drusen (hyaline bodies) of the optic disk. *Amer. J. Med. Sci., 210*:262, 1945.

1496. WAGENER, H. P.: Lesions of retina and optic nerve secondary to distant trauma. *Amer. J. Med. Sci., 228*:226, 1954.

1497. WAGENER, H. P.: Tumors of the optic papilla. *Amer. J. Med. Sci., 230*:213, 1955.

1498. WAGENER, H. P.: Central angiospastic retinopathy and central serous chorio-retinitis. *Amer. J. Med. Sci., 233*:220, 1957.

1499. WAGENER, H. P.: Some recent studies on Eales' disease. *Amer. J. Med. Sci., 236*:250, 1958.

1500. WAGENER, H. P.: Gliomas of the optic nerve. *Amer. J. Med. Sci., 237*:238, 1959.

1501. WAGENER, H. P.: Measurement of retinal arterial pressure. *Amer. J. Med. Sci., 238*:211, 1959.

1502. WAGENER, H. P.: Glaucoma following occlusion of the central retinal artery. *Amer. J. Med. Sci., 240*:253, 1960.

1503. WAGENER, H. P., AND HOLLENHORST, R. W.: The ocular lesions of temporal arteritis. *Amer. J. Ophthal., 45*:617, 1958.

1504. WAGENER, H. P., AND KEITH, N. M.: Diffuse arteriolar disease with hypertension and the associated retinal lesions. *Medicine, 18*:317, 1939.

1505. WAGENER, H. P., AND LOVE, J. G.: Fields of vision in cases of tumor of Rathke's pouch. *Arch. Ophthal., 29*:873, 1943.

1506. WAKSMAN, B. H.: *Experimental Allergic Encephalomyelitis and the "Auto-allergic" Disease.* Basil: S. Karger, 1959.

1507. WAKSMAN, B. H., AND ADAMS, R. D.: Infectious leukoencephalitis; a critical comparison of certain experimental and naturally-occurring viral leukoencephalitides with experimental allergic encephalomyelitis. *J. Neuropath. Exp. Neurol., 21*:491, 1962.

1508. VAN WALBEEK, K.: A family with dominant hereditary retinitis pigmentosa. *Ophthalmologica, 128*:246, 1954.

1509. WALD, G.: Pigments of retina; bull frog. *J. Gen. Physiol., 19*:781, 1936.

1510. WALD, G.: Photo-labile pigments of chicken retina. *Nature. (Lond), 140*: 545, 1937.

1511. WALD, G.: The photoreceptor process in vision. *Amer. J. Ophthal., 40*:18, 1955.

1512. WALD, G.: The photoreceptor process in vision. In *Handbook of Physiology-Neurophysiology I.* Washington: American Physiological Society 1959-60.

1513. WALD, G.: General discussion of retinal structure in relation to the visual process. In *The Structure of the Eye.* Ed. G. K. Smelser. N.Y.: Academic Press, 1961, p. 101-115.

1514. WALD, G., AND BROWN, P. K.: The role of sulfhydryl groups in the bleaching and synthesis of rhodopsin. *J. Gen. Physiol., 35*:797, 1951-1952.

1515. WALD, G., AND BROWN, P. K.: Human rhodopsin. *Science, 127*:222, 1958.
1516. WALD, G., BROWN, P. K., AND SMITH, P. H.: Iodopsin. *J. Gen. Physiol., 38*:623, 1954-55.
1517. WALDENSTROM, J.: Incipient myelomatosis or "essential" hyperglobulinemia with fibrinogenopenia—new syndrome? *Acta Med. Scand., 117*:216, 1944.
1518. WALKER, C. B., AND CUSHING, H.: Studies of optic-nerve atrophy in association with chiasmal lesions. *Arch. Ophthal., 45*:407, 1916.
1519. WALLNER, E. F., AND MOORSMAN, L. T.: Hemangioma of the optic disc. *Arch. Ophthal., 53*:115, 1955.
1520. WALLS, G. L.: The lateral geniculate nucleus and visual histophysiology. *Univ. of Calif. Publications in Physiology, 9*:1, 1953.
1521. WALSH, F. B.: Ocular importance of sarcoid. Its relation to uveoparotid fever. *Arch. Ophthal., 21*:421, 1939.
1522. WALSH, F. B.: In Symposium: Toxoplasmosis. Introduction of subject. *Trans. Amer. Acad. Ophthal. Otolaryng., 54*:177, 1950.
1523. WALSH, F. B.: In Symposium. Diseases of the optic nerve by Carroll, F. D.; Henderson, J. W.; Zimmerman, L. E.; Walsh, F. B., and Rucker, C. W. *Trans. Amer. Acad. Ophthal. Otolaryng., 60*:7, 1956.
1524. WALSH, F. B.: The ocular signs of tumors involving the anterior visual pathways. *Amer. J. Ophthal., 42*:347, 1956.
1525. WALSH, F. B.: *Clinical Neuro-ophthalmology,* 2nd. ed. Baltimore: Williams and Wilkins, 1957. a. p. 218; b. p. 349; c. p. 350; d. p. 644; e. p. 650; f. p. 657; g. p. 793; h. p.907.
1526. WALSH, F. B., AND FORD, F. R.: Central scotomas, their importance in topical diagnosis. *Arch. Ophthal., 24*:500, 1940.
1527. WALSH, F. B., AND GASS, J. D.: Concerning the optic chiasm. Selected pathologic involvement and clinical problems. *Amer. J. Ophthal., 50*:1031, 1960.
1528. WALSH, F. B., AND HEDGES, T. R.: Optic nerve sheath haemorrhage. *Trans. Amer. Acad. Ophthal. Otolaryng., 54*:29, 1950.
1529. WALSH, F. B., AND KING, A. B.: Ocular signs of intracranial saccular aneurysms, experimental work on collateral circulation through the ophthalmic artery. *Arch. Ophthal., 27*:1, 1942.
1530. WALSH, F. B., McMEEL, J. W., AND NEETENS, A.: Fractures of the skull: ophthalmological significance. *Bull. N.Y. Acad. Med., 36*:238, 1960.
1531. WALSH, F. B., AND SMITH, G. W.: Ocular complications of carotid angiography; ocular signs of thrombosis of internal carotid artery. *J. Neurosurg., 9*:517, 1952.
1532. WALSH, J. P., AND O'DOHERTY, D. S.: A possible explanation of the mechanism of ophthalmoplegic migraine. *Neurology, 10*:1079, 1960.
1533. WARBURG, M.: Norrie's disease: a new hereditary bilateral pseudotumor of the retina. *Acta Ophthal. (Kbh.), 39*:757, 1961.
1534. WARRINGTON, E. K.: The completion of visual forms across hemianopic field defects. *J. Neurol. Neurosurg. Psychiat., 25*:208, 1962.
1535. WARRINGTON, E., AND ZANGWILL, O. L.: Study of dyslexia. *J. Neurol. Psychiat., 20*:208, 1957.
1536. WEAVER, R. G., AND DAVIS, C. H.: Subhyaloid hemorrhage. *Amer. J. Ophthal., 52*:257, 1961.
1537. WEBER, J., AND SCHMIDT, R. M.: Zum Problem Stauungspapille und

Liquordrucksteigerung. *Arztl. Wschr.,* 10:1053, 1955. (Abst., *Excerpta Med. XII, 11*:#540, 1957.)

1538. WECHSLER, I. S.: Partial cortical blindness with preservation of color vision; report of case following asphyxia (carbon monoxide poisoning?); consideration of question of color vision and its cortical localization. *Arch. Ophthal., 9*:957, 1933.

1539. WEEKLEY, R. D., POTTS, A. M., REBOTON, J., AND MAY, R. H.: Pigmentary retinopathy in patients receiving high doses of a new phenothiazine. *Arch. Ophthal., 64*:65, 1960.

1540. WEIGELIN, E.: Schwerste periphlebitische Augenhintergrundsveränderungen bei einem Fall von multipler Skelrose. Presented at the 32nd meeting of Rhein-Mainischen Augenärzte, Nov. 28-29, 1959. (Abst., *Klin, Mbl. Augenheilk., 136*:574, 1960.)

1541. WEIMAN, C. G., McDOWELL, F. H., AND PLUM, F.: Papilledema in poliomyelitis. *Arch. Neurol. Psychiat., 66*:722, 1951.

1542. WEINBERGER, H. A., V.D. WOUDE, R., AND MAIER, H. C.: Prognosis of cortical blindness following cardiac arrest in children. *J.A.M.A., 179*: 126, 1962.

1543. WEINBERGER, L. M., GIBBON, M. H., AND GIBBON, J. H.: Temporary arrest of circulation to central nervous system; pathologic effects. *Arch. Neurol. Psychiat., 43*:961, 1940.

1544. WEINER, R. L., AND FALLS, H. F.: Intermediate sex-linked retinitis pigmentosa. *Arch. Ophthal., 53*:530, 1955.

1545. WEINSTEIN, E. A., AND KAHN, R. L.: *Denial of illness.* Springfield, Ill.: Charles C. Thomas, 1955.

1546. WEISENBERG, T. H., AND McBRIDE, K. E.: *Aphasia, A Clinical and Psychological Study.* London: Oxford University Press, 1935.

1547. WEIZENBLATT, S.: Metastatic disease of the optic nerve. *Amer. J. Ophthal., 47*:77, 1959.

1548. WELCH, K.: Homonymous hemianopsia following interruption of the parieto-occipital vein. *Neurology, 7*:69, 1957.

1549. WELCH, R. B., AND COOPER, J. C.: Macular edema, papilledema and optic atrophy after cataract extraction. *Arch. Ophthal., 59*:665, 1958.

1550. WELLER, T. H., MACAULEY, J. C., CRAIG, P. M., AND WIRTH, P.: Isolation of intranuclear inclusion producing agents from infants with illnesses resembling cytomegalic inclusion disease. *Proc. Soc. Exp. Biol. Med., 94*:4, 1957.

1551. WENDLAND, J. P.: Some instructive manifestations of chiasmal disease. *Arch. Ophthal., 54*:13, 1955.

1552. WENDLAND, J. P., AND NERENBERG, S.: Visual field studies after temporal lobectomy for epilepsy. *Arch. Ophthal., 64*:195, 1960.

1553. WERTHEIMER, P., DECHAUME, J., LECUIRE, J., AND MOULIN, J.: Réflexions sur la coexistence de neurinomes multiples, de méningiomes et de gliomes encéphaliques dans la maladie nerveuse de Recklinghausen; à propos des chitoneuromes. *Neurochirurgie (Par.), 3*:145, 1957.

1554. WEVE, H.: Über "Ablatio falciformis cong." *Arch. Augenheilk., 109*:371, 1936.

1555. WHITBOURNE, D.: Nutritional retrobulbar neuritis in children in Jamaica. *Amer. J. Ophthal., 30*:169, 1947.

1556. WHITE, J. C., AND ADAMS, R. D.: Combined supra- and infraclinoid aneurysms of internal carotid artery. *J. Neurosurg., 12*:450, 1955.

1557. WHITE, J. C., AND BALLANTINE, H. T.: Intrasellar aneurysms simulating hypophyseal tumours. *J. Neurosurg., 18*:34, 1961.

1558. WHITE, J. C., AND COBB, S.: Psychological changes associated with giant pituitary neoplasms. *Arch. Neurol. Psychiat., 74*:383, 1955.

1559. WHITE, L. E., AND FOLTZ, E. L.: Optic atrophy as isolated sign of unruptured carotid aneurysm. *Neurology, 7*:803, 1957.

1560. WHITING, M. H.: Retrobulbar optic neuritis in measles. *Trans. Ophthal. Soc. U.K., 71*:197, 1951.

1561. WHITTERIDGE, D., AND DANIEL, P. M.: The representation of the visual field on the calcarine cortex. In *The Visual System*. Ed. R. Jung and H. Kornhuber. Berlin: Springer-Verlag, 1961, pp. 223-227.

1562. WHITTY, C. W. M.: Neurologic implications of Behcet's syndrome. *Neurology, 8*:369, 1958.

1563. WILBRAND, H.: Ein Fall von Seelenblindheit und Hemianopsia mit Sectionsbefund. *Deutsch. Z. Nervenheilk., 2*:361, 1891.

1564. WILBRAND, H.: Über die Bedeutung kleinster homonym-hemianopischer Gesichtsfelddefekte. *Z. Augenheilk., 58*:197, 1926.

1565. WILBRAND, H.: Ueber die wissenschaftliche Bedeutung der Kongruenz und Inkongruenz der Gesichtsfeld-defekte. *J. Psychol. Neurol., 40*:133, 1930.

1566. WILDER, H. C.: Nematode endophthalmitis. *Trans. Amer. Acad. Ophthal. Otolaryng., 55*:99, 1950.

1567. WILDER, H. C.: Toxoplasma chorioretinitis in adults. *Arch. Ophthal., 48*: 127, 1952.

1568. WILDER, J.: Über Schief- und Verkehrtsehen. *Deutsch. Z. Nervenheilk., 104*:222, 1928.

1569. WILLIAMS, D., AND WILSON, T. G.: The diagnosis of the major and minor syndromes of basilar insufficiency. *Brain, 85*:741, 1962.

1570. WILLIAMS, M., AND PENNYBACKER, J.: Memory disturbances in third ventricle tumors. *J. Neurol. Neurosurg. Psychiat., 17*:115, 1954.

1571. WILLIAMSON-NOBLE, F. A.: Physiological cupping? *Trans. Ophthal. Soc. U.K., 81*:437, 1961.

1572. WILSON, R. P.: Crater-like holes in the disc. *Trans. Ophthal. Soc. N.Z., 8*: 35, 1955.

1573. WINCKLER, G.: L'innervation sensitive et motrice des muscles extrinsiques de l'oiel chez quelques ongules. *Arch. Anat., 23*:219, 1937.

1574. WINTROBE, M. M., AND BUELL, M. V.: Hyperproteinemia associated with multiple myeloma, with report of a case in which extraordinary hyperproteinemia was associated with thrombosis of retinal veins and symptoms suggesting Raynaud's disease. *Bull. Johns Hopkins Hosp., 52*: 156, 1933.

1575. WISE, B. L., BROWN, H. A., NAFFZIGER, H. C., AND BOLDREY, E. B.: Pituitary adenomas, carcinomas, and craniopharyngiomas. *Surg. Gynec. Obstet., 101*:185, 1955.

1576. WITT, J. A., MACCARTY, C. S., AND KEATING, F. R.: Craniopharyngioma (pituitary adamantinoma) in patients more than 60 years of age. *J. Neurosurg., 12*:354, 1955.

1577. WOLFF, E., AND DAVIES, F.: A contribution to the pathology of papilloedema. *Brit. J. Ophthal., 15*:609, 1931.

1578. VON WOLFFERSDORFF, H.: Beiderseitige Optikusatrophie durch Hypoxämie
infolge akuter schwerster Magenblutung. *Deutsch. Gesundh., 10*:530,
1955.

1579. WOLTER, J. R.: Regenerative potentialities of the centrifugal fibers of the
human optic nerve. *Arch. Ophthal., 64*:697, 1960.

1580. WOLTER, J. R.: Silver carbonate techniques for the demonstration of
ocular histology. In *Symposium on the Eye*. New York, International
Congress of Anatomy, 1960.

1581. WOLTER, J. R.: The rosettes of a neuroepitheliomatous retinoblastoma.
Amer. J. Ophthal., 52:497, 1961.

1582. WOLTER, J. R., AND PHILLIPS, R. L.: Secondary glaucoma following
occlusion of the central retinal artery. *Amer. J. Ophthal., 47*:335, 1959.

1583. WOODWARD, J. H.: The ocular complications of mumps. *Ann. Ophthal.,
16*:7, 1907.

1584. WOODWORTH, J. A., BECKETT, R. S., AND NETSKY, M. G.: A composite
of hereditary ataxias. A familial disorder with features of olivopontocere-
bellar atrophy, Leber's optic atrophy, and Friedreich's ataxia. *Arch.
Intern. Med., 104*:594, 1959.

1585. WORMS, G.: Syndrome oculo-hypophysaire consécutif a une sinusite
sphénoïdale suppurée: examen anatomo-pathologique. *Arch. Ophtal.
(Par.), 53*:207, 1936.

1586. WORTHAM, E., LEVIN, G., AND WICK, H. W.: Altitudinal anopsia following
thoracoplasty. *Arch. Ophthal., 47*:248, 1952.

1587. WRIGHT, P.: Meningocoele of the optic disc. *Brit. J. Ophthal., 44*:570,
1960.

1588. WUEST, F. C.: Bitemporal hemianopsia following a traumatic lesion of
the optic chiasm. *Arch. Ophthal., 63*:721, 1960.

1589. WYBAR, K. C.: Ocular manifestations of disseminated sclerosis. *Proc. Roy.
Soc. Med., 45*:315, 1952.

1590. WYBAR, K. C.: Anastomoses between the retinal and ciliary arterial
circulations. *Brit. J. Ophthal., 40*:65, 1956.

1591. WYBURN-MASON, R.: Arteriovenous aneurysm of midbrain and retina,
naevi, and mental changes. *Brain, 66*:163, 1943.

1592. WYKE, M., AND ETTLINGER, G.: Efficiency of recognition in left and
right visual fields. Its relation to the phenomenon of visual extinction.
Arch. Neurol., 5:659, 1961.

1593. YASKIN, H. E., AND ALPERS, B. J.: Foster Kennedy syndrome with post-
traumatic arachnoiditis of optic chiasm and base of frontal lobes. *Arch.
Ophthal., 34*:399, 1945.

1594. YASUNA, E. R.: Hysterical amblyopia in children and young adults. *Arch.
Ophthal., 45*:70, 1951.

1595. YOUMANS, J. R., AND SCARCELLA, G.: Extracranial collateral cerebral circulation. *Neurology, 11*:166, 1961.

1596. YOUNG, G.: The relation of the optic nerve to the sphenoidal and posterior
ethmoidal sinuses. *Brit. Med. J., 2*:1258, 1922.

1597. YOUNG, G. F., KNOX, D. L., AND DODGE, P. R.: Necrotizing encephalitis and chorioretinitis in a young infant: report of a case with rising herpes simplex antibody titers. *Arch. Nevro., 13*:15, 1965.

1598. YUHL, E. T., AND RAND, C. W.: Tuberculous opticochiasmatic arachnoiditis. Report of a case. *J. Neurosurg., 8*:441, 1951.

1599. ZANEK, J. AND BRIHAYE, J.: L'hemianopsie horizontale opto-chiasmatique. *Bull. Soc. Ophtal. Franc.*, p. 411, 1948.

1600. ZEITLIN, H., AND LEVINSON, S.: Intracranial chordoma. *Arch. Neurol. Psychiat., 45*:984, 1941.

1601. ZIMMERMAN, H.: cited by Chamlin, M. and Davidoff, L. M.: Ref. 238.

1602. ZIMMERMAN, H. M., AND NETSKY, M. G.: The pathology of multiple sclerosis. In *Multiple Sclerosis and the Demyelinating Diseases*. Proc. Assoc. Research in Nervous and Mental Diseases 28:271, 1950.

1603. ZIMMERMAN, L. E.: Pathology of the demyelinating diseases. In Symposium: diseases of the optic nerve. *Trans. Amer. Acad. Ophthal. Otolaryng.*, p. 46, 1956.

1604. ZIMMERMAN, L. E., AND GARRON, L. K.: Melanocytoma of the optic disc. In *Tumors of the eye and adnexa*. Ed. L. E. Zimmerman. Boston: Little, Brown & Co. 1962 pp. 431-440.

1605. ZINTZ, R.: Zur Frages der traumatischen Chiasmaschädigung. *Klin. Mbl. Augenheilk., 127*:539, 1955.

1606. ZOLLINGER, R., AND CUTLER, E. C.: Aneurysm of the internal carotid artery. *Arch. Neurol. Psychiat., 30*:607, 1933.

1607. ZOLOG, N., POPESCU, E., LEIBOVICI, M., AND ADRIAN, D.: [Ocular manifestations of tuberculous meningitis in adults and children]. *Stud. Cercet. Stiint., 6*:117, 1959. (Abst., *Excerpta Med. XII, 15*:#964, 1961.)

1608. ZOURABACHVILLI, A. D.: [The conception of brain centres and a few data regarding the development of nuclei of the optic layers in man]. *Zh. Nevropat. Psikhiat. Korsakov, 57*:701, 1957. (Abst., *Excerpta Med. XII, 12*:#1191, 1958.)

1609. ZULCH, K. J.: *Brain tumors, their biology and pathology*. Berlin: Springer, 1957.

1610. ZULCH, K. J., AND NOVER, A.: Die Spongioblastome des Sehnerven. *Graefe Arch. Ophthal., 161*:405, 1960.

INDEX